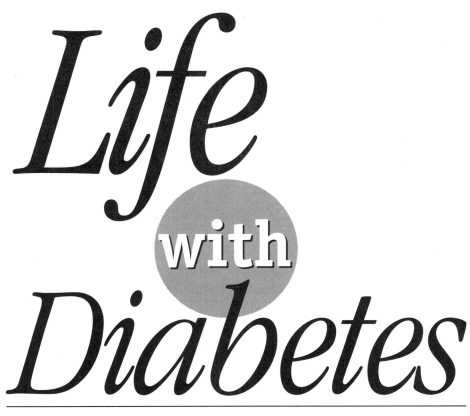

Life with Diabetes

THIRD EDITION

American Diabetes Association.
Cure • Care • Commitment®

Director, Book Publishing, John Fedor; *Associate Director, Professional Books,* Christine B. Charlip; *Editor,* Wendy M. Martin; *Associate Director, Book Production,* Peggy M. Rote; *Composition,* Circle Graphics, Inc.; *Cover Design,* Wickham & Associates, Inc.; *Illustrations,* Duckwell Productions; *Printer,* Port City Press, Inc.

Printed in the United States of America
3 5 7 9 10 8 6 4

The suggestions and information contained in this publication are generally consistent with the *Clinical Practice Recommendations* and other policies of the American Diabetes Association, but they do not represent the policy or position of the Association or any of its boards or committees. Reasonable steps have been taken to ensure the accuracy of the information presented. However, the American Diabetes Association cannot ensure the safety or efficacy of any product or service described in this publication. Individuals are advised to consult a physician or other appropriate health care professional before undertaking any diet or exercise program or taking any medication referred to in this publication. Professionals must use and apply their own professional judgment, experience, and training and should not rely solely on the information contained in this publication before prescribing any diet, exercise, or medication. The American Diabetes Association—its officers, directors, employees, volunteers, and members—assumes no responsibility or liability for personal or other injury, loss, or damage that may result from the suggestions or information in this publication.

♾ The paper in this publication meets the requirements of the ANSI Standard Z39.48-1992 (permanence of paper).

ADA titles may be purchased for business or promotional use or for special sales. To purchase this book in large quantities, or for custom editions of this book with your logo, contact Lee Romano Sequeira, Special Sales & Promotions, at the address below, or at LRomano@diabetes.org or call 703-299-2046.

American Diabetes Association
1701 North Beauregard Street
Alexandria, Virginia 22311

Library of Congress Cataloging-in-Publication Data

Life with diabetes: a series of teaching outlines by the Michigan Diabetes Research and
    Training Center / lead authors, Martha M. Funnell ... [et al.].—3rd ed.
        p. cm.
    Includes bibliographical references.
    ISBN 1-58040-205-4 (pbk)
        1. Diabetes—Outlines, syllabi, etc. 2. Diabetes—Study and teaching. 3. Patient education.
I. Funnell, Martha Mitchell. II. University of Michigan. Diabetes Research and Training
Center. III. American Diabetes Association.

RC660.L54 2004
616.4'62'0071—dc22
                                                    2004052185

Contents

➡ SUPPLEMENTARY OUTLINES

➡ SUPPORT MATERIALS

▶ ▶ ▶ ▶ ▶

These materials were originally developed under the direction of the Patient Education Committee of the Michigan Diabetes Research and Training Center. They were designed for use in teaching inpatients on the Diabetes Center Unit and were edited for their first publication in 1984 by Linda K. Strodtman, MS, RN; Patricia A. Barr, BS; John C. Floyd, Jr., MD; and me.

The second and third editions of these outlines were published in 1987 and 1991 by the Michigan DRTC after revisions to reflect both technological advances and changes in care and education. The American Diabetes Association took over publication of *Life with Diabetes* in 1997. This third edition of *Life with Diabetes* was revised to include current content areas necessary for meeting the National Standards for Diabetes Self-Management Education and for achieving Recognition from the American Diabetes Association Education Recognition Program. It also incorporates new therapies and new information about the prevention and treatment of diabetes.

Twenty years after the first publication of this resource, I am amazed by how many changes we have seen in diabetes care and diabetes education. The advances that have been made in the care and treatment of this devastating disease offer great benefit and hope. As impressive to me are the changes that we have seen in how we teach and think about people with diabetes. Diabetes education has clearly evolved from didactic content presentations to more theoretically-based empowerment models.

Beginning as early as 1984 and with each revision, we have made these materials more patient-centered and collaborative, reflecting the philosophy of educators at our center, including Bob Anderson, EdD, and our colleagues around the country. Our purpose is not just to provide knowledge but to help participants make informed choices about how they will live with diabetes. We have also incorporated psychosocial and behavioral issues and strategies into each of the content areas so that the instructor can better help participants integrate diabetes into their lives.

I believe that being an educator is the best job in the world because we have the opportunity to bring help and hope to people, which helps them live with diabetes more effectively and peacefully. I hope that you will find these materials helpful to you in your practice and in your work as you bring caring, compassion, and competence into the lives of people with diabetes.

Martha M. Funnell, MS, RN, CDE
Michigan Diabetes Research and
    Training Center
Ann Arbor, Michigan

Acknowledgments

▶ ▶ ▶ ▶ ▶

Many have contributed to the outlines in the past two decades. They have been the joint effort of many staff members of the Michigan Diabetes Research and Training Center Education Committee, the Clinical Implementation Core, the Educational Development and Evaluation Core, and the Continuing Education and Outreach Core. Martha M. Funnell, MS, RN, CDE; Marilynn S. Arnold, MS, RD, CDE; and Patricia A. Barr, BS, served as lead authors and editors of the first edition published by the American Diabetes Association, and Andrea J. Lasichak, MS, RD, CDE, joined them on the 2nd edition. Martha Funnell and Andrea Lasichak updated the text for this 3rd edition.

Additional contributors are listed as completely as memory permits:

Marilyn Allard, BSN
Diana Barlage, RN, CDE
Carol Barnett, MS, RN
Lucy Bauman, MS, RN
Marilyn Bowbeer, BA
Nugget Burkhart, MA, RN, CDE
Catherine Eichel, MS, RN
John Floyd, Jr., MD
Mary Frey, MS, RN
Margaret Howard, BSN
Patricia Johnson, MSN, RN, CDE
Ralph Knopf, MD
Catherine Martin, MS, RN, CDE
Patricia McNitt, BSN

Sandra Merkle, MS, RN
Mara Mesa, RN, MA, MSW
Lisa Root Parker, BSN
Patricia Rahe, BSN
Cecilia Sauter, MS, RD, CDE
Margaret Smith, RN, BA
Irene Soble, MS, RN
Martha Spencer, MD
Renate Starr, BSN
Linda Strodtman, MS, RN
Carolyn Templeton, MS, RD
Neil White, MD
Linda Zucker, BSN

Graphic Artists

Linda A. Alvira
Nancy Fortino Bates
Michele Dansereau
Holly Harrington
Christine Lux
Kathryn E. Simpson

Reviewers of Current and Previous Editions

Samuel L. Abbate, MD, CDE
Barbara Anderson, PhD
Connie Crawley, RD, BS, MS
John T. Devlin, MD
Charlotte Hayes, MS, RD, CDE
Lois Jovanovic, MD
Joseph B. Nelson, MA
Clara Schneider, MS, RD, RN, LD, CDE
Jacqueline Siegel, RN
Margie Fox, CDE
Neil White, MD

▶ ▶ ▶ ▶ ▶

PURPOSE

The primary purpose of *Life with Diabetes: A Series of Teaching Outlines by the Michigan Diabetes Research and Training Center* is to guide health professionals in the education of patients with diabetes mellitus. The outlines provide information on many diabetes-related topics. Although the content is generally for adults with either type 1 or type 2 diabetes, the information can easily be adapted for use with younger people, pregnant women, or those with special learning needs. The detail portions of the outlines are purposely worded to be brief so that the instructor can quickly scan the outline before teaching a session. The information included in the outlines comes from many sources and has been reviewed by content experts. In some cases, what has been included, and the way it has been stated or drawn, reflects our best compromise.

These outlines are only one component of an educational program and educational process. They are not a substitute for staff development and education nor are they intended to teach the instructor diabetes content or the how-tos of the teaching process. Health care professionals need to be educated in diabetes content and diabetes care as well as in the methods of behavior change, teaching, and counseling before they engage in diabetes education activities, if they are to be effective teachers.

A great deal has been learned in recent years about the effectiveness of diabetes education and about particular program and teaching strategies. As examples, multiple meta-analyses have shown that diabetes education is effective in producing positive outcomes, at least in the short-term. These studies have also shown that group education is effective and that patient participation and collaboration appear to produce more favorable results than didactic presentations. We have also learned that while no one education program is more effective than others, programs that incorporate the behavioral and affective aspects of diabetes produce better outcomes. We encourage you to use this information as you prepare your program and work with participants.

FORMAT AND TIPS FOR USE

For the first time, these outlines are bound into a book that allows you to more easily make copies of the pages. In addition, the book is accompanied by a full-content CD-ROM. Some educators find they use sections of these outlines exactly as they appear, but most prefer to use specific outlines, or portions, to develop individualized curricula. With the content on the CD, you can copy and combine the text, handouts, and graphics you specifically need for an education session. You are invited to use any of the materials in this book that are helpful to you in delivering patient education and to make any changes necessary to adapt the materials to meet specific needs. The

American Diabetes Association requests that any use of these materials be credited with a notification reading:

"These materials were adapted from *Life with Diabetes: A Series of Teaching Outlines by the Michigan Diabetes Research and Training Center.* 3rd Edition. American Diabetes Association, 2004."

Publication of these materials is not allowed without written permission from the American Diabetes Association. Duplication of patient handouts is allowed for classroom use.

The first section consists of core outlines that include the basic information generally taught to people with diabetes. The second section includes supplementary information that is useful for particular situations. It is not necessary to teach the sessions in the order that they are arranged in this book or to include all of the content from each outline in a session.

An approach that we have found to be effective is "ask the experts." In this format, session topics are generated by questions asked by participants. The instructor then builds on content generated by the responses to present related topics. Over the course of a program, a comprehensive curriculum can be presented. Keeping track of topics will help assure that this occurs and that all content areas are addressed. In addition, suggesting that participants try "behavioral experiments" between sessions gives them valuable experiences with behavior change. Beginning the following session with a discussion of what was learned from their experiment (regardless of its success or failure) can be used to generate topics and content areas to address at that session and helps to keep participants actively involved.

Each outline includes a statement of purpose; prerequisites that should be known by participants before attending a particular session; materials needed for teaching the session; a content outline that includes the general concepts to be covered, specific details, and instructor's notes or teaching tips; an evaluation and documentation plan; and suggested readings related to each topic. The content areas in the National Standards for Diabetes Self-Management Education were specifically written to allow for maximum flexibility and creativity in presentation style and method. Key behavioral and psychosocial aspects of each content area were incorporated to help participants to better integrate these aspects into their lives and self-management activities.

The material in each outline includes basic information about diabetes, diabetes self-care, and general health care practices. It does not include specific information for particular ethnic, cultural, or age-related groups, but it does make distinctions as to type 1 and type 2 diabetes. It is important to assess the individual and group needs of the participants because the effectiveness of education is enhanced by tailoring to the specific needs of the audience. Information may need to be added or deleted, depending on your population and their needs. Again, the content on the CD-ROM will enable just that.

It is particularly important to consider the literacy skills of your participants. Fully 25% of adults in the United States have difficulty reading even simple text, and their ability to understand complex information presented orally is also limited. Simplify concepts; use plain, straightforward language; and explain any unfamiliar words you use when teaching.

OVERVIEW OF NUTRITION OUTLINES

A significant portion of this curriculum addresses nutrition, often the most difficult aspect of diabetes self-care. Many different approaches to meal planning have been developed in recent years. Some are less rigid than earlier plans and may be less difficult for patients to use. However, the increase in meal-planning options presents an even greater challenge for educators, who need the information and skill to explain the choices to their participants and to further assist them in developing individual plans that help them to reach personal goals.

The nutrition outlines are based on the understanding that dietary changes are difficult to initiate and sustain and that the fewer the changes, the more likely they will be attempted and maintained. Fewer but more effective and reasonable changes can be developed when the participant and health care professional are aware of usual, cultural, and preferred eating patterns. The outlines provide activities intended to help class members become aware of when, how much, and what they are eating, before information about meal planning is given. People are often frustrated by changing dietary recommendations. Let class members know that the information provided is based on current interpretation of scientific findings—which do change.

Although there are many potential benefits that can occur as a result of food choices, blood glucose management is the benefit unique to diabetes. It contributes most to reducing acute and long-term complications and allows many people to feel better on a day-to-day basis. Therefore, the primary focus of the core nutrition outlines is blood glucose management. Although this is presented in the context of overall healthy food choices, it is important for the educator to distinguish between changes that benefit overall health and those that contribute directly to blood glucose management.

The sequence of topics has been chosen intentionally to help participants focus on one or two aspects of their diet at once and to encourage behavioral steps toward long-term goals. Blood glucose monitoring is encouraged to provide participants with information about the effects of different food choices on their blood glucose levels. The nutrition information to support blood glucose management is found in the Core Outlines section.

Additional content outlines are found in the Supplementary Outlines section. These include special issues and more intensive meal-planning approaches.

EVALUATION

The educational process is not complete without the evaluation of the outcomes achieved. This can be done in several ways. In terms of diabetes self-management skills and content, a conventional method is to assess the participant's preprogram knowledge, develop learning objectives based on the assessment, and then determine whether the participants met their learning objectives at the conclusion of the program. Diabetes self-care skills need to be evaluated by observation.

Application of knowledge is more difficult to evaluate than content learned. One method for evaluating behavior change is through personal goals, the development and implementation of a plan to achieve those goals, and goal attainment. In this approach, participants define and articulate meaningful and personal goals relevant to their diabetes care. It is generally most effective for participants to begin by choosing an overall or long-term goal related to their diabetes: for example, to lose 10 pounds over the next 4 months. They then choose short-term behavior-change goals that will be helpful in reaching their overall goal: for example, eat breakfast 5 days out of 7 for the next 2 weeks. They then rate how well they were able to achieve their short-term behavior-change goals. This rating is used as a basis for decision-making for additional goal-setting or problem-solving if the goal was not achieved. It can also be used to monitor the educational progress over time, i.e., over several encounters with the health care system.

In addition to achievement of individual learning objectives and behavioral goals, other outcome measures can be used to evaluate the program's effectiveness. Participant outcomes that can be measured include levels of metabolic control, acute complications, process measures for monitoring complications, hospitalizations related to diabetes, lost work or school days, and psychosocial indicators. The outcome measures selected depend on the program design, target population, resources, and goals.

RESOURCE MATERIALS

Additional information has been included to help you in using these teaching guides, including resources for audiovisual programs and written materials; lists of other resources, including health professional and patient organizations, publications, and Internet sources; and a list of supplemental readings.

DIABETES EDUCATION RECOGNITION PROCESS

The American Diabetes Association's Education Recognition Program is a national voluntary process that formally identifies diabetes self-management education programs that meet the National Standards for Diabetes Self-Management Education. For more information, visit http://www.diabetes.org/recognition/education or call 1-800-DIABETES.

Core
Outlines

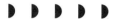

| #1 | What Is Diabetes? |

STATEMENT OF PURPOSE

This session is intended to provide information about the definition, pathophysiology, and treatment of diabetes.

PREREQUISITES

None.

OBJECTIVES

At the end of this session, participants will be able to:

1. identify diabetes as a chronic disorder of metabolism in which the body is unable to use food properly for energy, resulting in hyperglycemia;
2. identify the pancreas as the organ that makes the hormone, insulin;
3. state that the normal fasting plasma glucose is 70–100 mg/dl;
4. define *hyperglycemia* and list the symptoms;
5. state which of the two types of diabetes they have, type 1 or type 2;
6. list several factors that may contribute to the development of diabetes;
7. state that diabetes is a lifelong condition;
8. state that learning about diabetes and self-care is an important factor in the management of diabetes and prevention of complications;
9. list 3 components of the treatment of diabetes;
10. state the importance of their role in decision-making.

CONTENT

Diabetes Disease Process.

MATERIALS NEEDED

VISUALS PROVIDED	ADDITIONAL
1. Pancreas	■ Body model
2. Normal Glucose Metabolism	■ Video programs that provide an overview of the
3. How Insulin Works	pathophysiology and treatment of diabetes
4. Normal Blood Glucose and Insulin Levels	

MATERIALS NEEDED *continued*

VISUALS PROVIDED	ADDITIONAL

5. Glucose Metabolism in Diabetes
6. Oral Glucose Tolerance Test
7. Progression of Type 2 Diabetes
8. Insulin Resistance Due to Excess Weight

METHOD OF PRESENTATION

Start by introducing yourself and telling what you do. Ask participants to introduce themselves, say how long they have had diabetes, and how their diabetes is currently treated. Explain that the purpose of this session is to provide a basic overview of diabetes. Ask participants to identify what would be useful areas for discussion.

Present material in a question/discussion format. Show one of the videotapes, if desired, or encourage participants to "ask the expert" and provide content in response to questions.

CONTENT OUTLINE

CONCEPT	DETAIL	INSTRUCTOR'S NOTES
1. Definition of diabetes mellitus	1.1 Define *diabetes mellitus*.	*Diabetes* = running through *Mellitus* = sweet
	1.2 Diabetes is a disorder of metabolism.	Ask, "What is diabetes? How would you explain it to another person? What questions or concerns do you have about diabetes?"
	1.3 There is insufficient insulin activity in the body. Insulin is made by the pancreas. Insulin is needed to use the food we eat for energy.	
2. Pancreas	2.1 The pancreas is a large, elongated gland located behind the stomach.	Show pancreas on the body model or Visual #1, Pancreas.
	2.2 The pancreas has two functions:	
	a. Secretion of pancreatic juice that aids in digestion (exocrine function).	This is done by 99% of the pancreas.
	b. Secretion of hormones that control various body processes (endocrine function). Insulin is a hormone made by beta cells in the pancreas. Insulin regulates carbohydrate metabolism.	Only 1% of the pancreas—the islets of Langerhans—performs this job.

CONTENT OUTLINE

CONCEPT	DETAIL	INSTRUCTOR'S NOTES
3. Normal food metabolism	3.1 To understand and manage diabetes, you need to know what happens when you eat. Food is broken into simple forms by enzymes (chemicals) in the digestive system.	Some of these enzymes are produced by the pancreas.
	3.2 Most of the food you eat is broken down into glucose and other simple sugars.	
	3.3 Glucose is absorbed into the bloodstream to be used by cells for energy. Cells need glucose to work.	Use Visual #2, Normal Glucose Metabolism. Some of the non-glucose simple sugar is converted to glucose by the liver.
	3.4 Blood glucose rises promptly after food is eaten. Insulin is released from the pancreas as blood glucose levels go up.	
	3.5 Cells have receptor sites on the outside. When insulin attaches to the receptor sites, a passageway is made and glucose goes into the cell. Insulin "opens" the cells, like a key.	Most cells need insulin for glucose to enter. Brain, liver, and kidney cells do not; these cells receive glucose even though there is little insulin activity. Use Visual #3, How Insulin Works.
	3.6 Because glucose goes out of the blood and into the cells, plasma blood glucose levels stay in the normal range of 70–100 mg/dl.	Ask, "What are normal blood glucose levels?" Use Visual #4, Normal Blood Glucose and Insulin Levels.
	3.7 Excess food is generally converted into fat and stored.	Usually blood glucose rises to <140 mg/dl and returns to normal 2 hours after beginning to eat.
4. Food metabolism in diabetes	4.1 Food is broken down in the normal way.	
	4.2 Digestive enzymes act in the normal way.	The digestive enzymes produced by the pancreas are not affected by diabetes.
	4.3 Glucose is absorbed into the bloodstream in the normal way.	
	4.4 But, there is not enough insulin action.	The key to the cells (insulin) is missing.

CONTENT OUTLINE

CONCEPT	DETAIL	INSTRUCTOR'S NOTES
	4.5 Without insulin action, glucose can't get into most cells to be used for energy.	
	4.6 Glucose stays in the blood. There is not enough insulin action to maintain a normal blood glucose level.	Use Visual #5, Glucose Metabolism in Diabetes.
	4.7 Blood glucose level rises, leading to *hyperglycemia*.	Insulin maintains euglycemia by allowing glucose to move into the cells.
	4.8 Most cells are drowning in glucose on the outside and starving for it on the inside.	
5. Signs and symptoms of hyperglycemia	5.1 The symptoms are caused by high glucose levels and by your body's efforts to get rid of the extra sugar.	Ask, "What symptoms did you have before you found out you had diabetes?" *hyper* = high *glyc* = sugar *emia* = blood
	5.2 The kidneys work as filters to remove waste products from the blood, including excess glucose. The higher the glucose levels in the blood, the more glucose will appear in the urine, and the harder the kidneys have to work.	Glucose leaving the body in the urine is called *glycosuria*. In some patients, hyperglycemia must be extreme before glycosuria develops. The renal threshold is the level at which glycosuria develops.
	5.3 This leads to extra urine production. Your body must make more urine to get rid of the extra glucose. This is called *polyuria*.	High levels of glucose in the urine increases urination correspondingly, as your body dilutes the sugar.
	5.4 When you urinate a lot, your body needs more water. This increases your thirst. Increased thirst is called *polydipsia* and is due to polyuria.	
	5.5 *Polyphagia* (increased hunger) is due to starvation of the cells because glucose stays in the blood and is not available to the cells.	Loss of glucose through the urine means loss of calories.
	5.6 Dehydration, weight loss, weakness, and fatigue also happen.	Other factors, such as anorexia, may contribute to weight loss.

CONTENT OUTLINE

CONCEPT	DETAIL	INSTRUCTOR'S NOTES
	5.7 Blurred vision results from hyper-glycemia. Sugar accumulates in the lens of the eye, causing the lens to swell and distort vision. As blood glucose returns to normal, the lens usually recovers its shape and vision changes again.	Participants need to wait 6–8 weeks after blood glucose levels are regulated before under-going vision testing for glasses. Reassure participants that these changes are not related to blind-ness (retinopathy) from diabetes.
	5.8 Another symptom of high blood glucose is itching, especially in the genital area.	Itching can be caused by dry skin from dehydration, or an overgrowth of microorganisms.
	5.9 Slow or confused thinking can occur if hyperglycemia and dehydration are marked; coma and cerebrovascular accident can result.	The brain cannot function well if fluids are unbalanced.
6. Tests used to diagnose diabetes	6.1 One test to diagnose diabetes is called the fasting plasma glucose test. A blood sample is taken after a 10–12 hour fast, usually before breakfast. A normal result is 70–100 mg/dl. Values above 126 mg/dl more than once are diagnostic of diabetes.	Ask, "How was your diabetes diagnosed? Were you ever told you had pre-diabetes?" Pre-diabetes is defined as a fast-ing plasma glucose value ≥100 and ≤126 or a 2-hour plasma glucose value ≥140 and <200.
	6.2 Another test is called the random serum glucose test. A nonfasting plasma glucose level of >200 mg/dl along with classic symptoms is diagnostic.	
	6.3 A third test is the oral glucose toler-ance test (OGTT). After a 10- to 12-hour fast, a blood sample is taken. A glucose dose is then given and blood samples are taken every half hour for 2–5 hours. This test is done if there is a question of pre-diabetes or diabetes and the fasting plasma glucose level is not diagnostically elevated.	Use Visual #6, Oral Glucose Tolerance Test, if patients have had this test and are interested. An adequate carbohydrate diet before the test is necessary for the results to be reliable.
	6.4 A 2-hour postprandial plasma glucose test is often used for diagnostic purposes. A high-carbohydrate meal may be given before the test, especially to children.	

CONTENT OUTLINE

CONCEPT	DETAIL	INSTRUCTOR'S NOTES
7. Type 1 diabetes	7.1 There are several types of diabetes. The two most common types are type 1 and type 2.	
	7.2 In type 1, the pancreas makes little or no insulin.	Old names for type 1 are insulin-dependent, juvenile-onset, ketosis-prone, unstable, or brittle diabetes.
	7.3 People with type 1 are prone to develop ketosis.	Ketosis will be explained later.
	7.4 People with type 1 need insulin in order to stay alive.	
	7.5 Type 1 can begin at any age, but it usually occurs in children and young adults.	The incidence of type 2 diabetes among children and adolescents is increasing.
8. Type 2 diabetes	8.1 The pancreas is producing insulin, but the amount is not adequate, or the insulin is not effective in lowering blood glucose because the cells are resistant.	Old names for type 2 are maturity-onset, adult onset, and insulin-resistant diabetes. Use Visual #7, Progression of Type 2 Diabetes.
	8.2 With insulin resistance, the pancreas produces more insulin than usual, but the cells are unable to use the insulin because there are fewer receptors.	The insulin also remains in the bloodstream.
	8.3 People with type 2 are unlikely to develop ketosis.	
	8.4 Onset is possible at any age, but type 2 is more commonly diagnosed after age 30.	Type 2 diabetes may occur at younger ages in high-risk populations.
	8.5 The treatment for type 2 diabetes is done in phases or stages: nutrition therapy and exercise, and oral medications and/or insulin.	Exercise and weight loss may help decrease insulin resistance. Meal planning and exercise are important during all phases.
	8.6 Because pancreatic function declines over time, insulin is often needed to achieve blood glucose goals.	Emphasize that people with type 2 often progress to insulin and that it is not a failure or a sign that their diabetes is worse. Clarify the difference between type 1 and type 2 diabetes.

CONTENT OUTLINE

CONCEPT	DETAIL	INSTRUCTOR'S NOTES
9. Factors contributing to the development of diabetes	9.1 The exact cause of diabetes is unknown. Heredity is a factor in both types of diabetes, but is more often associated with type 2. If one parent has type 2, the risk is 10–15% that children will get it as adults. If one parent has type 1, the risk is 2–5%.	You don't catch diabetes or get it from eating sweets. Studies show that if one identical twin gets type 1, the other doesn't always (25–50%). This indicates that something in the environment has brought out the diabetes in one twin. If one twin gets type 2, the other usually does too (60–75%). The Diabetes Prevention Program (DPP) demonstrated that modest weight loss (5–10% body weight) and activity (150 minutes/week) is effective to delay/prevent the onset of type 2 diabetes for people of all ages and ethnic groups with pre-diabetes. Stress the importance of preventing type 2 diabetes among their children and grandchildren.
	9.2 Being overweight is a factor in developing diabetes. More and larger body cells require energy. Also, cells are more resistant to insulin than normal because, as cells get larger, receptor sites are lost. Thus, more insulin is needed for both reasons.	The most common precipitating factor in type 2 is that 80–90% are obese at the time of diagnosis. Use Visual #8, Insulin Resistance Due to Excess Weight. Note the larger body cell with fewer receptor sites. The insulin molecule cannot attach to the cell; therefore, the glucose molecule cannot attach to the insulin molecule.
	9.3 Stresses, both emotional and physical, may precipitate or aggravate type 1 and type 2: ■ pregnancy (gestational diabetes) ■ illness or surgery ■ medications such as glucosteroids (e.g., prednisone) 9.4 Age is a factor (incidence of diabetes increases with age).	Gestational diabetes may go away after the pregnancy, but may reappear as type 2 diabetes later in life.

CONTENT OUTLINE

CONCEPT	DETAIL	INSTRUCTOR'S NOTES
	9.5 Injury to the pancreas (infection, surgery, tumor, or trauma) may lead to diabetes, even in low-hereditary-risk groups.	People with diabetes as a result of pancreatectomy are considered to have type 1 diabetes.
	9.6 Ethnic background can contribute (Native Americans, Hispanic Americans, and African Americans have a higher incidence of type 2 diabetes).	
	9.7 In combination with hereditary factors predisposing to the development of type 1 are the following: ■ immunologic factors (antibodies against the islet cells that produce insulin) ■ viral factors (post-mumps, rubella, or coxsackie)	
10. Treatment of diabetes mellitus	10.1 Diabetes is a serious, lifelong condition. It is not curable, but it is treatable.	Stress the seriousness of both types of diabetes.
	10.2 Most (95–99%) of the daily care of diabetes is self-care. You make many decisions each day that affect your blood glucose levels and long-term outcomes.	Stress the importance of the role of the person with diabetes as a care provider.
	10.3 Most problems in diabetes are linked to blood glucose levels that are too high or too low. One of the most important things you can do is to learn about diabetes and how to manage blood glucose levels.	
	10.4 The first step is to decide your **personal** blood glucose goal. Treatment, including self-care, is then based on working toward this goal.	Keeping blood glucose levels near normal helps decrease symptoms and reduces the risks for the acute and long-term complications of diabetes.
	10.5 The treatment of type 1 diabetes always includes insulin. The intensity (number of shots each day, meal plan, and exercise) of the treatment is based on blood glucose and other goals.	

CONTENT OUTLINE

CONCEPT	DETAIL	INSTRUCTOR'S NOTES
	10.6 The treatment of type 2 diabetes is usually done in stages or phases— starting with meal planning and exercise, then oral medicines (if needed), and then insulin, alone or with oral medications (if needed). Each stage will be tried for 3–6 months. Effectiveness is evaluated based on blood glucose goals.	Stress that they may stay in one phase or stage for awhile, but that they should not stay with a form of treatment that is not effective. Remind participants that treatment failures are not personal failures.
	10.7 A meal plan for glucose control distributes carbohydrate, protein, and fat throughout the day to smooth out blood glucose levels and balance with insulin or oral medicines, if taken.	They will design their diabetes meal plan in collaboration with a dietitian.
	10.8 A meal plan for weight control reduces calorie intake within the framework of glucose control.	Even a small weight loss (5–10%) can lower blood glucose significantly for two reasons: receptor sites return, and there is less metabolic demand on the body.
	10.9 Exercise usually lowers blood glucose because exercise increases the rate of burning of blood glucose (metabolism). It also provides a sense of well-being, aids the vascular system, and helps in weight reduction.	
	10.10 Medication involves oral agents (which are **not** insulin) and/or insulin.	Stress the need to use meal plans and exercise along with medications.
11. Self-Care	11.1 Caring for diabetes is different than caring for other illnesses. You provide most of your own daily care. The choices and decisions you make each day affect both how you feel today and your long-term health.	Ask, "How is caring for diabetes different? What are some choices you make that affect your diabetes?"
	11.2 Caring for diabetes is not easy. It may mean changing the habits of of a lifetime.	
	11.3 Diabetes causes many feelings that can affect how you care for yourself.	

CONTENT OUTLINE

CONCEPT	DETAIL	INSTRUCTOR'S NOTES
	11.4 It is unrealistic to think that you can make all of the changes at one time. Many people find choosing long-term blood glucose and other goals and then choosing and reaching short-term goals is helpful.	Ask participants to select a long-term goal related to diabetes and an appropriate short-term goal that can be achieved by the next class. Examples: If the long-term goal is to lose 30 lb, the short-term goal could be to eat 1½ sandwiches for lunch instead of 2. If the long-term goal is a lower A1C level, then the short-term goal may be to walk three times a week for 20 minutes. The purpose of this is to give participants a chance to experiment and learn by trying to make a behavior change.
	11.5 Reward yourself when you accomplish your short-term goals.	
	11.6 These classes will also offer tips to carry out needed care.	

SKILLS CHECKLIST

None.

EVALUATION PLAN

Knowledge will be evaluated by achievement of learning objectives and by responses to questions during the session. The ability to apply knowledge will be evaluated by the recognition of feelings about diabetes, the development of personal self-care goals, the development and implementation of a plan to achieve those goals and through program outcome measures.

DOCUMENTATION PLAN

Record class attendance and achieved objectives as appropriate.

SUGGESTED READINGS

AADE White Paper. White paper on the prevention of type 2 diabetes and the role of *The Diabetes Educator*. 2002;28:964–970.

American Diabetes Association and National Institute of Diabetes, Digestive and Kidney Diseases. The prevention or delay of type 2 diabetes. *Diabetes Care*. 2002;25:742–749.

American Diabetes Association. *Annual Review of Diabetes*. Alexandria, VA: American Diabetes Association, 2003.

American Diabetes Association. Clinical practice recommendations. *Diabetes Care*. 2004;27(Suppl 1):1–150.

American Diabetes Association. *The Complete Guide to Diabetes*, 3rd Edition. Alexandria, VA: American Diabetes Association, 2003.

American Diabetes Association. Consensus Statement. Type 2 diabetes in children. *Diabetes Care*. 2000;23:381–338.

American Diabetes Association. *Diabetes A to Z*, 5th Edition. Alexandria, VA: American Diabetes Association, 2003.

American Diabetes Association. *Diabetes Ready-Reference Guide for Health Care Professionals*, 2nd Edition. Alexandria, VA: American Diabetes Association, 2004.

American Diabetes Association. Diagnosis and classification of diabetes mellitus. *Diabetes Care*. 2004;27(Suppl 1):S5–S10.

American Diabetes Association. *Medical Management of Type 1 Diabetes*, 4th Edition. Alexandria, VA: American Diabetes Association, 2003.

American Diabetes Association. *Medical Management of Type 2 Diabetes*, 5th Edition. Alexandria, VA: American Diabetes Association, 2004.

American Diabetes Association. Prevention or delay of type 2 diabetes. *Diabetes Care*. 2004;27(Suppl 1):S47–S54.

American Diabetes Association. Screening for type 2 diabetes. *Diabetes Care*. 2004;27(Suppl 1):S11–S14.

American Diabetes Association. Standards for medical care in diabetes. *Diabetes Care*. 2004;27(Suppl. 1):S15–S35.

American Diabetes Association. *A Field Guide to Type 1 Diabetes*. Alexandria, VA: American Diabetes Association, 2000.

American Diabetes Association. *Therapy for Diabetes Mellitus and Related Disorders*, 4th Edition. Alexandria, VA: American Diabetes Association, 2004.

Brown JB, Nichols GA, Glauber HS, Bakst AW. Type 2 diabetes: incremental medical care costs during the first 8 years after diagnosis. *Diabetes Care*. 1999;22:1116–1124.

Buse JB. Progressive use of medical therapies in type 2 diabetes. *Diabetes Spectrum*. 2000;13:211–220.

Clark CM Jr. Meeting the challenges of NIDDM. *Diabetes Spectrum*. 1996;9:23–62.

Clark W. Treatment options for type 2 diabetes: finding what's best for you. *Diabetes Self-Management*. 2002;19(2):6–13.

Clement S. Spring cleaning diabetes style. *Diabetes Forecast*. 2003;56(5):70–71.

Egede LE, Ye Z, Zheng D, Silverstein MD. The prevalence and pattern of complementary and alternative medicine use in individuals with diabetes. *Diabetes Care*. 2002;25:324–329.

Engelgau MM, Narayan KMV, Herman WH. Screening for type 2 diabetes: a technical review. *Diabetes Care*. 2000;23:1563–1580.

Engelgau MM, Thompson TJ, Herman WH, Boyle JP, Aubert RE, Kenny SJ, Badran A, Sous ES, Ali MA. Comparison of fasting and 2-hour glucose and HbA_{1c} levels for diagnosing diabetes. *Diabetes Care*. 1997;20:785–791.

Ernst E. Complementary medicine: it's hidden risks. *Diabetes Care*. 2001;24:1486–1488.

Expert Committee on the Diagnosis and Classification of Diabetes Mellitus: Report of the Expert Committee on the Diagnosis and Classification of Diabetes Mellitus. *Diabetes Care*. 1997;20:1183–1197.

Franz MJ, Hunt C, Kulkarni K, Polonsky WH, Yarborough PC, Zamudio J, Eds: *A Core Curriculum for Diabetes Educators*, 4th Edition. Chicago, IL: American Association of Diabetes Educators, 2001.

SUGGESTED READINGS *continued*

Funnell MM, Merritt JH: The older adult with diabetes. *Nurse Practitioner Forum.* 1998;9:98–107.

Guthrie DW, Guthrie RA, eds. *Nursing. Management of Diabetes Mellitus,* 5th Edition. Springer Publishing Company, 2001.

Hagopian W, Hirsch IB. Demystifying diabetes type. Practical Diabetology. 2004;23(1):30–32.

Harris JI, Klein R, Welborn TA, Knuiman MW. Onset of NIDDM occurs at least 4–7 years before clinical diagnosis. *Diabetes Care.* 1992;15:815–819.

Harris MI. Health care and health status and outcomes for patients with type 2 diabetes. *Diabetes Care.* 2000;23:754–764.

Institute of Medicine of the National Academies. New eating and physical activity targets to reduce chronic disease risk factors. *The Diabetes Educator.* 2003;29:76–79.

Jorgensen WA, Polivka BJ, Lennie TA. Perceived adherence to prescribed or recommended standards of care among adults with diabetes. *The Diabetes Educator.* 2002;28:989–998.

Koro CE, Bowlin SJ, Beourgeois N, Fedder DO. Glycemic control from 1988 to 2000 among US adults diagnosed with type 2 diabetes: a preliminary report. *Diabetes Care.* 2004;27:17–20.

Lindstrom J, Tuomilehto J. The diabetes risk score. *Diabetes Care.* 2003;26:725–731.

Narayan KMV, Boyle JP, Thompson TJ, Sorensen SW, Williamson DF. Lifetime risk for diabetes mellitus in the US. *JAMA.* 2003;290:1884–1890.

National Diabetes Information Clearinghouse. *The Diabetes Dictionary.* Bethesda, MD: National Diabetes Information Clearinghouse, 2003.

Nichols GA, Hillier TA, Javor K, Brown JB. Predictors of glycemic control in insulin-using adults with type 2 diabetes. *Diabetes Care.* 2000;23:273–277.

O'Connell B, Hieronymus L. What is diabetes? *Diabetes Self-Management.* 2003;20(5):93–97.

Payne C. Complementary and integrative medicine: emerging therapies for diabetes. *Diabetes Spectrum.* 2001;14:129–171.

Riddle MC. Managing type 2 diabetes over time: lessons from the UKPDS. *Diabetes Spectrum.* 2000;13:194–223.

Sacks DB, Brtuns DE, Goldstein DE, Macaren MK, McDonald JM, Parrott M. Guidelines and recommendations for laboratory analysis in the diagnosis and management of diabetes mellitus. *Diabetes Care.* 2001;24:750–786.

Saddine JB, Engelgau MM, Beckles GL, Gregg EW, Thompson TJ, Narayan KMV. A diabetes report card for the US: quality of care in the 1990s. *Annals of Internal Medicine.* 2002;136:565–574.

Saudek CD, Loman K. 10 tips for better blood sugar control. *Diabetes Forecast.* 2001;54(10):58–62.

Service RJ, Rizza RA, Zimmerman BR, Dyck PJ, O'Brien PC, Melton LJ: The classification of diabetes by clinical and c-peptide criteria. *Diabetes Care.* 1997;20:198–201.

The QuED Study Group. The relationship between physicians' self-reported target fasting blood glucose levels and metabolic control in type 2 diabetes. *Diabetes Care.* 2001;24:423–429.

Touchette N: *The Diabetes Problem Solver.* Alexandria, VA: American Diabetes Association, 1999.

Vinicor, F, Burton B, Foster B, Eastman, B. Healthy people 2010: diabetes. *Diabetes Care.* 2000;23:853–855.

Wagner EH, Grothaus LC, Sandhu N, Galvin MS, McGregor M, Artz K, Coleman, EA. Chronic care clinics for diabetes in primary care. *Diabetes Care.* 2001;24:695–700.

Weir GC, Nathan DM, Singer DE. Standards of care for diabetes: a technical review. *Diabetes Care.* 1994;17:1514–1522.

Weiss R, Caprio S. Type 2 diabetes in children and adolescents. *Practical Diabetology.* 2004;22(4):19–23.

➡ Pancreas

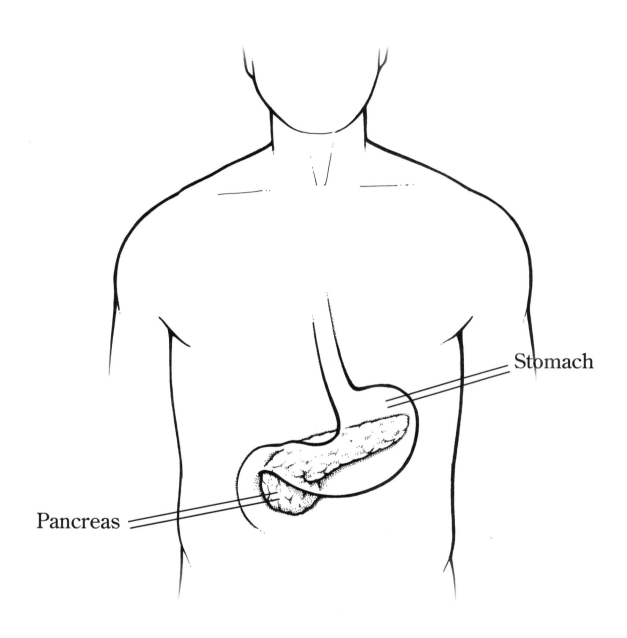

Stomach

Pancreas

➜ Normal Glucose Metabolism

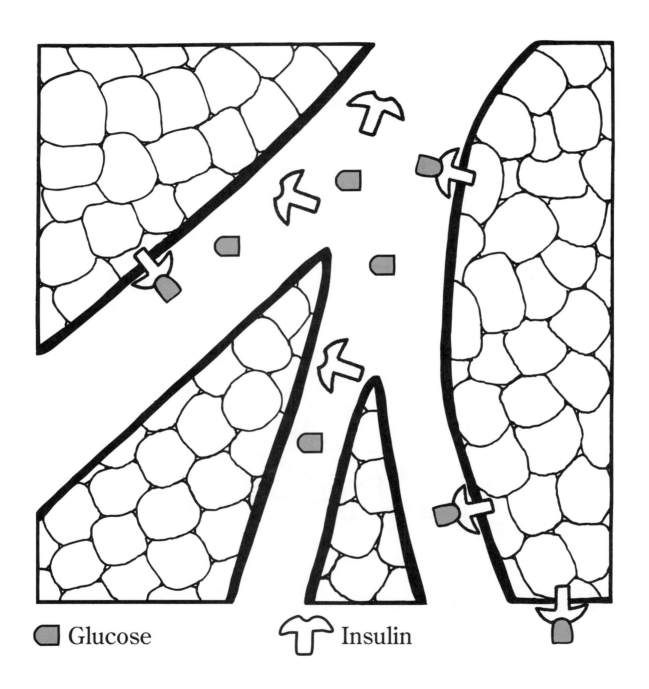

Glucose   Insulin

➲ How Insulin Works

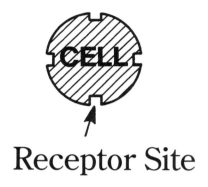

Receptor Site

Insulin Fills Receptor Sites

Insulin

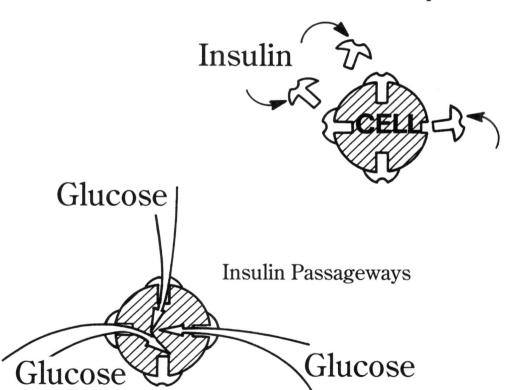

Glucose

Insulin Passageways

Glucose   Glucose

⮕ Normal Blood Glucose and Insulin Levels

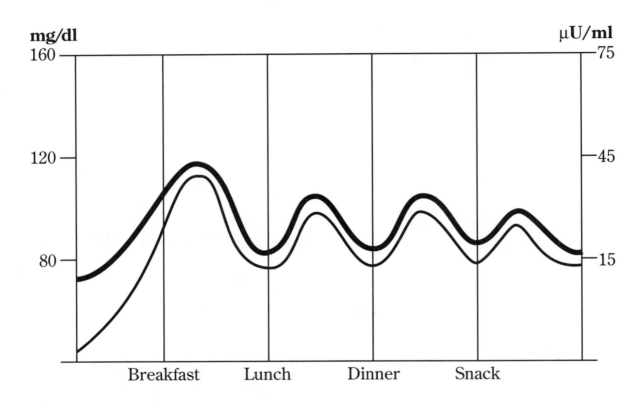

mg/dl   **μU/ml**

160 ———————————————————————— 75

120 ———————————————————————— 45

80 ———————————————————————— 15

Breakfast   Lunch   Dinner   Snack

▬▬▬ Blood Glucose Level

—— Plasma Insulin Level

➡ Glucose Metabolism in Diabetes

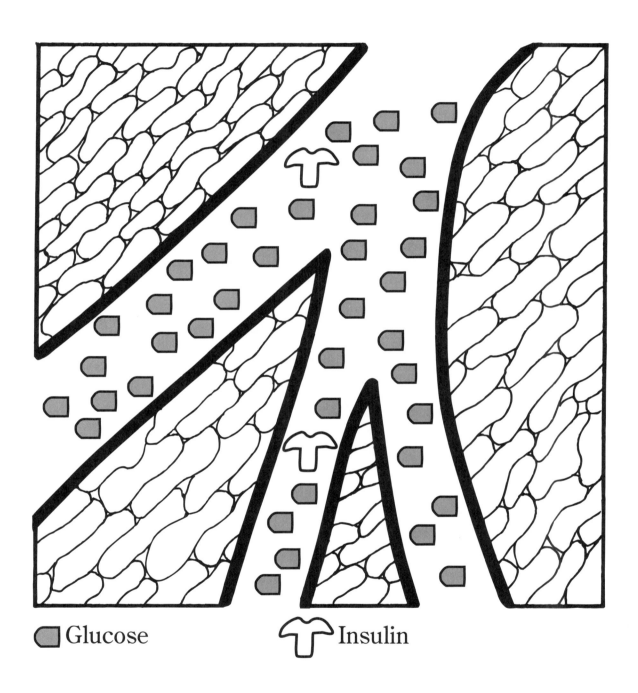

⬟ Glucose   ⬥ Insulin

➔ Oral Glucose Tolerance Test

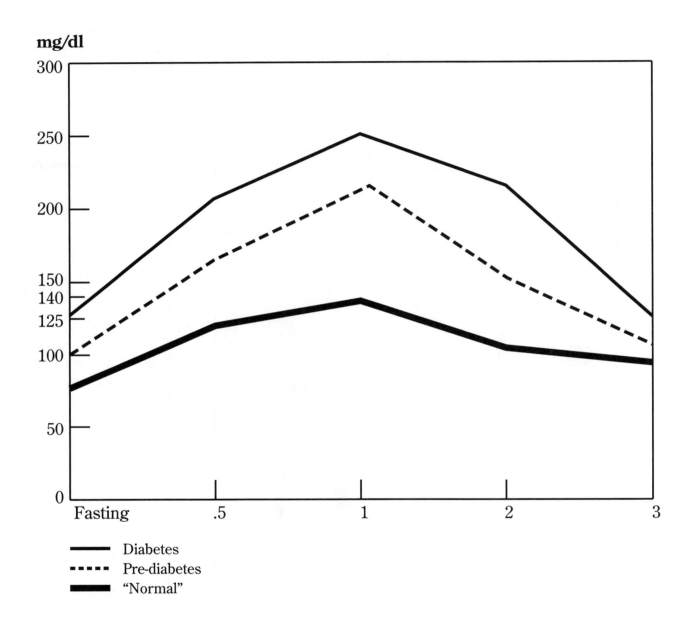

mg/dl

Diabetes
Pre-diabetes
"Normal"

➥ Progression of Type 2 Diabetes

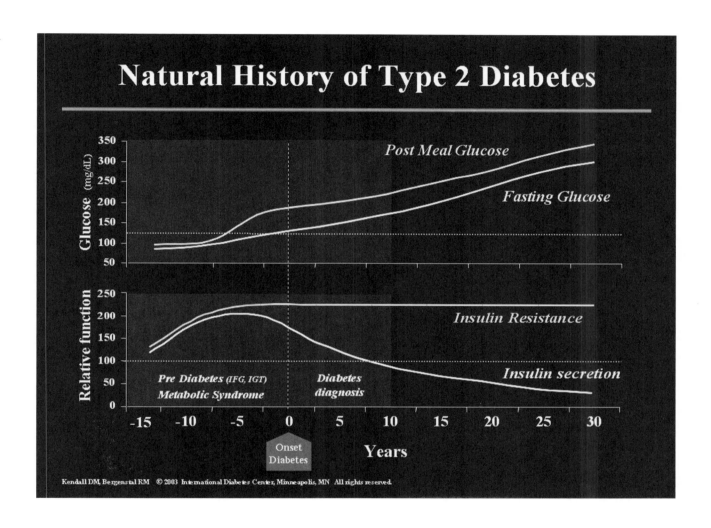

➔ Insulin Resistance Due to Excess Weight

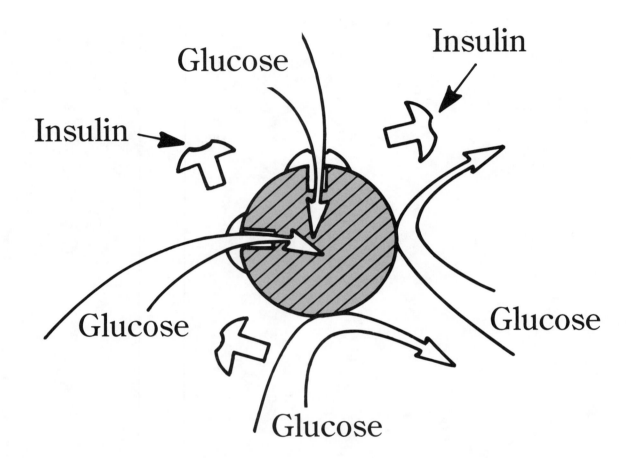

| #2 | **Learning to Live with Diabetes** |

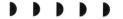

STATEMENT OF PURPOSE

This session is intended to encourage people with diabetes and their significant others to recognize and express feelings about having diabetes and how it affects their lives.

PREREQUISITES

None.

OBJECTIVES

At the end of this session, participants will be able to:

1. express the effects diabetes has had or may have on their way of life and the lives of their families;

2. state who they have told about their diabetes, and state who needs to be told and why;

3. express feelings about having diabetes;

4. share experiences, personal successes, and problems in coping with diabetes;

5. identify a source of emotional support, or state one way to increase support.

CONTENT

Psychosocial Adjustment.

MATERIALS NEEDED

VISUALS PROVIDED	ADDITIONAL
None.	■ Information about local diabetes support groups and other local resources ■ "Trigger" videotapes to initiate discussion of these issues

METHOD OF PRESENTATION

Start by introducing yourself and telling what you do. Ask participants to introduce themselves. Explain that the purpose of this session is not only to give information, but to provide a time for participants to express their thoughts about living with diabetes. You may wish to use a videotape as an introduction to the topic, and then facilitate a group discussion.

It is important to acknowledge and validate any feelings expressed by participants. If parents or other family members are present, you can draw them into the discussion by asking about their thoughts and concerns. One option is to close with an exercise from Outline #16, *Putting the Pieces Together*, such as situation two, three, and/or ten.

CONTENT OUTLINE

CONCEPT	DETAIL	INSTRUCTOR'S NOTES
1. Diabetes as a chronic illness	1.1 Diabetes is a lifelong condition.	Feelings are a critical component of diabetes self-management and need to be acknowledged and incorporated throughout the educational program.
	1.2 As such, it affects many aspects of a person's life.	
2. Possible effects on the way one lives	2.1 Some of the effects diabetes may have on your life are: ■ the need for a regular schedule ■ a change in eating habits ■ daily medication and monitoring ■ possible changes in recreational or occupational pursuits ■ possible changes in relationships with people ■ fear of future effects on life and health	Ask, "What effect has diabetes had on your life?" Acknowledge the difficulties of living with diabetes every day.
3. Identification of self as a person with diabetes	3.1 Who has been told?	
	3.2 Does everyone need to know?	Ask, "How have others reacted when you've told them you have diabetes? How would you like others to respond?"

CONTENT OUTLINE

CONCEPT	DETAIL	INSTRUCTOR'S NOTES
	3.3 Who needs to know and why (family, school, employer, or responsible adult)?	School personnel need preparation to accommodate the child with diabetes. Other classmates need reassurance that diabetes isn't contagious.
4. **Feelings about having diabetes**	4.1 Everyone has feelings or thoughts about having diabetes.	Ask, "What were your feelings (thoughts) when you first found out you had diabetes? What are your feelings (thoughts) now about diabetes? What are your fears or concerns about diabetes? What's the worst thing about diabetes for you?"
	4.2 Feelings may vary from day to day and change over time.	It is important for the instructor to realize that feelings are not problems to be solved. The instructor's role is to assist participants to acknowledge and clarify feelings with questions such as, "You felt *(feeling)* because of *(reason)*?" It is unlikely that participants will resolve their feelings by the end of this class session.
	4.3 Fear or worry about long-term effects of diabetes is also common.	
	4.4 Your feelings and stress levels affect your blood glucose levels, and your blood glucose levels affect your mood and your ability to cope with stress.	
	4.5 Family members, expecially parents, may feel guilty. Adult children may worry about getting diabetes, and siblings may feel jealous of the attention paid to the family member with diabetes.	
	4.6 It is common to go through stages of the grieving process: denial, anger, depression, and adaptation.	

CONTENT OUTLINE

CONCEPT	DETAIL	INSTRUCTOR'S NOTES
	4.7 **Denial.** People may find it hard to believe they have diabetes, that they really have to take care of it or that certain aspects of their treatment are needed.	Learning may be difficult at this stage. When a participant is experiencing denial, it is important to support the person without supporting his or her denial. An appropriate response might be, "I can see you are sincere in your belief about _____, but can I tell you why I'm concerned about you?"
	4.8 **Anger.** People may wonder, "Why me?" or act angrily to family and friends. They are really angry about having diabetes.	Ask, "Do you find that you get angry more easily?" Anger about an illness can be expressed as anger toward other people. Again, it is essential to continue accepting the participants as he or she is. Statements such as, "You sound angry about _____" can let him or her know that you are a concerned, willing listener.
	4.9 **Depression.** Anger, bottled up inside over time, can lead to feeling very sad and blue—even hopeless.	Ask, "What are signs of depression?" Accepting the participant and actively listening can be positive interventions. Statements such as, "It sounds as if you're sad about _____" can help the participant talk about the issue.
	4.10 People with diabetes are twice as likely to suffer from depression. While everyone feels sad now and then, clinical depression is a serious medical problem. Feeling sad most of the time for more than 2 weeks may indicate clinical depression. This type of depression can be successfully treated with a combination of medication and counseling.	Screening questions for clinical depression are: "Over the past 2 weeks, have you felt down, depressed, and hopeless?" and "Over the past 2 weeks, have you felt little interest or pleasure in doing things?"

CONTENT OUTLINE

CONCEPT	DETAIL	INSTRUCTOR'S NOTES
	4.11 The direct effects of depression on glycemic control are not known, but many people find it hard to care for themselves when they are depressed.	Point out the similarity of symptoms of high blood glucose and diabetes.
	4.12 **Acceptance.** Gradually, most people adjust or adapt. They still wish they did not have diabetes, but they are better able to live with it.	Ask, "Have you ever had any of these feelings? How did they affect you? How did they affect your ability to care for your diabetes? How did they affect your relationships with family and friends?" This adjustment process can take time. If participants are "stuck" at a particular stage, it may be a sign that additional help is needed. Remember that this process may be repeated if other diabetes-related problems occur (e.g., starting on insulin, complications).
5. Coping with feelings	5.1 Feelings do not happen in a particular order. They come and go, and you may have two or more of these feelings at once.	Feelings change from day to day—it's normal to have more than one feeling at a time.
	5.2 These are common responses to problems. The way you have handled your feelings in the past can help you deal with your feelings now.	Point out that this process is the same as for other problems or losses. Ask, "How have you handled difficulties in the past?" Ask participants what they believe will be helpful, based on these past coping strategies. Ask participants to identify coping strategies. Coping strategies are more likely to be meaningful and implemented if identified by the person with the problem.
	5.3 Feelings also affect behavior because thoughts influence feelings, which influence motivation.	Point out that although they didn't choose to have diabetes, they can choose how they respond to and care for it.

CONTENT OUTLINE

CONCEPT	DETAIL	INSTRUCTOR'S NOTES
	5.4 For example, people who think of diabetes as a disaster or burden feel and behave differently from those who view it as a challenge or opportunity.	Ask, "How do you view diabetes?" Point out that to change their emotional response, motivation, or behavior, they first need to evaluate the influence of their thoughts.
	5.5 It is important to recognize personal need for support.	
	5.6 The role of the health care team is to provide information, strategies to help you change behavior, and support.	
6. Getting the support you want	6.1 Most people find a support person helpful when living with diabetes.	Ask, "What have you found helpful in living with diabetes? Who do you turn to when you have a problem? Could he or she help you with your diabetes?"
	6.2 Support can come from family, friends, your health care team, and/or others with diabetes.	Support groups may be particularly helpful for those with limited family support.
	6.3 Families and friends generally want to be supportive, but may not know how.	Ask, "How have your family and friends responded to your diabetes? How do you feel about their responses?"
	6.4 Family and friends need to know about diabetes and what you want them to do to help you.	Ask the group to brainstorm ideas for ways others can be supportive. Write these on the board. (Examples: exercise or diet with you, notice positives rather than negatives, go to a support group with you, listen to your concerns, etc.)
	6.5 Also, family and friends may have feelings about your having diabetes. You need to recognize these feelings and their impact on support.	

CONTENT OUTLINE

CONCEPT	DETAIL	INSTRUCTOR'S NOTES
	6.6 Some find it helpful to join a diabetes support group, or to talk with a counselor or another person with diabetes.	Ask, "Has anyone been in a support group? Did you find it helpful?" Provide information about local support groups or other resources. Ideas for resources include the American Diabetes Association, Community Mental Health Centers, Crisis Counseling Centers, Catholic Social Services, Jewish Family Services, and Pastoral Counseling Services.
	6.7 Living with diabetes is difficult, but help and support are available.	You may want to close by discussing situations two, three, and/or ten from Outline #16, *Putting the Pieces Together*. Ask participants to share a thought, feeling, or experience that has helped them to live with diabetes.

SKILLS CHECKLIST

None.

EVALUATION PLAN

Knowledge will be evaluated by achievement of learning objectives, by responses to questions during the session, and by the ability to acknowledge thoughts or feelings about diabetes. The ability to apply knowledge will be evaluated by the development of personal self-care goals, by the development and implementation of a plan to achieve those goals, and through program outcome measures.

DOCUMENTATION PLAN

Record class attendance and achieved objectives as appropriate.

SUGGESTED READINGS

Affeninto SG, Backstrand JR, Welch GW, Lammi-Keefe CJ, Rodriguez NR, Adams CH: Subclinical and clinical eating disorders in IDDM negatively affect metabolic control. *Diabetes Care.* 1997;20:182–184.

American Diabetes Association: *Winning with Diabetes.* Alexandria, VA: American Diabetes Association, 1997.

Anderson BJ, Rubin RR. *Practical Psychology for Diabetes Clinicians,* 2nd Edition.

SUGGESTED READINGS *continued*

Alexandria, VA: American Diabetes Association, 2002.

Anderson RJ. The prevalence of comorbid depression in adults with diabetes: a meta-analysis. *Diabetes Care.* 2001:24:1069–1078.

Anderson RM, Barr PA, Edwards GJ, Funnell MM, Fitzgerald JT, Wisdon K: Using focus groups to identify psychosocial issues of urban black individuals with diabetes. *The Diabetes Educator* 1996;22:28–33.

Anderson RM, Fitzgerald JT, Gruppen LD, Funnell MM, Oh MS. The diabetes empowerment scale-short form (DES-SF). *Diabetes Care.* 2003;6:1641–1643.

Anderson RM, Funnell MM, Fitzgerald JT, Marrero DG. The diabetes empowerment scale: a measure of psychosocial self-efficacy. *Diabetes Care.* 2000;23:739–743.

Arroo C, Hu FB, Ryan LM, Kawachi I, Colditz GA, Speizer FE, Manson J. Depressive symptoms and risk of type 2 diabetes in women. *Diabetes Care.* 2004:27:129–133.

Brown LK. Clinical aspects of drug abuse in diabetes. *Diabetes Spectrum.* 1991;4:45–47.

Butler D. For family members only. *Diabetes Self-Management.* 2002;19(1):7–10.

Chalmers KA, Gallagher S. Should you be eating that? *The Diabetes Educator.* 1994;20:66–69.

Coffey JT, Brandle M, Zhou H, Mariott D, Burke R, Tabaei BP, Engelgau MM, Kaplan RM, Herman WH. Valuing health-related quality of life in diabetes. *Diabetes Care.* 2002;25:2238–2243.

Davis R, Magilvy JK. Quiet pride: the experience of chronic illness by rural older adults. *Journal of Nursing Scholarship.* 2000; 32:385–390.

DCCT Research Group: Influence of intensive diabetes treatment on quality-of-life outcomes in the Diabetes Control and Complications Trial. *Diabetes Care.* 1996;19:195–203.

Deatcher J. Spiritual self-care and the use of prayer. *Diabetes Self-Management.* 2002; 19(6):57–59.

De Groot M, Anderson R, Freedland KE, Clouse RE, Lustman PJ. Association of depression and diabetes complications: A meta-analysis. *Psychosom Med.* 2001;63: 619–30.

Dunning PL, Petrie R. Exploring the psychosocial side of diabetes: the yellow ball. *The Diabetes Educator.* 1994; 20:64–65.

Egede LE. Diabetes, major depression, and functional disability among US adults. *Diabetes Care.* 2004;27:421–428.

Fabricore AN, Wadden TA. Psychological functioning of obese individuals. *Diabetes Spectrum.* 2003;16:245–252

Faulkner MS, Clark FS: Quality of life for parents of children and adolescents with type 1 diabetes. *The Diabetes Educator* 1998;24:721–727.

Fitzgerald JT, Anderson RM, Davis WK. Gender differences in diabetes attitudes and adherence. *The Diabetes Educator.* 1995;21:523–529.

Gary TL, Crum RM, Cooper-Patrick L, Ford D, Brancati FL. Depressive symptoms and metabolic control in African-Americans with type 2 diabetes. *Diabetes Care.* 2000;23:23–29.

Glasgow RE, Ruggiero L, Eakin EG, Dryfoos J, Chobanian L. Quality of life and associated characteristics in a large national sample of adults with diabetes. *Diabetes Care* 1997;20:562–567.

Golden SH, Williaims JE, Ford DE, Yeh H-C, Sanford CP, Nieto FJ, Brancati FL. Depressive symptoms and the risk of type 2 diabetes. *Diabetes Care.* 2004;27:429–435.

Gottlieb SH. Lost in darkness: depression, diabetes and heart disease. *Diabetes Forecast.* 2003;56(5):44–46.

Handron DS. COPE: Early psychosocial intervention for chronic illness. *Nurse Practitioner.* 1995;20(5):6–13.

Hernandez CA. The experience of living with insulin-dependent diabetes: lessons for the diabetes educator. *The Diabetes Educator.* 1995;21:33–37.

Himmelfarb L. Body image: how you see yourself. *Diabetes Self-Management.* 2003;20(1):19–25.

Jacobson AM, Hauser ST, Willett JB, Wolfsdorf JI, Dvorak R, Herman L, DeGroot M: Psychological adjustment to IDDM: 10-year

SUGGESTED READINGS *continued*

follow-up of an onset cohort of child and adolescent patients. *Diabetes Care.* 1997;20:811–818.

Jacobson AM. The psychological care of patients with insulin-dependent diabetes mellitus. *The New England Journal of Medicine.* 1996;334:1249–1252.

Jost KE. Psychosocial care: document it. *American Journal of Nursing.* 1995; 95(7):46–49.

Lustman P, Anderson RJ, Freedland KE, de Groot M, Carney RM, Clouse RE. Depression and poor glucose control: a review of the literature. *Diabetes Care.* 2000;23:934–942.

Lustman PJ, Clouse RE. Treatment of depression in diabetes: impact on mood and medical outcomes. *Journal of Psychosomatic Research.* 2002;53:917–924.

MacLean HM, Goldman JB. A decade of qualitative research on diabetes: a review and synthesis. *Canadian Journal of Diabetes Care.* 2000;24(2)54–63.

Nelson JB. Big boys don't cry. *Diabetes Self-Management.* 2004;21(2):19–24.

Nichols GA, Brown JB. Unadjusted and adjusted prevalence of diagnosed depression in type 2 diabetes. *Diabetes Care.* 2003;26:744–749.

Paterson B. The myth of empowerment in chronic illness. *Journal of Advanced Nursing.* 2001;574–581.

Perry SJ. My spouse has diabetes. *Diabetes Forecast.* 2000;53(6):118–121.

Peyrot M, Rubin RR: Levels and risks of depression and anxiety symptomatology among diabetic adults. *Diabetes Care* 1997;20:585–590.

Pibernik-Okanovic M, Prasek M, Poljicanin-Flipovic T, Pavlic-Renar I, Metelko Z. Effects of an empowerment-based psychosocial intervention on quality of life and metabolic control in type 2 diabetic patients. *Patient Education and Counseling.* 2004;52:193–199.

Polonsky WH: *Diabetes Burnout.* Alexandria, VA: American Diabetes Association, 1999.

Polonsky WH. Listening to our patients' concerns: understanding and addressing diabetes-specific emotional distress. *Diabetes Spectrum.* 1996;9:8–11.

Polonsky WH, Parkin CG. Depression in patients with diabetes: seven facts every health-care provider should know. *Practical Diabetology.* 2001:20(4):20–30.

Polonsky WH. The role of emotional distress in diabetes. *Practical Diabetology.* 2003; 22(3):34–39.

Rappaport WS: *When Diabetes Hits Home.* Alexandria, VA: American Diabetes Association, 1999.

Restinas J. Type 2 diabetes: adjusting to the diagnosis. *Diabetes Self-Management.* 2003;20(3):27–30.

Roszler J. In sickness and health. *Diabetes Forecast.* 2003;56(1):30–32.

Rubin RR: Diabetes and quality of life. *Diabetes Spectrum.* 2000;13:21–48.

Schafer LC. Lifestyle and behavior: fostering quality of life in individuals with diabetes. *Diabetes Spectrum.* 2000;13:50–55.

Seevers RJ. Diabetes support groups: structure, function, and professional roles. *The Diabetes Educator.* 1991;17:399–401.

Soeken KL, Carson, VJ. Responding to the spiritual needs of the chronically ill. *Nursing. Clinics of North America.* 1987;22:603–612.

Spero D. Halt in the name of health. *Diabetes Self-Management.* 2003;20(2):93–42.

Spero D. With a little help from our friends. *Diabetes Self-Management.* 2004;20(6):57–63.

Talbot F, Nouwen A. A review of the relationship between depression and diabetes in adults: is there a link? *Diabetes Care.* 2000;23:1556–1562.

Testa MA, Simonson DC: Health economic benefits and quality of life during improved glycemic control in patients with type 1 diabetes. *JAMA* 1998;280:1490–1496.

Trief PM, Wade MJ, Britton KD, Weinstock RS. A prospective analysis of marital relationship factors and quality of life for diabetes. *Diabetes Care.* 2002;25:1154–1158.

UK Prospective Diabetes Study Group: Quality of life in type 2 diabetic patients is affected by complications but not by intensive policies to

SUGGESTED READINGS *continued*

improve blood glucose or blood pressure control (UKPDS 37). *Diabetes Care* 1999;22:1125–1136.

Van der Does FEE, De Neeling JND, Snoek FJ, Kostense PJ, Grootenhuis PA, Bouter LM, Heine RJ. Symptoms and well-being in relation to glycemic control in type II diabetes. *Diabetes Care.* 1996;19:204–210.

van der Ven NCW, Weinger K, Yi J, Pouwer F, Adèr H, van der Ploeg HM, Snoek FJ. The confidence in diabetes self-care scale: psychometric properties of a new measure of diabetes-specific self-efficacy in Dutch and U.S. patients with type 1 diabetes. *Diabetes Care.* 2003;26:713–717.

Wallhagen MI. Social support in diabetes. *Diabetes Spectrum.* 1999;12:254–256.

Watkins CE. Coping with your diagnosis. *Diabetes Forecast.* 2002;55(5):58–61.

Watkins CE. Depression and anxiety in the person with diabetes. *Practical Diabetology.* 1998;17(4):16–20.

Weiss MA, Funnell MM. Beyond the numbers. *Diabetes Forecast.* 2004;57(5):53–54.

Welch GW, Jacobon AM, Polonsky WH. The problem areas in diabetes scale. *Diabetes Care.* 1997;20:760–766.

Wysocki T: *The Ten Keys to Helping Your Child Grow Up with Diabetes.* Alexandria, VA: American Diabetes Association, 1999.

| #3 | The Basics of Eating |

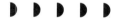

STATEMENT OF PURPOSE

This session is intended to emphasize the critical role of macronutrient intake in diabetes management. The composition of food groups and their impact on blood glucose are discussed, and participants are asked to consider how they most want to benefit from meal planning. The effects of composition, timing, and amount of food intake on blood glucose are addressed. Practice in measuring food is included. Encourage participants to have the person who prepares their food attend the nutrition sessions with them. Participants are asked to assess their own eating by keeping a food diary before the next session.

PREREQUISITES

None.

OBJECTIVES

At the end of this session, participants will be able to:

1. identify three macronutrients and their impact on blood glucose;

2. state the most important personal reason they might use a meal plan;

3. state how the timing of food can help them reach their blood glucose goals;

4. state how the composition of their meal plans can help them reach their blood glucose goals;

5. state how monitoring the amount of food eaten can help them reach their blood glucose or weight goals;

6. demonstrate how to measure liquid and dry ingredients;

7. describe how to keep a food diary;

8. identify one action they could take during the coming week to space the timing or modify the amount or type of food eaten.

CONTENT

Nutritional Management.

MATERIALS NEEDED

VISUALS PROVIDED	ADDITIONAL
1. Reasons for Meal Planning	■ Food models
	■ Measuring cups and spoons
Handouts (one per participant)	■ Food scale
1. Food Diary Example	■ Chalkboard and chalk
2. Food Diary	■ Colored water and clear glasses
	■ Cereal and cereal bowls
	■ Other food as desired (see section 6)

METHOD OF PRESENTATION

Start by introducing yourself and telling what you do. Ask participants to introduce themselves. Explain that the purposes of this session are to discuss the role of diet in the treatment of diabetes and provide basic guidelines for eating.

Ask how they did with their short-term goal and what they learned from it. Present material in a question/discussion format. If appropriate, explain that although the information provided is useful for people with type 1 and people with type 2 diabetes, it is important to realize that the dietary recommendations may be different.

CONTENT OUTLINE

CONCEPT	DETAIL	INSTRUCTOR'S NOTES
1. Definition of diabetes mellitus	1.1 Diabetes mellitus is a disorder in which the body either does not produce enough insulin (type 1) or is unable to use the insulin that it makes (type 2).	Review definition by asking: ■ What is diabetes? ■ What does insulin do? ■ Where does blood glucose come from? ■ What happens if blood glucose cannot enter the cell?
	1.2 Food is composed of protein, fat, carbohydrate, vitamins, minerals, and water.	Ask, " What questions or concerns do you have about diabetes and food?"
	1.3 When food is eaten and digested, it is broken down into simple substances—one of which is glucose (a form of sugar).	
	1.4 Glucose is needed by the cells for energy.	
	1.5 Insulin enables glucose to enter body cells.	
	1.6 If insulin is not available or effective, the glucose cannot enter the cells.	

CONTENT OUTLINE

CONCEPT	DETAIL	INSTRUCTOR'S NOTES

1.7 If glucose cannot enter the cells, it builds up in the blood, causing hyperglycemia (high blood glucose).

2. Role of diet

2.1 Food raises blood glucose. What, when, and how much food you eat affects how much the blood glucose increases. The more you know about what is in food, the better you'll understand how it affects your blood glucose. This helps you make decisions about what, when, and how much to eat.

Instructor's Notes: Each person's glycemia response to foods varies. Blood glucose monitoring helps people learn about their individual responses. General guidelines are presented here.

2.2 Learning ways to balance food, diabetes medicines, and activity helps to keep blood glucose levels in your target range.

Instructor's Notes: Ask, "How do food, insulin, and activity each affect blood glucose?"

2.3 Many people with type 2 diabetes can keep their blood glucose in their target range with meal planning alone. However, meal planning is basic for the treatment of all types of diabetes, even when oral agents or insulin need to be taken.

3. Reasons for meal planning

3.1 The reasons for meal planning include:

Maintain blood glucose as close to your target range as possible.

Blood glucose management is the main reason for meal planning. It is also one reason that is different for people with diabetes than for people without diabetes. The closer to normal blood glucose levels can be safely kept, the lower the risk for eye, kidney, and nerve damage for people with diabetes.

Most of the other reasons for meal planning apply to everyone.

Instructor's Notes: Ask, "What are your reasons for paying attention to food choices?" Use Visual #1, Reasons for Meal Planning.

See Outline #11, *Managing Blood Glucose.*

Point out that nutrition is a growing science, so advice will change from time to time.

CONTENT OUTLINE

CONCEPT	DETAIL	INSTRUCTOR'S NOTES

3.2 Maintain cholesterol (blood fats) and blood pressure levels as close to your target as possible.

People with diabetes havegreater risk of developing h a eart and blood vessel disease, especially when blood glucose and blood pressure levels are high for a period of time. High blood pressure levels also increase the risk for microvascular complicaitons

Diet to normalize cholesterol and other types of fat in the blood may help reduce the risk of heart disease. Information about reducing total fat is provided in Outline #4, *Food and Blood Glucose.* More information about this topic is in Outline #18, *Eating for a Healthy Heart.*

3.3 Prevent, delay, or treat diabetes-related complications.

Long-term complications with dietary implications include renal disease, gastroparesis, hypertension, and lipid abnormalities. Additional recommendations for protein, fiber, and sodium may be needed. See Outline #14, *Long-Term Complications*, and Outline #18, *Eating for a Healthy Heart.*

3.4 Improve health through food choices.

Like everyone, eating a variety of foods each day helps provide the many different vitamins and minerals your body needs.

Optimal nutrition helps avoid fatigue and increases resistance to infectious diseases. The diet for diabetes is a healthy diet for nearly everyone. Additional vitamins and minerals are not generally recommended at this time. Specifically for people with diabetes, women who plan to become pregnant need to take folate and should also take calcium to prevent bone loss. People with chronically high glucose levels may benefit from supplementing the B vitamins lost with polyuria. It is important to assess vitamin, herbal, and nutritional supplement use by asking, "What vitamins, minerals, other supplements, or alternative therapies do you use?" The

CONTENT OUTLINE

CONCEPT	DETAIL	INSTRUCTOR'S NOTES
		American Medical Association recently recommended that all adults take a multivitamins daily.
	3.5 **Meet individual nutritional needs.** Food meets both physical and psycho-social needs and is an expression of our cultures and families.	Address individual needs including lifestyle, personal, and cultural preferences and desire to make changes.
	3.6 Calories are needed for: ■ reasonable body weight ■ normal growth and development ■ pregnancy and lactation ■ energy to work/play—physical activity	Caloric needs for pediatric patients are based on RDAs. Growth is plotted on a growth basis.
	3.7 Weight loss in an overweight person with diabetes may help reduce blood glucose, blood fats, and blood pressure. Losing 10–20 lb or 5–10% of usual body weight can help.	Very high- or low-calorie diets can be disruptive to blood glucose levels. Moderate weight loss of 1–2 lb/week is recommended.
	3.8 A reasonable weight goal is one that: ■ you choose and discuss with your health care team ■ you can achieve and maintain ■ you can stick with over time	Weight management is covered in Outline #4, *Food and Blood Glucose.* Help the group identify the costs and benefits of weight loss. Write on the chalkboard.
	3.9 Some reasons may be more important to you than others.	Ask, "What is the most important reason for you to plan meals?"
4. Timing	4.1 Three things that directly affect blood glucose levels are timing of intake, portion sizes, and food composition.	
	4.2 The more you eat at one time, the more insulin you need. If you eat smaller amounts throughout the day, you will need less insulin. Eating a lot of carbohydrate at one time also increases your need for insulin. It takes more insulin to bring down a high blood glucose level than to keep a normal level in range.	

CONTENT OUTLINE

CONCEPT	DETAIL	INSTRUCTOR'S NOTES
	4.3 Basic guidelines are:	These guidelines are starting points. The more information participants learn about food and diabetes care, the more flexible they can be and still reach their goals.
	■ Eat at least three times throughout the day. Small meals throughout the day help keep glucose levels more even.	Ask, "How many times do you eat each day?" A minimum of three meals a day is usually encouraged, but two meals and a snack may accomplish the same goal.
	■ Eat each meal and snack at about the same time each day.	Ask, "What times do you usually eat? Do they change from day to day?"
	■ Eat about the same amount at each meal each day. (Each breakfast should have about the same amount of food, and each lunch, etc.). Day-to-day consistency is especially important for people who take one or two insulin shots per day.	Consistency is less important for those treated with multiple insulin injections who learn to use carbohydrate/insulin ratios.
	■ Do not skip meals. Carry food with you if a meal is delayed or if you are more active than usual. Skipping a meal after taking insulin or some diabetes medications greatly increases the risk of low blood glucose levels. It may also mean that you overeat later, which makes it harder to manage both blood glucose and weight.	Ask, "What happens if you skip a meal?" Discuss occasions when a meal might be delayed. Attempting to skip meals early in the day often leads to over-eating in the evening. This prevents hunger in the morning, perpetrating the cycle.
	■ Eat breakfast. Research shows that eating early in the day helps to set an increased metabolic rate, promotes weight loss, and helps you control overall intake.	Some people feel that eating breakfast increases hunger. After a few days, however, the body adjusts and regulates caloric intake so that late-evening hunger is diminished.
	■ Learn to balance the time you take medicine for your diabetes with the time you eat. Insulin	Explain problems associated with not doing this (e.g., taking insulin on rising without eat-

CONTENT OUTLINE

CONCEPT	DETAIL	INSTRUCTOR'S NOTES
	and some diabetes medications work to lower blood glucose better if you take them at the right time.	ing breakfast or taking short-acting insulin immediately before a meal). Some experts recommend a nighttime snack to maintain blood glucose levels for people who take insulin.
5. Portion size	5.1 Too much food at one time raises blood glucose levels. Too much total food increases body weight.	
	5.2 If your blood glucose is high after some meals or if your weight is going up, eating less may help.	Ask, "How do you know you are eating too much?" Encourage blood glucose monitoring to evaluate the effect of different meals on blood glucose levels.
	5.3 Some ways to eat less are: ■ Choose smaller portions (one piece of toast for breakfast or one sandwich for lunch instead of two). ■ Eat only one serving. No seconds. ■ Use a small plate instead of a large plate. ■ Eat more slowly so you are the last one to finish the meal. ■ Serve plates in the kitchen instead of putting serving dishes on the table. ■ Keep tempting foods out of sight or out of the house. ■ Share dessert. ■ Put your fork down between each bite. ■ Reduce the amount you eat gradually. Find out exactly how much you are eating of a food and make a plan to eat a little less the next week. For example, eat 6 oz of meat instead of 8 oz, or 1½ cups of potatoes instead of 2 cups. ■ Ask someone else to do the tasting when you are cooking. ■ Eat smaller meals and low-calorie snacks to prevent hunger.	Ask, "Can you think of other ways to eat less food?" Brainstorm. Different ideas work for different people. (This section is not appropriate for growing children.)

CONTENT OUTLINE

CONCEPT	DETAIL	INSTRUCTOR'S NOTES
6. Weighing and measuring food	6.1 Many people do not know how much they eat.	Demonstrate the differences between perceived and actual amounts of food with activities such as the following: ■ Hold up glasses of colored water and ask how much is in each. Pour into a measuring cup to see. ■ Ask three participants to pour a serving of cereal into a bowl (a different size/shape for each) and tell the amount. Measure each. ■ Pass around a piece of bread spread with margarine and jam. Ask participants to estimate the amount of each in teaspoons. Give answers. ■ Using food models, ask participants to estimate the ounces of different-sized meat portions.
	6.2 Weighing or measuring food is the way to know the amount you actually eat.	Introduce measuring as a tool to help participants become more aware of how they eat now. Suggest that participants weigh or measure usual portions at home to get an idea of actual intake. The appropriate amount and the need for precision will vary from person to person and is reviewed in later sessions.
	6.3 Use measuring cups and spoons to measure items that take the shape of the container, such as liquids and noodles.	Rice, noodles, soups, casseroles, vegetables, beverages, and condiments are usually measured by volume.
	6.4 Use any easy-to-read food scale to weigh fruits, bread, baked goods, and meat.	If possible, demonstrate and allow time for participants to practice weighing and measuring.

CONTENT OUTLINE

CONCEPT	DETAIL	INSTRUCTOR'S NOTES

6.5 Weigh and measure foods after cooking; the amount can change.

Instructor's Notes: Use Handout #1 from Outline #20, *Diabetes Exchange Lists*, if needed to answer questions.

6.6 With practice, you will learn to estimate the amount of food in your dishes at home without measuring.

Instructor's Notes: Most people do not weigh and measure all the time and do not need to do so.

6.7 You can also learn to estimate serving sizes.

- A 1-cup serving carbohydrates, including fruit, vegetables, pasta, or rice, is about the size of your fist.
- One 3-oz serving of protein, such as meat, fish, or poultry, is equivalent to the size of a deck of playing cards or the palm your hand.
- A 1-oz serving of cheese is equal to the size of your thumb.
- A teaspoon-size serving of mayonnaise or margerine is about the size of your thumb-tip.
- A 2-oz serving of a snackfood is about the size of a handful.
- A 1-cup serving of yogurt or fresh greens is about the size of a tennis ball.

6.8 You may need to weigh and measure your foods when:
- you're just learning about portion sizes or making a change in your meal plan
- you lose or gain weight
- your blood glucose goes out of target range
- you change your medication doses or exercise level
- you want to avoid "portion-size creep," when portion sizes gradually increase without you noticing

Instructor's Notes: Measuring helps you to be sure food intake is consistent so other changes can be better understood and evaluated.

CONTENT OUTLINE

CONCEPT	DETAIL	INSTRUCTOR'S NOTES
7. Assessing how you eat now	7.1 You (and your health care team) need to know what you are eating now so you can see what changes would help you. People are often not aware of what they eat during the day.	The fewer changes a person makes, the more likely he or she is to maintain those changes. Making fewer changes that can be sustained is more useful than short-lived radical or multiple changes.
	7.2 A food diary shows exactly what you are eating. It shows you the kinds, times, and amounts of foods you eat.	Ask, "What is a food diary?" Distribute Handout #1, Food Diary Example.
	7.3 A food diary is a record of what you eat during the day. It shows: ■ what foods you eat and drink ■ amounts of food ■ the times you eat ■ the way you usually eat	Ask, "How can a food diary help you?" A food diary can benefit both the patient and the health care team in several ways. The following can be identified: ■ total intake ■ meal timing and location ■ food preparation patterns ■ food preferences ■ emotional eating Changes to improve blood glucose or reduce calories can be easily determined.
	7.4 Decide which days to keep the diary. Choose both weekdays and weekend days. Write down: ■ the food you eat and drink (even small bites) ■ the amount in teaspoons, tablespoons, cups, and ounces ■ the time ■ the place ■ your thoughts and feelings about eating	Ask, "How do you keep a food diary?" Acknowledge that the task has cost (work) and benefit (learning about yourself).
	7.5 Write down the foods when you eat them so you don't forget. Keep the diary where you can see it, such as on the refrigerator.	Encourage participants to record how the food is prepared.
	7.6 Try writing down what you plan to eat and drink before you actually do—this may help with portion control.	Studies have shown this to be a most effective weight loss and maintenance method.

CONTENT OUTLINE

CONCEPT	DETAIL	INSTRUCTOR'S NOTES
	7.7 Let's review some food diary examples.	See examples on Handout #1. Ask, "What do you notice?"
	7.8 Include information about where you were and what you were doing and feeling. This helps to identify specific situations that are hard for you.	If possible, have participants practice recording their most recent meals or snacks.
	7.9 Remember to write down the amount of each food you eat (the portion size). Include liquids. Remember that all the little bites of food you eat while you are cooking need to be recorded.	Remind them to record the parts of a sandwich as: <u>1 sandwich:</u> bread, 2 slices regular roast beef, 2 oz mayonnaise, 1 tsp lite lettuce, tomato
	7.10 Note how the food was prepared.	
	7.11 Be sure to write down salad dressings, condiments, and any other added items (e.g., nondairy creamer to coffee).	Distribute Handout #2, Food Diary. Participants can use this to keep their own food diaries.
	7.12 Keep the food diary for at least 3 days before the next nutrition session. The food diary will be most helpful if you try to eat in your usual way while keeping it.	Write the date of that session on the chalkboard. The days selected should be typical of their eating pattern and reflect weekdays and weekend days.
8. Getting started	8.1 Lasting eating changes usually come in steps, not all at once. Steps are actions you can measure. For example, you could: ■ carry lunch to work one day ■ drink ½ cup instead of 1 cup of juice for breakfast ■ test before and after a snack if you would like to see how that snack affects your blood glucose	Ask class members to identify one eating change to try during the next week that would help them move toward their long-term blood glucose or weight goals. Reviewing the *Healthy Eating Brochure* may be helpful for some participants who are ready to initiate a simple approach to food choices. See Outline #5, *Planning Meals*. Reducing blood glucose or weight are long-term goals or outcomes, not actions a person can take. Help participants identify action steps as behavior-change goals. See Outline #15, *Changing Behavior*.

SKILLS CHECKLIST

Each participant will be able to weigh and measure food and keep a food diary.

EVALUATION PLAN

Knowledge will be evaluated by achievement of learning objectives and by responses to questions during the session. The ability to apply knowledge will be evaluated by the development of personal meal-planning goals, by implementation of changes in the amount or timing of food intake, and through program outcome measures.

DOCUMENTATION PLAN

Record class attendance and achieved objectives as appropriate.

SUGGESTED READINGS

American Diabetes Association. *Eating Healthy with Diabetes*. Alexandria, VA: American Diabetes Association, 1998.

American Diabetes Association. Eating right with diabetes. (Patient Information Sheet.) *Diabetes Spectrum*. 1996;9(2)139–140.

American Diabetes Association. Nutrition recommendations and principles for people with diabetes mellitus. *Diabetes Care*. 2004;27 (Suppl 1):S36–S46.

American Diabetes Association. Translation of the diabetes nutrition recommendations for health care institutions. *Diabetes Care* 2004;27(Suppl 1):S55–S57.

Brown JE, Glasgow RE, Toobert DJ. Integrating dietary self-management counseling into the regular office visit. *Practical Diabetology* 1996;15(4):16–22.

Chalmers KH, Peterson AE. *16 Myths of the Diabetic Diet*. Alexandria, VA: American Diabetes Association, 1999.

Franz MF, Battle JP. *ADA Guide to Medical Nutrition Therapy*. Alexandria, VA: American Diabetes Association, 1999.

Franz MJ. 2002 Nutrition recommendations: grading the evidence. *The Diabetes Educator*. 2002;28:756–766.

Franz MJ. Diabetes nutrition recommendations for 2002. *Practical Diabetology*. 2002; 21(2):15–18.

Franz MJ. So many nutrition recommendations—contradictory or compatible? *Diabetes Spectrum*. 2003;16:65–62.

Franz MJ, Bantle JP, Beebe CA, Brunzell JD, Chiasson J-L, Garg A, Holzmeister LA, Hoogwerf B, Mayer-Davis E, Mooradian AD, Purnell JQ, Wheeler M. Evidence-based nutrition principles and recommendations for the treatment and prevention of diabetes and related complications: a technical review. *Diabetes Care*. 2002;25:148–198.

Geil PB, Holzmeister LA. *101 Nutrition Tips for People with Diabetes*. Alexandria, VA: American Diabetes Association, 1999.

Glasgow RE, Toobert DJ, Hampson SE. Effects of a brief office-based intervention to facilitate diabetes dietary self-management. *Diabetes Care*. 1996;19:834–842.

Hagberg L. Making sense of dietary recommendations. *Diabetes Self-Management*. 2003; 20(4):53–63.

Pastors JG, Warshaw H, Daly A, Franz, M, Kulkarni K. The evidence of the effectiveness

SUGGESTED READINGS *continued*

of medical nutrition therapy in diabetes. *Diabetes Care.* 2002;25:608–613.

Powers MA, ed. *Handbook of Diabetes Nutritional Management.* 2nd Edition. Rockville, MD: Aspen Publishers, 1996.

Schafer RG, Bohannon B, Franz M, Freeman J, Holmes A, McLaughlin S, Haas LB,

Kruger DF, Lorenz RA, McMahon MM. Translation of the diabetes nutrition recommendations for health care institutions. *Diabetes Care.* 1997;20:96–105.

Warsaw HS. Estimating food portions? Easy! *Diabetes Forecast.* 2002;53(9):84–87.

➲ Reasons for Meal Planning

- Maintain blood glucose as close to your target range as possible.

- Maintain cholesterol (blood fats) as close to your target range as possible.

- Maintain blood pressure as close to your target level as possible.

- Prevent, delay, or treat diabetes-related complications.

- Improve health through food choices .

- Meet individual nutritional needs.

➥ Food Diary Example

Time	Place	Thoughts and Feelings	Foods and How Prepared	Amount
8:15 am	Home	Hungry, in a hurry	Egg, poached Orange juice Toast Margarine	1 ½ cup 1 slice 1 tsp
10:00 am	Work		Coffee	1 cup
12:30 pm	Home	Hungry, ate alone	Sandwich: Bread Roast beef Mayonnaise Lettuce, tomato Sugar cookies Low-fat (1%) milk	 2 slices reg. 2 oz 1 Tbsp lite 2 1½ cups
6:00 pm	Restaurant	Enjoyed friends, got too full	Fried chicken Coleslaw Mashed potatoes Gravy Apple pie Lemonade	1 leg and thigh ½ cup 1 cup ¼ cup 1 piece 1½ cups
10:00 pm	Movie	Tired, popcorn smelled good	Buttered popcorn Diet cola	2 cups 2 cups (16 oz)

➲ Food Diary

NAME _____ DAY _____ DATE _____

Time	Place	Thoughts and Feelings	Foods and How Prepared	Amount

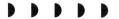

#4	Food and Blood Glucose

STATEMENT OF PURPOSE

This session is intended to provide an understanding of how different foods affect blood glucose levels and lay the groundwork for approaches to meal planning. Participants are asked to review their food diaries and look for relationships between their food intake and blood glucose levels. To help participants predict the likely impact of individual foods, the general effects of carbohydrate, protein, and fat on blood glucose are presented; food groups are introduced; and the nutrients present in foods from each group are identified. Participants are encouraged to use blood glucose monitoring to evaluate the actual effects of different foods on their blood glucose levels. The need for all nutrients and the benefits of including all food groups to promote overall health are stressed. This approach to diabetes nutrition education emphasizes outcomes and encourages experimentation. Access to monitoring supplies is helpful. Select the material from this outline that is appropriate for your audience.

The impact of food on weight and the cardiovascular system is expanded in Outline #17, *Food and Weight*, and Outline #18, *Eating for a Healthy Heart*. Encourage the participants to bring the person who prepares their food to this and other nutrition sessions.

PREREQUISITES

It is recommended that participants have attended Session #3, *The Basics of Eating*, or have achieved those objectives. Ask participants to bring their completed food diaries to this session.

OBJECTIVES

At the end of this session, participants will be able to:

1. discuss what they learned from keeping a food diary;

2. name the six basic groups of food;

3. name several foods in each group;

4. state that the body needs foods from all the groups to stay healthy;

5. name the three nutrients in food that contain calories and affect blood glucose;

6. describe how each nutrient affects blood glucose;

7. state that blood glucose monitoring is a way to find out how specific foods affect blood glucose;

8. name the food groups high in carbohydrate, protein, and fat;

9. identify one behavior change they could make during the coming week to move closer to their blood glucose goals.

CONTENT

Nutritional Management.

MATERIALS NEEDED

VISUALS PROVIDED	**ADDITIONAL**
1. Reasons for Meal Planning	■ Food models
2. Nutrients in Food	■ Commercial food product containers or labels that illustrate types of food
	■ Chalkboard and chalk
Handouts (one per person)	■ *The First Step in Diabetes Meal Planning, Eating Healthy with Diabetes,* and *Exchange Lists for Meal Planning* (available from the American Diabetes Association, 800-232-6733)
1. Food Groups	
2. Nutrients in Food Groups	
	■ *Guide to Good Eating* (one-page flyer with color pictures of foods in each of five groups; available from the National Dairy Council)

METHOD OF PRESENTATION

Start by introducing yourself and telling what you do. Ask participants to introduce themselves. Explain that the purposes of this session are to provide information about different groups of foods, the nutrients in each group, and the effects these nutrients have on blood glucose and overall health. The information can be used by participants to make food choices that help them reach personal goals.

Present material in a question/discussion format. Begin by asking how they did with their short-term goal and what they learned from it.

CONTENT OUTLINE

CONCEPT	DETAIL	INSTRUCTOR'S NOTES
1. Review	1.1 The purpose of meal planning is to help you reach blood glucose, weight, and other long-term goals.	Review reasons for meal planning using Visual #1, Reasons for Meal Planning. Ask participants to identify the reason that is most important to them.
2. Food diary	2.1 Keeping a food diary can help you become more aware of how you eat.	Ask participants to look over their food diaries and discuss what they found. Ask questions like, "Did you discover anything? How far apart were the times you ate? Were there some days you ate later than others? Did you eat large amounts at some meals or on some days and much smaller amounts other times? Did keeping the record affect your food choices?"
	2.2 If you notice what you eat and monitor your blood glucose at home, you can discover how food choices affect your blood glucose.	Ask, "Did you notice any differences in your blood glucose when you ate differently?" Explore this neutrally; allow participants to find (or not find) links between their eating and blood glucose levels.
	2.3 Your food diary can help you figure out what is easy and hard for you about food choices and what foods you want to keep in your plan and which foods you can easily do without.	Assessment is essential before making plans for change. Ask, "Did you identify any changes you want to make based on your food diaries?"
	2.4 Learning about food and how it affects you can also help.	
3. What are food groups?	3.1 For decades, foods with similar nutritional value have been sorted into groups.	Some people will remember the Basic 4 or even the Basic 7 food groups. The food guide pyramid and the exchange systems for meal planning build on the use of food groups.

CONTENT OUTLINE

CONCEPT	DETAIL	INSTRUCTOR'S NOTES

3.2 Grouping foods can make it easier to think about how different foods affect your blood glucose, weight, heart, and overall health.

3.3 At the present time, foods are divided into six groups:

- starch
- vegetable
- fruit
- meat
- milk
- fat

Ask, "What are the six food groups used today?" List the six groups on the chalkboard. Acknowledge different ways to group foods.

3.4 Foods in each group include:

- **Starch.** Bread, rolls, pasta, rice, cereal, and dried beans and starchy vegetables such as potatoes, corn, peas, and winter squash.
- **Fruit.** Apples, oranges, bananas, and all other fruits—fresh, frozen, canned, or juiced.

Ask, "What foods belong in the starchy vegetables, grains, and bread group?" Use food models or pictures to illustrate which foods belong to each group. Allow time for participants to practice assigning foods to groups. For a more complete listing, refer to Exchange Lists for Meal Planning. Repeat for each food group.

Use Handout #1, Food Groups, The First Step in Diabetes Meal Planning, or the Guide to Good Eating from the National Dairy Council.

- **Vegetable.** Carrots, green beans, broccoli, beets, greens, and other crunchy vegetables.

Fat added to vegetables needs to be counted in the fat group.

- **Milk.** All milk and some yogurts.

Plain or artificially sweetened yogurt has about the same nutrients as a glass of milk. Extra sugar is added to fruit-flavored and frozen yogurts. Some diet hot chocolate mixes may fit in this group.

- **Meat.** Beef, fish, poultry, cheese, cottage cheese, eggs, tofu, and wild game.

Note that the meat group includes fish, meat substitutes, and other high-protein foods.

- **Fat.** Butter, margarine, cream, oils, salad dressings, sour cream,

Some foods do not obviously fit in one of these groups. The

CONTENT OUTLINE

CONCEPT	DETAIL	INSTRUCTOR'S NOTES
	cream cheese, fatback, bacon, nuts, olives, and avocados. Alcohol is included in this group.	grouping rationale is addressed later.
	3.5 Your body needs food from all six groups. Each group contains different nutrients.	The amount of food needed from each group is discussed in Outline #5, *Planning Meals.*
4. Nutrients in food	4.1 Your body needs nutrients to live. You have to take in nutrients because your body cannot make them.	Ask, "What is a nutrient?"
	4.2 Some foods make your blood glucose go up more and faster than others. Knowing about the nutrients in food can help you predict what different foods will do to your blood glucose.	
	4.3 Nutrients in food are carbohydrate, protein, fat, vitamins, minerals, and water.	Ask, "What are the major nutrients in food?" As the class names the nutrients, list them on the chalkboard, or use Visual #2, Nutrients in Food.
	4.4 Carbohydrate, protein, and fat contain calories. Only carbohydrates directly affect blood glucose levels.	Ask, "Which nutrients directly affect blood glucose levels?"
	4.5 Vitamins, minerals and water do not contain calories or raise blood glucose but are necessary for optimal health.	Some vitamins and minerals are required for the body to use glucose for energy.
5. What is carbohydrate?	5.1 Carbohydrate is another term for sugar and starch. Starch is a chain of sugar molecules. All starch is broken down into sugar. Starch is like a string of beads, where each single bead is sugar.	In terms of glycemia, the total amount of carbohydrte is more important than the source or type.
	5.2 Your body burns carbohydrate for energy and needs more of this nutrient than any other.	Clarify the difference between starch as a nutrient (one component of food) and starch as a food group.

CONTENT OUTLINE

CONCEPT	DETAIL	INSTRUCTOR'S NOTES
	5.3 Starch, fruit, and milk are the food groups high in carbohydrate. Small amounts of carbohydrate are present in foods from the vegetable group.	See Handout #2, Nutrients in Food Groups. To illustrate that sugar is not inherently bad for people with diabetes, note that the carbohydrate in fruit and milk is in the form of a sugar.
	5.4 Foods that include ingredients from those three food groups contain carbohydrate. Some examples are casseroles, soups, stews, pizza, and snacks (chips, pretzels, and french fries). Sweets (ice cream, cake, cookies, and pie) and some alcoholic beverages (beer and sweet wine) also contain carbohydrate.	Ask participants to review their food diaries and find foods that contain carbohydrate. Most of these foods contain fat, and some also contain protein.
6. What is protein?	6.1 Protein is also a nutrient in food. Protein builds and repairs muscles, skin, and every cell in the body.	Ask, "What is protein?"
	6.2 Protein breaks down into amino acids.	The body needs insulin to use protein.
	6.3 Nitrogen from the breakdown of amino acids must be filtered by the kidney. Reducing protein is often recommended for people with diagnosed nephropathy.	The recommended daily allowance (RDA) for protein is 0.8 gm/kg. For a 150-lb person, this is 55 gm, which is provided by 4 oz meat, 1 cup milk, 6 slices of bread, and ½ cup vegetables. Many people eat more than this each day.
	6.4 Milk and meat groups are high in protein. Smaller amounts are found in foods from the starch and vegetable groups. Including ½ cup milk and 3–4 oz meat per day, within a balanced diet, will provide the RDA for protein.	Refer to Handout #2, Nutrients in Food Groups. Ask participants to review their food diaries and find foods that contain protein. Note how cheese, eggs, and peanut butter can be substituted for meat. Point out that more milk products are needed to provide the RDA for calcium.

CONTENT OUTLINE

CONCEPT	DETAIL	INSTRUCTOR'S NOTES
7. What is fat?	7.1 Fat is an essential nutrient that supplies energy, maintains healthy skin, and carries the fat-soluble vitamins A, D, E, and K.	Ask, "What is fat?" A very small amount (1 tsp corn oil) is required to prevent fatty acid deficiency. More fat (18% of calories) is needed to transport fat-soluble vitamins.
	7.2 Fat contributes flavor and texture. Without fat, beef and lamb would taste about the same.	
	7.3 Too much saturated fat increases the risk for heart and blood vessel disease.	A low-fat, high-carbohydrate diet elevates triglycerides in some people. A diet with 20–40% calories from fat may be optimal. Saturated fat contributes most to cardiovascular disease. Types of fat are discussed in Outline #18, *Eating for a Healthy Heart.*
	7.4 Fat is high in calories. Foods with fat contain more calories per bite than foods without fat. All fats have the same number of calories, even though some are better than others for your heart and blood vessels.	Each gram of fat has 9 calories. This is more than twice the 4 calories per gram in carbohydrate and protein.
	7.5 The nutrient fat is, of course, high in the fat food group. Several (but not all) foods in the milk and meat group also provide fat.	Refer again to Handout #2, Nutrients in Food Groups. Examples: A cup of whole milk or a regular hot dog contain 8 gm of fat (equal to about 1½ pats of butter). Skim milk and some reduced-fat hot dogs contain less than 1 gm of fat.
	7.6 Fat is present in most combination, convenience, snack, and sweet items.	Ask, "What other foods contain fat?" Ask participants to review their food diaries to find foods that contain fat.
8. Effects of carbohydrates, on blood glucose levels	8.1 As much as 100% of the carbohydrate you eat may be changed into glucose in your body.	You may want to use the word *metabolism*—the process by which energy is made available for body functions.

CONTENT OUTLINE

CONCEPT	DETAIL	INSTRUCTOR'S NOTES
	8.2 All absorbable carbohydrate foods turn to sugar in the blood. In equal amounts, sugar and starch affect blood glucose in a similar way.	Starch, a string of glucose molecules, may be absorbed more quickly than sucrose (table sugar), a combination of glucose and fructose. Fructose is absorbed more slowly than glucose.
	8.3 Most carbohydrate is digested and absorbed within 2 hours after eating.	
	8.4 Liquids are even more quickly digested and absorbed than solid food.	You may want to suggest limiting fruit juice to ½ cup and milk to 1 cup at a time with food.
	8.5 Other sweet liquids, such as regular soft drinks, lemonade, punch, and cider, will also raise your blood glucose quickly, as will sherberts and sorbets.	These items may be used to treat a low blood glucose reaction.
	8.6 Foods with added sugar, such as cookies and candy, contain a lot of carbohydrate per bite. It is easy to eat more carbohydrate than you think you are eating.	
	8.7 Compact foods like Grape Nuts or dried fruit are also higher in carbohydrate per bite than similar foods that contain more air and/or water. Eating the same amount of cereal every morning does not always mean eating the same amount of carbohydrate.	Compare the volume of different cereals with 30 gm of carbohydrate. Ask, "Which cereal would you choose?" There is no "right" answer. Ask participants to pour out three different cereals in same-size bowls. Ask them to calculate the grams of carbohydrate based on the nutrition label information.
	8.8 If you divide carbohydrate among all your meals and snacks, your body can use the glucose more easily and keep your blood glucose levels more even. This does not necessarily mean eating less total carbohydrate.	Ask participants to use food models to show a day's menu that does (and does not) distribute carbohydrate-containing foods throughout the day.

CONTENT OUTLINE

CONCEPT	DETAIL	INSTRUCTOR'S NOTES
	8.9 Fat may take all day to be digested and absorbed. Because fat leaves the stomach more slowly, it slows down how fast carbohydrate (including sugar) reaches the bloodstream.	High-sugar, high-fat foods like regular ice cream may not cause an immediate or noticable post-prandial increase in blood glucose.
9. Finding balance	9.1 Your body needs all the nutrients to feel good, repair itself, and fight disease. We all need carbohydrate, protein, and fat every day.	Meals that include carbohydrate plus protein and/or fat delay the absorption of glucose into the bloodstream and may delay hunger.
	9.2 But too much carbohydrate makes blood glucose too high, too much fat contributes to weight gain and heart and blood vessel disease, and too much protein may increase the chance for kidney problems. Eating too much food of any kind can give your body more carbohydrate, protein, fat, and calories than it needs.	
	9.3 Eating meals that contain carbohydrate, protein, and fat helps keep your blood glucose levels more even.	Point out that substituting a low-fat or fat-free food may cause blood glucose levels to rise more quickly.
	9.4 A sample meal would include: ■ 2–3 starch choices (such as 2–3 slices of bread or 1–1½ cups of potato, pasta, or rice) ■ 1 piece of fruit and/or 1 cup of plain vegetables ■ 1 cup of milk and/or 1–3 oz of meat, poultry, fish, or cheese	Help the class develop several meals that fit these criteria. One possibility is to write a meal on the chalkboard and ask the class what is missing.
	9.5 Foods with added sugar or fat can make your meal plan more enjoyable. Knowing the nutrients in food can help you make choices about how much and how often you want to eat these foods.	
	9.6 In general, everyone also benefits from: ■ spacing meals and eating regularly ■ controlling portion sizes ■ eating at least three meals per day	Refer to Outline #3, *The Basics of Eating*.

CONTENT OUTLINE

CONCEPT	DETAIL	INSTRUCTOR'S NOTES
10. Planning for change	10.1 The following are food choices that could help you lower your blood glucose after a meal: ■ Eat less carbohydrate at the meal and include some fat or protein in the meal. ■ Eat more fiber at the meal.	Ask, "What is your blood glucose target? At what times of the day is your blood glucose higher or lower than you want it to be? What food changes might help you lower or raise your blood glucose at that time?"
	10.2 To eat less carbohydrate at a meal: ■ Choose fewer high-carbohydrate foods. You could have orange juice, toast, and peanut butter instead of orange juice, cereal, milk, and banana. Or, choose baked potato, green beans, and tossed salad instead of baked potato, corn, and a roll. ■ Eat smaller portions. Drink ½ cup juice instead of 1 cup, or have one roll instead of two. ■ Eat foods with less carbohydrate per bite. Choose 1 cup of Cheerios instead of 1 cup of granola, or 1 cup of broccoli instead of 1 cup of peas. ■ Drink a diet soft drink instead of a regular one. ■ Skip dessert or eat a small portion. ■ Eat a less sweet dessert. Choose plain ice cream instead of a hot fudge sundae.	Ask, "What are ways to eat less carbohydrate at a meal?" Refer to concept 8 in this section. *Note:* Substituting carbohydrate foods with items from the meat or fat group is a way to reduce postprandial blood glucose levels and still satisfy hunger and meet caloric needs.
	10.3 Check blood glucose regularly to see if you are reaching your goals and to see how different foods affect your blood glucose.	
	10.4 Treat a low blood glucose reaction with the right amount of carbohydrate to bring your blood glucose level up to the normal level without going too high.	Refer to Outline #11, *Managing Blood Glucose*, for information about treating hypoglycemia.

CONTENT OUTLINE

CONCEPT	DETAIL	INSTRUCTOR'S NOTES
	10.5 Choose one change you want to make this week to help you reach your goal(s).	Although overall health is not the primary focus in this session, some participants may be interested in adding foods from a food group (such as milk or vegetables) they currently omit.
		Participants may prefer to continue working on spacing meals or limiting portion sizes as discussed in Outline #3, *The Basics of Eating*.

SKILLS CHECKLIST

None.

EVALUATION PLAN

Knowledge will be evaluated by achievement of learning objectives and by responses to questions during the session. The ability to apply knowledge will be evaluated by development of personal meal-planning goals to improve blood glucose levels and through program outcome measures.

DOCUMENTATION PLAN

Record class attendance and achieved objectives as appropriate.

SUGGESTED READINGS

Anderson EJ, Richardson M, Castle G, Cercone S, Delahanty L, Lyon R, Mueller D, Snetselaar L (The DCCT Research Group). Nutrition interventions for intensive therapy in the Diabetes Control and Complications Trial. *Journal of the American Dietetic Association*. 1993;93: 768–772.

Bassous V. Forbidden fruit? *Diabetes Forecast*. 1997;50(8):38–40.

Bolderman KM, Mersey JH. Faithful fasting. *Diabetes Forecast*. 1996;49(9):48–50.

Delahanty L, ed. Challenges and lessons from the Diabetes Control and Complications Trial. *On the Cutting Edge*, Diabetes Care and Education Practice Group newsletter, The American Dietetic Association. 1994;15(2):1–24.

Franz MJ. Protein controversies in diabetes. *Diabetes Spectrum*. 2000;13:132–141.

SUGGESTED READINGS *continued*

Gillespie S. Implementing liberalized carbohydrate guidelines: nutrition free-for-all or
more rational approach to carbohydrate con-
sumption. *Diabetes Spectrum.* 1996;9:165–167.

Gillespie SJ. A carbohydrate is a carbohydrate
is a carbohydrate: is the ban on sugar really
lifted? *The Diabetes Educator.* 1996;
22:449–452, 457.

Glasgow RE, Toobert DJ, Hampson SE. Effects
of a brief office-based intervention to facilitate
diabetes dietary self-management. *Diabetes
Care.* 1996;19:834–842.

Kulkarni K. Nutrition counseling for Indian and
Pakistani patients. *Practical Diabetology.*
1996;15(2):19–20.

Magnus MH. What's your IQ on cross-cultural
nutrition counseling? *The Diabetes Educator.*
1996;22:57–62.

Markowski DM, Larsen JL, McElligott MC,
Walter GA, Miller SA, Risbie K, Stratta RJ.
Diet after pancreas transplantation. *Diabetes
Care.* 1996;19:735–738.

Valmadrid CT, Klein R, Moss SE, Klein BE,
Cruickshanks, NJ. Alcohol intake and the
risk of coronary heart disease mortality in
persons with older-onset diabetes mellitus.
JAMA. 1999;282:239–246.

Vessby B. Dietary carbohydrates. *American
Journal of Clinical Nutrition.* 1994;59
(Suppl 3):742–746.

Wheeler M, Mazur ML. Sugars and diabetes.
Diabetes Forecast. 1997;50(2):38–42.

➲ Reasons for Meal Planning

- Maintain blood glucose as close to your target range as possible.

- Maintain cholesterol (blood fats) as close to your target range as possible.

- Maintain blood pressure as close to your target level as possible.

- Prevent, delay, or treat diabetes-related complications.

- Improve health through food choices.

- Meet individual nutritional needs.

➲ Nutrients in Food

Nutrient	Contains Calories
Carbohydrate	☑
Protein	☑
Fat	☑
Vitamins	☐
Minerals	☐
Water	☐

➲ Food Groups

Starch	Bread, rolls, bagels, English muffins, tortillas, pita bread, naan, crackers, matzoh
	Rice, pasta, noodles, spaghetti, macaroni
	Cereal, dry or cooked
	Legumes: lentils, dried or canned beans (garbanzo, kidney, black, or butter beans), dried peas (split peas or black-eyed peas), miso
	Starchy vegetables: potatoes, corn, green peas, squash, taro root, yams
Fruit	Apples, oranges, bananas, and all other fruits except avocado—fresh, frozen, canned, or juiced
Milk	All milk products
	Yogurt (plain or artificially sweetened)
Vegetable	Carrots, green beans, wax beans, broccoli, beets, greens, okra, and all other crunchy vegetables
Meat	Beef, pork, lamb, chicken, turkey, fish
	Peanut butter, cheese, cottage cheese, eggs, tofu
Fat	Butter, margarine, cream, oil, salad dressing, mayonnaise
	Sour cream, cream cheese, coffee creamer
	Bacon, lard, fatback, nuts, seeds

➡ Nutrients in Food Groups

Food Group	Nutrient(s)	Effect on Blood Glucose	Rate of Effect on Blood Glucose
Starch	**Carbohydrate** Protein	Large	Fast
Fruit	**Carbohydrate**	Large	Fast
Milk	**Carbohydrate** Protein Fat	Large	Fast (slower if reduced fat [2%] or whole milk)
Vegetable	**Carbohydrate** Protein	Small	Fast
Meat	**Protein** Fat	—	—
Fat	**Fat**	—	—

| #5 | **Planning Meals** |

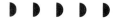

STATEMENT OF PURPOSE

This session builds on the information in Outline #3, *The Basics of Eating*, and Outline #4, *Food and Blood Glucose*, and provides information and practice in planning menus using *Healthy Food Choices, The First Step in Diabetes Meal Planning, Eating Healthy with Diabetes, Month of Meals,* and the plate method. Information about the basics of carbohydrate counting is also included in this outline. The purpose of this session is to present a variety of options for meal planning. Omit discussion of approaches that do not meet the needs of your audience. Sections on eating out, the use of alcohol, and selecting cookbooks are included. More advanced carbohydrate counting and the exchange system for meal planning are covered in later sessions.

The choice of the meal-planning approach depends on the personal goals, abilities, and lifestyle needs of each participant and the type and status of his or her diabetes. Encourage participants to consider which approach they could most easily use on a consistent basis.

PREREQUISITES

This session will be more useful for those who complete and bring a food diary to the session. It is recommended that each participant have attended sessions #3, *The Basics of Eating*, and #4, *Food and Blood Glucose*, or have achieved those objectives. If they have a meal plan, ask that participants bring it to class with them.

OBJECTIVES

At the end of this session, participants will be able to:

1. using the food diary, compare their food choices with the basic guidelines;

2. describe five different approaches to planning meals;

3. use one of these approaches to plan a menu for 1 day;

4. plan one restaurant meal that fits with their usual plans;

5. describe how alcohol may affect a person with diabetes;

6. identify three guidelines for the use of alcohol (if they use alcohol);

7. explain how at least three cookbook recipes would fit into their meal plans.

CONTENT

Nutritional Management.

MATERIALS NEEDED

VISUALS PROVIDED	ADDITIONAL

VISUALS PROVIDED
1. The Diabetes Food Pyramid
2. Plate Method: Breakfast
3. Plate Method: Lunch or Dinner

Handouts (one per participant)
1. The Diabetes Food Pyramid
2. Counting Carbohydrate Servings
3. Tips for Counting Carbohydrate Grams
4. Eating Away From Home
5. Guidelines for Use of Alcoholic Drinks
6. Cookbooks for People with Diabetes

ADDITIONAL
- Chalkboard, chalk
- Food models or pictures of food
- *The First Step in Diabetes Meal Planning* and *Eating Healthy with Diabetes* (booklets available from the American Diabetes Association, 800-232-6733)
- The *Month of Meals* series (books available from the American Diabetes Association—use several)
- *Basic Carbohydrate Counting* (booklet available from the American Diabetes Association)
- Restaurant menus (obtain from restaurants popular with the participants)
- Examples of diabetes cookbooks, including appropriate ethnic cookbooks

METHOD OF PRESENTATION

Start by introducing yourself and telling what you do. Ask participants to introduce themselves. Begin by asking about their short-term goal and what they learned from it. Review food diaries by asking if they made any discoveries while they were keeping it.

Family members and significant others, especially those who shop or prepare meals for the person with diabetes, should be encouraged to attend. Present material in a question/discussion format. Include time for participants to practice meal planning by creating menus they could use at home and at a restaurant.

CONTENT OUTLINE

CONCEPT	DETAIL	INSTRUCTOR'S NOTES
1. Basic guidelines	1.1 These basic guidelines offer a starting point for meal planning: ■ Eat at least three meals or snacks spaced throughout the day. ■ Eat each meal and snack at about the same time each day.	Ask, "What questions or concerns do you have about planning meals?" Review the guidelines discussed in Outline #3, *The Basics of Eating*. Ask to what extent they use these guidelines.

CONTENT OUTLINE

CONCEPT	DETAIL	INSTRUCTOR'S NOTES

■ Do not skip meals.
■ Eat about the same amount at each meal each day.
■ Notice how much you eat.

Allow time for participants to share their experiences and ask questions. Day-to-day variation leads to uneven glucose patterns.

1.2 The purpose of meal planning is to help you reach your personal blood glucose or weight goals. Some can reach their goals by spacing their food intake and limiting portion sizes. Others benefit from a more specific meal plan.

Review reasons for meal planning in Outline #3, *The Basics of Eating*. Ask participants if they can identify their personal blood glucose and weight goals.

1.3 Knowing what and when you eat now is the first step in deciding what changes might help you.

Assessment is essential to identify patterns, meal components, and areas of difficulty. Consider self-determined blood glucose, lipid and weight goals; medical needs; weight history; food preferences; psychosocial needs; interest in change; and available resources.

1.4 Keeping a food diary can help you become more aware of how you eat now. It may also help you understand how certain foods affect your blood glucose when combined with your monitoring record.

Ask participants to look over their food diaries. Ask, "How did your choices compare with the basic guidelines? What did you learn about yourself and your eating habits? Did you find anything you would like to change?"

1.5 There are many different ways to plan meals for diabetes. Approaches presented in this session are:
■ healthy food choices
■ the food guide pyramid
■ preplanned menus
■ the plate method
■ basic carbohydrate counting

An overview of carbohydrate counting may be introduced in this session. It is discussed in more detail in Outline #19, *Carbohydrate Counting*. A dietitian may work with someone to count calories or fat grams (methods often used for weight loss), but these methods are not detailed in these outlines.

1.6 Different plans work for different people. You may use different approaches over time or in different situations. Think about which approaches might work for you.

Any method that helps participants to focus on meal planning is helpful. Refer participants to a dietitian who is a diabetes educator.

CONTENT OUTLINE

CONCEPT	DETAIL	INSTRUCTOR'S NOTES
2. Healthy Food Choices	2.1 *Healthy Food Choices* is a guide for simplifying diabetes meal planning. It has two main parts: "Healthy Food Choices" and "Food Servings," a meal planning section.	
	2.2 "Healthy Food Choices" gives eight guidelines: ■ Eat a variety of foods. ■ Avoid skipping meals. ■ Eat healthy carbohydrates. ■ Watch serving sizes. ■ Eat less fat. ■ Be at a healthy weight. ■ Be physically active. ■ Choose a healthy lifestyle.	Ask participants to read each section. Refer to their food diary or ask them to write down everything they ate since yesterday at this time or just think about the food they eat each day. Ask participants to think about how much exercise they get each week.
	2.3 One idea under EAT HEALTHY CARBOHYDRATES says: "Avoid regular soft drinks. One can has 9 teaspoons of sugar!" It also has 150–200 calories.	Other ideas include eating fewer sweet foods and using sugar-free soft drinks/powdered drinks, sparkling water, club soda, sugar-free iced tea, or a slice of lemon in plain water. Ask, "What other changes can you make to eat healthier carbohydrates?"
	2.4 Then look at the ideas under EAT LESS FAT. The first idea talks about how meat is cooked. Another strategy is to choose lower-fat meat and other foods.	Ask, "How can you eat less fat? If you eat 8 oz of meat at dinner, could you eat 5 or 6 oz instead?" Other ideas include having a meatless meal a few times a week; buying veggie burgers, lean hamburger, or ground round; using less butter, cream, and salad dressing; and drinking skim or low-fat milk instead of whole milk.
	2.5 The "Food Servings" section helps you to plan meals using foods from six food groups and two specialty sections. The six food groups are: ■ starch ■ fruits ■ milk ■ nonstarchy vegetables ■ meat and meat substitutes ■ fats	Space for developing menu ideas that fit into the participants' meal plan is given on the back of the pamphlet. It is better for the participants and instructor to design a meal plan to fit individual food preferences and calorie needs. Any plan should include a variety of foods from each group. Eating a food high in vitamin C

CONTENT OUTLINE

CONCEPT	DETAIL	INSTRUCTOR'S NOTES
	The specialty sections are "Other Foods" and "Free Foods."	every day and a food high in vitamin A three or four times a week is recommended. Calcium requirements also need to be considered, particularly for post-menopausal women.
	2.6 You can design your own meal plan or work with a dietitian to help you plan the number of servings from each group. Each person's needs (calories, nutrients), likes, and dislikes are different.	
	2.7 In each food group, each food listed is one serving. For example: 1 serving of starch = ⅓ cup pasta (noodles), **or** 1 small potato, **or** 1 slice of bread, **or** 3 cups popcorn Read the foods listed in each group. If there are foods you like that aren't listed, ask your dietitian to tell you how to count them.	If your plan has four servings from the starch group, you could either choose four different foods or eat four servings of one food (such as four slices of bread). Note the spaces to write in menu ideas. Some of your favorite foods may be combination foods (one, two, or more different food groups in one serving), such as pizza or casseroles. Exchange values of foods are available in *Exchange Lists for Meal Planning* and other books. Calorie, carbohydrate, protein, and fat values for additional foods are available in commercial product information or texts, such as Pennington and Church's *Food Values of Portions Commonly Used.*
	2.8 Here are some tips about food groups: ■ **Fruits**. No sugar or syrup is added. ■ **Milk**. 1% and 2% milk counts as reduced fat. Skim and ½% milk counts as low fat. Plain yogurt counts as milk.	Note that calories vary in different kinds of milk, but the amount of carbohydrate, protein, and calcium are the same. If syrup or juice from canned fruit is used in cooking, it is counted as fruit juice.

CONTENT OUTLINE

CONCEPT	DETAIL	INSTRUCTOR'S NOTES

■ **Vegetables**. Use without sauce or added fat. (Choose from fat group if desired.)

■ **Protein**. Servings are given in ounces. Add up the total ounces per day. One egg or ¼ cup tuna counts as 1 oz of protein.

■ **Fats**. Ask your dietitian how to plan for high-fat foods.

Protein servings are likely to be smaller than participants usually eat. Illustrate with models.

Other examples of high-fat foods are bacon and powdered coffee creamer.

2.9 At the bottom of the "Food Servings" page, "Other Foods" shows how to include combination foods, which include more than one food group in a single serving.

Examples:
Casserole (1 cup) = 2 starch servings + 2 protein servings + 0–2 fat servings
Cream soup (1 cup) = 1 starch serving + 1 fat serving

2.10 "Free Foods" lists foods with less than 20 calories per serving that can be eaten with meals or between meals. Limit these foods to one or two servings per day. Remember that even low-calorie foods can add up to weight gain if you eat a lot of them.

It is important to weigh the costs and benefits when choosing these foods. Examples:
1 stick diet gum = 5–10 calories
½ cup diet Jell-O = 8 calories
1 Tbsp diet syrup = 10 calories
1 Tbsp diet salad dressing = 6–16 calories

Some people eat large amounts of "free" vegetables with diet salad dressing. The calories add up. Too many free foods can slow weight loss. If participants eat a lot of free foods, their calorie level may need to be increased. A meal plan that is too hard to stay on without overeating free foods won't last long and may not provide adequate nutrients.

2.11 Use the "Menu Ideas" space on the back to write the times of your meals/snacks and menu ideas.

When discussing meal times, keep in mind that consistency is more important for people who take insulin than for those who don't. It is desirable, however, for all participants to spread foods out over the day. For par-

CONTENT OUTLINE

CONCEPT	DETAIL	INSTRUCTOR'S NOTES
		ticipants who take insulin, the number of servings planned for each meal can be included to the left of the sample meals to help ensure consistency. Encourage participants to plan sample meals using the information in the pamphlet.
	2.12 Now that you have some ideas for food choices, it is time to think about your goals. Choose what is important to you and do what is possible. Use the space under "Guidelines for Healthy Food Choices" to write down your goals.	Suggested steps: ■ Choose one way to change eating habits to work toward goals. ■ Write a sample menu using *Healthy Food Choices*.
3. Food guide pyramid	3.1 The kinds and amounts of foods to eat are illustrated by the food guide pyramid. Foods for people with diabetes are healthy choices for everyone and do not need to cost more.	Use *The First Step in Diabetes Meal Planning*, a version of the food guide pyramid modified for people with diabetes. If not available, use Visual #1 and Handout #1, The Diabetes Food Pyramid.
	The food guide pyramid for diabetes is the same as the standard food guide pyramid except that foods are grouped by the way they are likely to affect blood glucose levels.	In the standard pyramid, potatoes are in the vegetable group and cheese is in the milk group. Alcohol is not included in the standard pyramid.
	3.2 Foods are divided into six groups: ■ Starch (including grains, beans, and starchy vegetables) ■ Fruit ■ Milk ■ Vegetables ■ Meat ■ Fats, sweets, and alcohol	Review the six groups by listing on the chalkboard or on newsprint. Using food models or pictures, have participants practice assigning foods to a group. Note that alcohol and sugar have been added to the fat group. These foods are similar in that they add flavor but few nutrients.
	3.3 Each group contains different nutrients and affects your blood glucose in a different way. Your body	This approach is often adequate to aid in blood glucose control. This is a general, flexible method

CONTENT OUTLINE

CONCEPT	DETAIL	INSTRUCTOR'S NOTES

needs food from all six groups, but you can see on the pyramid that you need more food from the larger sections on the bottom (bread, cereal, rice, vegetables, and fruit) than from the smaller sections near the top (milk, meat, and fats).

to manage composition, carbohydrate intake, and portion size.

3.4 These are the recommended number of servings from each group:
- Starch — 6 or more
- Fruit — 2–4
- Milk — 2–3
- Vegetables — 3–5
- Meat and meat subtitutes — 4–6 oz
- Fats, sweets, alcohol (no minimum amount) — Limit

Staying within the recommended number of servings for each group helps provide a diet low in sugar, fat, and calories and high in nutrients.

Ask, "How many choices are recommended from the starch group and the fruit, vegetable, protein, and milk groups?" Use Handout #1, The Diabetes Food Pyramid, or *The First Step in Diabetes Meal Planning*.

3.5 Fruits and vegetables contain many important vitamins and minerals including antioxidants.

Routine supplementation with antioxidants is not advised for people with diabetes. Plants also contain other antioxidants. Oil, wheat germ, and nuts are rich in vitamin E.

3.6 The serving size for each group varies depending on the food. For example, in the starch group, one serving can be 1 slice of bread, ⅓ cup pasta or rice, ¼ bagel, or 1 small potato.

Serving sizes for the other groups are:
- Fruit: 1 small piece, ½ cup
- Vegetables: ½ cup cooked, 1 cup raw
- Milk: 1 cup
- Meat: 2–3 oz (2 Tbsp peanut butter)
- Fat: 1 tsp butter, margarine, oil, or mayonnaise; 1 Tbsp cream cheese or salad dressing; 10 peanuts

Use food models and measuring cups and spoons to show the amount of food in a serving. (Note that many people require more than one serving per meal.) Take special note of the meat serving size, which differs from the exchange system.

Limit sweets and alcohol.

CONTENT OUTLINE

CONCEPT	DETAIL	INSTRUCTOR'S NOTES
	3.7 Look at your food diary again. Count the number of servings you ate in each group each day. How does your intake compare with the recommended number of servings? Too much of any food can make your blood glucose or your weight go up. If you eat too few servings from any food group, you may miss needed nutrients.	Ask, "Are there any foods you need to eat more of? Less of?" Record suggestions. Ask patients to check things they are already doing and circle things they might want to change. If time is a problem, do this exercise for one meal or one to three food groups. Participants may need help assigning foods to groups.
	3.8 Including the following at each meal will help you to meet the recommended number of servings for the day: ■ 2–3 starches ■ 1 fruit and/or 1–2 vegetables ■ 1 milk and/or 1–3 meats	This simple plan was introduced in Outline #4, *Food and Blood Glucose*. If possible, allow time during class for individuals or small groups to plan a day's menu using a recommended number of servings from each group.
	3.9 Combination foods like stew, chili, and goulash can be used in the diet.	For example, stew would fill your need for both meat and starch choices. Combination foods make it easier to eat more like the pyramid: more starch and less meat.
	3.10 *Eating Healthy with Diabetes* lists examples of one serving from each of the food groups for various meals.	In groups, ask participants to plan a menu for a day that they would be willing to prepare and eat.
4. Preplanned menus	4.1 Using preplanned menus is another way to structure eating. The *Month of Meals* series presents menus with 28 breakfasts, 28 lunches, and 28 dinners. The pages of the books are divided so that each breakfast can go with any lunch and dinner.	Show a book from the *Month of Meals* series, and demonstrate the variety of menus that could be planned. These menus offer a resource for participants who say, "Just tell me what to eat," and others interested in using preplanned menus and recipes.
	4.2 The three meals plus a planned snack provide 1500 calories. Instructions are included to increase or decrease the calorie level to match your needs.	Point out the snack lists in the back of the book. Show how to adjust the calorie level.

CONTENT OUTLINE

CONCEPT	DETAIL	INSTRUCTOR'S NOTES
	4.3 Simple recipes are printed with the menus. Most recipes make one to four servings.	In groups (depending on the number of copies of *Month of Meals* books available), ask participants to plan a menu for a day that they would be willing to prepare and eat.
5. The plate method	5.1 The plate method is a way to plan meals with no measuring. You fill your plate to match the amount of vegetables, starch, and meat in a sample picture, then add a piece of fruit and/or a glass of milk.	This is a simple method used first in Europe. It is especially appropriate for older adults, those with low literacy skills, and those who do not choose more structured approaches. Some patients who use other approaches may find this method helpful when eating away from home (e.g., at potlucks, restaurants, or dinner parties).
	5.2 Divide your plate into fourths. At breakfast, ½ is for starches and ¼ for meat. No vegetables are eaten and protein is optional, so the entire plate is not used.	Use Visual #2, Plate Method: Breakfast. Using food models, ask participants to create breakfast meals using Visual #2 as a guide. If participants eat cereal for breakfast, mark a disposable bowl with a line showing a serving size of the cereal they like to take home.
	5.3 At lunch and dinner, use ¼ for starches, ¼ for meat, and ½ for vegetables.	Use Visual #3, Plate Method: Lunch or Dinner. Create other lunch and dinner meals (including a potluck or restaurant meal) using Visual #3 as a guide. Use food models on a plastic plate with sections or a marked paper plate. For those unwilling to eat a lot of vegetables, use ½ of the plate for the fruit serving instead of vegetables.

CONTENT OUTLINE

CONCEPT	DETAIL	INSTRUCTOR'S NOTES
	5.4 Filling a dinner (9-inch) plate without snacks will provide 1200–1500 calories per day, depending on serving size.	
6. Basic carbohydrate counting	6.1 Carbohydrate counting is another meal-planning approach. As you remember, carbohydrate affects blood glucose more than any other nutrient.	Review the effects of carbohydrate, protein and fat on blood glucose from Outline #3, *The Basics of Eating*, as needed.
	6.2 The starch, fruit, milk, and sweets and desserts groups have similar amounts of carbohydrate.	Use *Basic Carbohydrate Counting* or review carbohydrate-containing foods from Outline #4 as needed. Ask the group to practice identifying which foods do and do not contain carbohydrate. Note that vegetables contain 5 gm carbohydrate, but that amount is so small it can be ignored unless three or more servings are eaten.
	6.3 Each serving of starch, fruit, or milk is counted as one carbohydrate serving.	
	6.4 Each carbohydrate serving provides about 15 gm carbohydrate. You can count either carbohydrate servings or grams. If you know the carbohydrate content, all foods can be worked into this plan.	Use food labels or reference books to determine the amounts of foods often eaten by participants that equal 15 gm carbohydrate.
	6.5 You first need to decide how many servings or grams of carbohydrates to have at each meal. You can then make choices about the specific carbohydrate foods you will eat to match the number of servings. This provides flexibility and variety in your meals.	The carbohydrate level and distribution is determined by each person, based on food preferences, blood glucose records, caloric needs, and triglyceride levels. Stress the importance of pre- and postmeal blood glucose monitoring.

CONTENT OUTLINE

CONCEPT	DETAIL	INSTRUCTOR'S NOTES
	Examples of meals providing five carbohydrate servings each: 1 sandwich 1 cup milk 1 small apple 1 oz potato chips OR 1 cup spaghetti 2 slices garlic bread OR ½ cup juice 1 cup oatmeal 2 Tbsp raisins 1 slice toast	Using food models, show how to use different carbohydrate food items to create different meals with similar carbohydrate content. Use the *Basic Carbohydrate Counting* booklet and Handouts #2 and #3 to reinforce these concepts.
7. Eating away from home	7.1 Many people enjoy eating in restaurants, but the food is different than you might fix at home.	Ask, "Do you enjoy eating at restaurants? Why?" Discuss reasons for eating out (other than food).
	7.2 Review reasons for meal planning. Your most important personal goal may be to improve blood glucose levels, cholesterol levels, or weight.	Ask participants to identify their most important nutritional goal.
	7.3 Possible barriers to eating in a restaurant: ■ temptation to overeat ■ foods don't fit your meal plan ■ methods of food preparation make it hard to tell what's in the food ■ mealtime may be early or late	Ask, "Do you expect any problems taking care of your diabetes when eating away from home?" Use responses to discuss the barriers. Enlist ideas from participants.
	7.4 Tips for eating out: ■ Know what is important to you about eating out. ■ Remember the reasons you use a meal plan. ■ Know your meal plan. ■ Choose kinds and amounts of food that best fit into your meal plan. ■ Choose plain food. Avoid foods that have been sweetened,	Distribute Handout #4, Eating Away from Home. Review content and answer questions. Plain foods have fewer calories per bite. Choosing plain foods

CONTENT OUTLINE

CONCEPT	DETAIL	INSTRUCTOR'S NOTES
	breaded, or fried or are in sauces or gravies. It is hard to predict the nutrient value of combination foods.	makes it possible to eat more without overeating.
	■ Plan ahead—call the restaurant or hostess if you are unsure of the menu.	Collect sample menus to review at home.
	■ Substitute an extra starch for a fruit or milk choice if milk or fruit are not available.	Bread or rolls are often more available than unsweetened fruit or fat-free (skim) milk, and the carbohydrate content is similar.
	■ Look for free foods or plain vegetables to increase amount of food without raising blood glucose.	Raw or plain cooked vegetables should not greatly affect blood glucose or calorie levels.
	■ Ask how foods are prepared—breaded, fried, sugar added?	Ask, "How comfortable are you with asking questions or asking for an item that's not on the menu?" Role-playing may help people become more assertive in asking for what they want in a restaurant.
	■ Ask if foods are available even if they are not listed on the menu: fresh fruit, juice, fat-free (skim) milk, vegetables, margarine, and diet drinks.	
	7.5 The following are requests you might make:	
	■ Serve salad dressing, sour cream, and butter on the side so you can control your portion.	
	■ Prepare vegetables and meat without added fat.	Examples: Broiled fish instead of fried fish; baked potato instead of french fries.
	■ Substitute plain vegetable, starch, or fruit for a sweetened menu item.	Examples: Fresh fruit instead of fruit cocktail; toast instead of a sweet roll.
	7.6 Activity: Select a restaurant dinner using the food guide pyramid and/or the plate method.	Distribute the restaurant menus. Use the plate method as a guide to choosing foods from the menu, not a literal "filling-the-plate" unless selecting from a buffet.
	Choose the main dish first. Notice the foods that would most easily fit into a meal plan.	Ask, "What items are missing that you might request?"

CONTENT OUTLINE

CONCEPT	DETAIL	INSTRUCTOR'S NOTES
	Consider changes you might make to your usual plan.	Discuss possible changes in the meal plan. If you have time, have each participant plan a restaurant meal using his or her own meal plan.
	7.7 It is possible to adjust insulin to cover increases in food if you know the amount of carbohydrate in the food.	
8. Guidelines for altered mealtimes	8.1 If the meal is delayed: ■ 1 hour—eat a piece of fruit or bread from dinner at the regular time; subtract them from dinner ■ 2–3 hours—eat the evening snack at dinnertime and dinner at snack time	Delayed meals may cause hypoglycemia if you take medicine (particularly insulin) for diabetes.
	Each person responds differently to changes in meal timing, depending on insulin, activity, etc. Blood glucose monitoring can help you adjust your meal schedule and keep your blood glucose level where you want it to be.	Ask participants what changes have worked for them. For some, a delay of 1 hour does not cause a problem.
	8.2 If the meal is early: ■ 1 hour—follow regular eating pattern (or use next option) ■ 2–3 hours—save one starch from meal and eat it as a snack at your regular mealtime	Stress that guidelines for delayed and early meals will vary depending on the individual meal plan.
9. Use of alcoholic drinks	9.1 Alcohol is not a food. It provides no carbohydrate, protein, fat, or vitamins. It does provide 7 calories per gram.	Ask, "How could drinking alcohol affect your diabetes?" Write down answers on the board.
	9.2 Alcohol is treated as a poison by the body. Your liver works to get rid of the alcohol and is less able to help regulate your blood glucose. You may have a low blood glucose reaction after drinking alcohol. This is of particular concern for people who take insulin or certain diabetes medications.	The liver may not be able to counterregulate during hypoglycemia because alcohol blocks gluconeogenesis. This effect can last 8–12 hours.

CONTENT OUTLINE

CONCEPT	DETAIL	INSTRUCTOR'S NOTES

9.3 Alcohol is a depressant. You may not be able to tell the difference between early effects of alcohol and early symptoms of hypoglycemia.

Alcohol itself does not improve cholesterol. It is other compounds in the ingredients of an alcoholic beverage that are beneficial.

9.4 Alcohol during pregnancy can harm the developing baby.

9.5 Alcohol is not recommended with some types of medication. Alcohol changes the action of many drugs.

Alcohol may cause flushing, nausea, or vomiting when taken with chlorpropamide.

9.6 Because it provides calories without other nutrients and stimulates appetite, alcohol can make weight control more difficult.

The additional calories in alcoholic beverages counted as fats in the exchange system. Twelve ounces of regular beer has 150 calories and counts as 1 starch and 2 fat exchanges. Twelve ounces of nonalcoholic beer has 60 calories and counts as 1 starch exchange.

9.7 Guidelines for using alcohol include:
- Alcohol can be safely used only when your blood glucose is well controlled. Discuss its use with your provider.

Distribute Handout #5, Guidelines for Use of Alcoholic Drinks. Ask, "How can alcohol be enjoyed safely?"

- Because alcohol can lower blood glucose, drink only with meals or snacks containing carbohydrate.

Name some carbohydrate snacks. Note that peanuts, cheese, or boiled eggs do not provide carbohydrate.

- Drink in moderation.
- Avoid sweet wine, liqueurs, and sweetened mixed drinks because of their high sugar content.

Moderation is defined as one equivalent for women and two for men per day. Equivalent =
- 1½ oz distilled spirits
- 4 oz dry wine
- 12 oz beer

- Mixers such as water, soda water, and sugar-free carbonated drinks are free; unsweetened fruit or vegetable juices can be counted as fruit or vegetable exchanges.

Wine spritzer made with club soda is a better choice than a wine cooler, which is made with fruit juice or sweetened mixers.

- Sip slowly.
- Do not drink before, during, or after vigorous exercise.

Both alcohol and exercise can lower blood glucose. In combination, reactions are more likely.

CONTENT OUTLINE

CONCEPT	DETAIL	INSTRUCTOR'S NOTES
10. Recipes	10.1 Most recipes can be adapted to provide low-fat, low-sugar foods that still taste similar.	As an activity, ask for favorite recipes and show how to adapt them.
	10.2 Try reducing the amount of fat you add to your favorite recipe, or substitute a nonfat or lite product. The sugar in baked products can often be reduced by $\frac{1}{4}$ to $\frac{1}{2}$ of the original recipe without major changes in taste.	Ask, "Have you tried to lower the fat or sugar content of a familiar recipe? How did it work?"
	10.3 Several cookbooks provide low-fat, low-sugar recipes and provide information about nutrient content.	Distribute Handout #6, Cookbooks for People with Diabetes. Show sample cookbooks. *Note:* Not all recipes from a cookbook for people with diabetes fit all meal plans.
	10.4 Keep in mind that no single food or dish is good or bad. The combination of all the food you eat helps or hinders your diabetes care.	Practice by selecting recipes and stating how that dish might fit into an overall plan. Choose a short-term goal to try before the next session.

SKILLS CHECKLIST

Participants will be able to create a menu that helps to meet their goals and will be able to identify items on a restaurant menu that fit with their meal plans.

EVALUATION PLAN

Knowledge will be evaluated by achievement of learning objectives and by responses to questions during the session; skills will be evaluated by observation. The ability to apply knowledge will be evaluated by the development of personal meal-planning goals, by development and implementation of a plan to achieve those goals, and through program outcome measures.

DOCUMENTATION PLAN

Record class attendance and achieved objectives as appropriate.

SUGGESTED READINGS

American Diabetes Association, The American Dietetic Association. *The First Steps in Diabetes Meal Planning.* Chicago, IL: The American Dietetic Association; Alexandria, VA: American Diabetes Association; 1995.

American Diabetes Association, The American Dietetic Association. *Eating Healthy with Diabetes.* Chicago, IL: The American Dietetic Association; Alexandria, VA: American Diabetes Association; 1998.

American Diabetes Association, The American Dietetic Association. *Healthy Food Choices.* Chicago, IL: The American Dietetic Association; Alexandria, VA: American Diabetes Association; 1998 (Spanish version available).

American Diabetes Association. *Magic Menus for People with Diabetes.* Alexandria, VA: American Diabetes Association, 1998.

American Diabetes Association. *Month of Meals,* Revised Editions. Alexandria, VA: American Diabetes Association, 1999.

The American Dietetic Association, American Diabetes Association. *Ethnic and Regional Food Practices Series: Food Practices, Customs and Holidays for Jewish, Mexican American, Chinese American, Hmong, Navajo, Alaska Native, Filipino American, Soul and Traditional Southern, Cajun and Creole.* Chicago, IL: The American Dietetic Association; Alexandria, VA: American Diabetes Association, 1986.

Anderson EJ, Richardson M, Castle G, Cercone S, Delahanty L, Lyon R, Mueller D, Snetselaar L (The DCCT Research Group). Nutrition interventions for intensive therapy in the Diabetes Control and Complications Trial. *Journal of the American Dietetic Association.* 1993;93: 768–772.

Barner CW, Wylie-Rosett J, Gans K. WAVE: A pocket guide for a brief nutrition dialogue in primary care. *The Diabetes Educator.* 2001; 27:352–362.

Booth SM. Using the nondiet approach to diabetes meal planning. *The Diabetes Educator.* 2002;28:530–534.

Davis D, Lipps J. Alcohol use. *Diabetes Forecast.* 2000;53(9):57.

Diabetes Care and Education Practice Group; Elisberg T (Project Chair). *Selected Diabetes and Nutrition Education Resources: For the Person With Diabetes.* Chicago, IL: The American Dietetic Association, 1994.

Franz MJ. *Exchanges for All Occasions.* 3rd Edition. Minneapolis, MN: Chronimed Publishing, 1993.

Gottlieb SH. A drink a day. *Diabetes Forecast.* 2004;52(5):56–57.

Idaho Diabetes Care and Education Practice Group. *Plate Method Posters.* (Order from Julie C. Harker, P.O. Box 441, Rexburg, ID 83440–0441.)

McCabe RE, Mills JS, Polivy J. Ditch your diet. *Diabetes Forecast.* 2000;53(1):49–53.

Pastors JG, Holler HJ, eds. *Meal Planning Approaches for Diabetes Management.* 2nd Edition. Chicago, IL: The Diabetes Care and Education Practice Group of The American Dietetic Association, 1994.

Peterson AE, Maryniuk MD. Using a nutrition assessment to determine a nutrition prescription. *The Diabetes Educator.* 1996;22:205–210.

Powers MA, ed. *Handbook of Diabetes Nutritional Management.* 2nd Edition. Rockville, MD: Aspen Publishers, 1996.

Tinker LF. Measuring up: the food guide pyramid. *Diabetes Spectrum.* 1995;8: 200–202.

Wakabayashi I, Kobaba-Wakabayashi R, Masuda H. Relation of drinking alcohol to atherosclerotic risk in type 2 diabetes. *Diabetes Care.* 2002;25:1223–1228.

Wilson C, Brown T, Acton K, Gilliland S. Effects of clinical nutrition education and educator discipline on glycemic control outcomes in the Indian Health Service. *Diabetes Care.* 2003;26:2500–2504.

Ziemer DC, Berkowitz KJ, Panayioto RM, El-Kebbi IM, Musey VC, Anderson LA, Wanko NS, Fowke ML, Brazier CW, Dunbar VG, Slocum W, Bacha GM, Gallina DL, Cook CB, Phillips LS. A simple meal plan emphasizing healthy food choices is as effective as an exchange-based meal plan for urban African Americans with type 2 diabetes. *Diabetes Care.* 2003;26:1719–1724.

➜ The Diabetes Food Pyramid

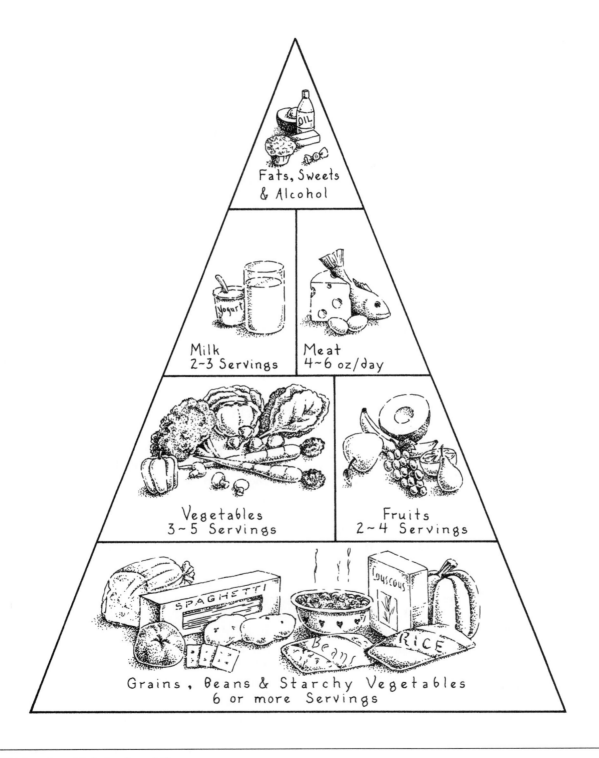

Fats, Sweets
& Alcohol

Milk
2~3 Servings

Meat
4~6 oz/day

Vegetables
3~5 Servings

Fruits
2~4 Servings

Grains, Beans & Starchy Vegetables
6 or more Servings

➡ **Plate Method: Breakfast**

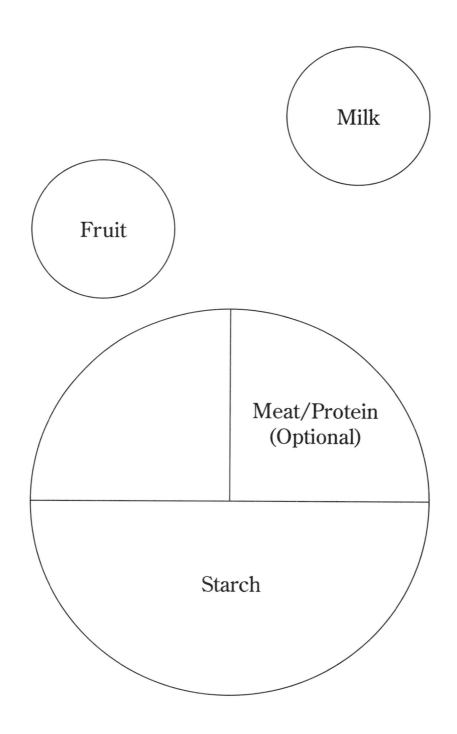

➡ Plate Method: Lunch/Dinner

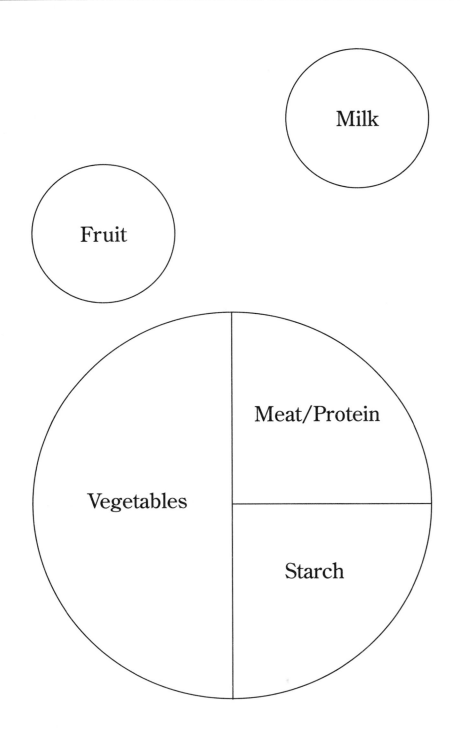

➡ The Diabetes Food Pyramid

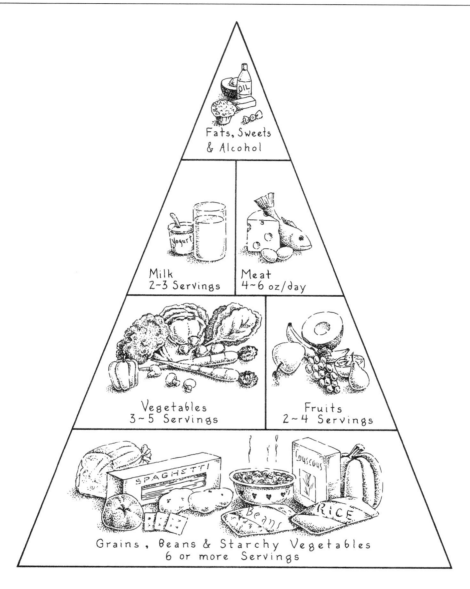

The food guide shows you the kinds and amounts of food you need to be healthy. The large bottom section shows bread, cereal, rice, and pasta. Your body needs more of the foods in this group. The small top section shows fats: margarine, butter, oil, gravy, salad dressing, and sweets. Your body needs less of the foods in the fat group. It is important to include food from each group in your daily diet.

Compare what you eat now with the foods on the chart. How are your food choices like the chart? How are they different? Are there changes you want to make in your food choices?

THE DIABETES FOOD PYRAMID *continued*

STANDARD FOOD GUIDE

Foods To Eat	Number of Servings Each Day	What Is a Serving?

Starches and Breads	6–11	1 slice bread
		⅓ cup rice or noodles
		½ cup cooked cereal
		¾ cup dry cereal
		    (Eat whole grain, fortified, or enriched
		    starches, breads, and cereals.)

Vegetables	3–5	½ cup vegetables, cooked 1 cup vegetables, raw

Fruits	2–4	½ cup fruit
		½ cup fruit juice
		    (Choose fruits and juices that are
		    fresh, frozen, or canned without sugar.)
		1 medium piece of fresh fruit

Milk and Milk Products	2–3	1 cup fat-free (skim) or low-fat (1%) milk ¾ cup plain or artificially sweetened yogurt

Meat and Meat Substitutes	4–6 oz/day	Cooked lean meat, fish, or poultry
		1 oz meat is equal to:
		    1 egg
		    1 oz cheese
		    1 oz tuna, salmon, or cottage cheese
		    1 Tbsp peanut butter

Fat	Use little	1 tsp margarine 1 Tbsp salad dressing 1 tsp oil or mayonnaise

Based on *Food Guide Pyramid: A Guide to Daily Food Choices*. Bulletin #249. Washington, DC: U.S. Government Printing Office, 1992.

If you choose the fewest number of servings from each food group and choose low-fat milk and lean meat, you will eat about 1200 calories each day. This is the lowest amount of calories suggested for women. The lowest calorie level suggested for men is 1500 calories.

If you choose the largest number of servings from each food group and use higher-fat milk and meat, you will eat about 2400 calories each day.

➡ Counting Carbohydrate Servings

Meal Time _____:_____

_____ carbohydrate servings OR

_____ grams carbohydrate

_____ meat or meat substitutes

_____ fats

Snack Time _____:_____

_____

_____

Meal Time _____:_____

_____ carbohydrate servings OR

_____ grams carbohydrate

_____ meat or meat substitutes

_____ fats

Snack Time _____:_____

_____

_____

Meal Time _____:_____

_____ carbohydrate servings OR

_____ grams carbohydrate

_____ meat or meat substitutes

_____ fats

Snack Time _____:_____

_____

_____

➲ Tips for Counting Carbohydrate Servings

Grams of usable carbohydrate	Count as
0–5 gm	Do not count
6–10 gm	½ carbohydrate serving or ½ starch, fruit, or milk serving
11–20 gm	1 carbohydrate serving or 1 starch, fruit, or milk serving
21–25 gm	1½ carbohydrate serving or 1½ starch, fruit, or milk servings
26–35 gm	2 carbohydrate servings or 2 starch, fruit, or milk servings

Know what you are eating. Measure or weigh your foods to help you learn what carbohydrate servings look like. The foods I will measure are:

_____

The food labels I will check are:

_____

Feel good about what you already do. If you decide to make food changes, choose only one or two changes to make. This is what I will do:

_____

_____

Counting carbohydrate in your food allows you more flexibility in food choices and helps keep your blood glucose levels within target range.

➜ Eating Away From Home

- ■ Know what is important to you about eating out.
- ■ Know your goals and your meal plan.
- ■ Choose the kinds and amounts of food that best fit your meal plan.
- ■ Plan ahead—call the restaurant or hostess if unsure of the menu.*
- ■ Consider using the plate method as a guideline.

EATING IN RESTAURANTS

Choose

- ■ *Appetizers*
  Broth or bouillon, unsweetened fruit or vegetable juice, fresh fruit, or raw vegetables

- ■ *Salads*
  Tossed vegetable or fresh fruit salads served with low-fat dressing or dressing that is on the side

- ■ *Main Course*
  Any main dish item that does not contain large amounts of gravy, cream sauce, breading, or fat and contains ingredients that can be easily identified

- ■ *Vegetables*
  Stewed, steamed, or boiled

- ■ *Starches*
  Baked potatoes, plain noodles, rice, hard rolls, melba toast, bread sticks, matzoh, or other plain breads

- ■ *Desserts*
  Fresh fruits or artificially sweetened Jell-O

- ■ *Drinks*
  Water, unsweetened coffee or tea, fat-free (skim) milk, juices, diet soft drinks, or soda or sparkling waters

---

* This is especially important for vegetarians looking for nonmeat menu items.

EATING AWAY FROM HOME *continued*

Request

- Salad dressings, butter, sour cream, gravies, or sauces to be served on the side so you can control how much you use

- Vegetables and main dishes to be served plain, without butter, margarine, or sauces

- Tomato or other juice (usually available if the restaurant has a bar or serves breakfast)

- Low-calorie salad dressing and artificially sweetened Jell-O, if available

- Fresh fruit and fat-free (skim) milk (usually available even though not listed on the menu)

Choose less often

- Cream soups[1]

- Salads with dressing already added, such as potato salad or cole slaw[1]

- Foods that are breaded, deep-fat fried, creamed, or scalloped[1,2]

- Casseroles or mixed dishes, unless you can easily identify the types and amounts of ingredients[1,2]

- Desserts, pastries, sweetened fruits or juices, and regular gelatin desserts or salad[1,2]

---

[1] These items contribute extra fat that interferes with control of weight and blood fats.
[2] These items contribute large or hard-to-measure amounts of carbohydrate that interfere with blood glucose control.

➔ Guidelines for Use of Alcoholic Drinks

- Discuss use of alcohol with your health care team. Consider drinking only if your diabetes is well controlled and you are not pregnant. Alcohol can make some problems worse.

- Alcohol initially lowers your blood glucose level. If you use insulin or certain diabetes medications, you are more likely to have a low blood glucose reaction when you drink alcohol.

- Drink alcohol with meals or snacks containing carbohydrate, such as pretzels, bread sticks, or crackers.

- Alcohol makes insulin reactions harder to recognize. It also interferes with some medicines.

- Use alcohol in moderation (up to 1 equivalent for women and 2 for men per day).

    Equivalent = 1½ oz distilled spirits
    4 oz dry wine
    12 oz beer

- Mix alcohol with:

Free	Fruit/Vegetable Exchange
• water	• fruit juice (1 fruit)
• club soda*	• tomato juice (4 oz = 1 vegetable)
• seltzer*	• V8 juice (4 oz = 1 vegetable)
• diet soft drinks	

- Avoid sweet wine, liqueurs, and sweetened mixed drinks. Try a wine spritzer made with club soda rather than a wine cooler, which is usually made with a sweetened, fruit-flavored mix.

- Drink with someone who recognizes and knows how to treat a low blood glucose reaction.

- Note the differences in calories and carbohydrates among alcoholic drinks.

* Carbonation makes alcohol enter the bloodstream more quickly.

ALCOHOLIC DRINKS

Beverage	Amount	Calories	Carbohydrates
Beer:			
regular	12 oz	150	13
light	12 oz	100	5
nonalcoholic	12 oz	75	16
Cocktails:			
Distilled spirits (80 proof): gin, rum, scotch, vodka, whiskey	1½ oz	100	trace
Martini	5 oz	310	4
Wines			
Red	4 oz	80	2
White	4 oz	80	1
Hard lemonade	12 oz	250	37

➡ Cookbooks for People with Diabetes

Cookbooks written for people with diabetes may add variety to your meal planning. Choose a cookbook that:

- lists the serving size and number of servings per recipe
- lists the carbohydrate content and food exchange value for each serving
- contains recipes with acceptable ingredients (evaluate each recipe before you use it)

Many diabetes cookbooks are available. Check your local bookstore or library. The following cookbooks can be obtained from the American Diabetes Association by calling 800-232-6733 or by visiting http://store.diabetes.org.

At Home with Gladys Knight: Her Personal Recipe for Living Well, Eating Right, and Loving Life.
by Gladys Knight

Cooking with the Diabetic Chef
by Chris Smith

Diabetes Meal Planning Made Easy, 2nd Edition
by Hope Warshaw

Diabetes Quickflip Cookbook
by Eileen Faughey

Diabetic Cooking for Latinos
by Olga V. Fuste

Diabetic Cooking for Seniors
by Kathleen Stanley

Diabetic Meals in 30 Minutes—or Less!
by Robyn Webb

Express Lane Diabetic Cooking
by Robyn Webb

Forbidden Foods Diabetic Cooking
by Maggie Powers and Joyce Hendley

Last Minute Meals for People with Diabetes
by Nancy Hughes

COOKBOOKS FOR PEOPLE WITH DIABETES *continued*

More Diabetic Meals in 30 Minutes—or Less!
by Robyn Webb

One Pot Meals for People with Diabetes
by Ruth Glick and Nancy Baggett

Quick & Easy Diabetic Recipes for One
by Kathleen Stanley and Connie Crawley

Quick & Easy Low-Carb Cooking for People with Diabetes
by Nancy S. Hughes

The Diabetes Food & Nutrition Bible
by Hope S. Warshaw and Robyn Webb

The Diabetes Snack Munch Nibble Nosh Book, 2nd Edition
by Ruth Glick

The Healthy HomeStyle Cookbook
by Ruth W. McGary

The New Soul Food Cookbook for People with Diabetes
by Fabiola Demps Gaines and Roniece Weaver

Also by the American Diabetes Association:

Brand-Name Diabetic Meals in Minutes
Cook'n for Diabetes (recipe software)
Guide to Health Restaurant Eating, 2nd Edition
How to Cook for People with Diabetes
Magic Menus for People with Diabetes
Mix 'n Match Meals in Minutes for People with Diabetes
Month of Meals: All-American Fare
Month of Meals: Classic Cooking
Month of Meals: Festive Latin Flavors
Month of Meals: Meals in Minutes
Month of Meals: Old-Time Favorites
Month of Meals: Soul Food Selections
Month of Meals: Vegetarian Pleasures
Mr. Food's Every Day's a Holiday Diabetic Cookbook
Mr. Food's Quick & Easy Diabetic Cooking
The Complete Quick & Hearty Diabetic Cookbook
The NEW Family Cookbook for People with Diabetes

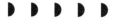

#6	Stocking the Cupboard

STATEMENT OF PURPOSE

This session is intended to help participants plan grocery lists that include the foods they need to use their meal plans discussed in session #5, *Planning Meals*. Label reading and the use of food products modified to be low in sugar, fat, or salt (including the use of sugar and fat substitutes) are discussed.

PREREQUISITES

It is recommended that participants have attended sessions #3, *The Basics of Eating*, and #5, *Planning Meals*, or have achieved those objectives. Ask participants who have them to bring their meal plans to class. Ask participants to bring food labels for a few items they like to eat.

OBJECTIVES

At the end of this session, participants will be able to:

1. plan a shopping list that includes the foods needed to use their meal plans;

2. read a food label to find the ingredients, the serving size, and the carbohydrate, fat and salt content of each serving;

3. use a food label to decide where, if, and how the food fits into their meal plans;

4. name the sugar and fat substitutes available and how they might be used in their meal plans;

5. state the guidelines for choosing free foods and how they might be used in their meal plans.

CONTENT

Nutritional Management.

MATERIALS NEEDED

VISUALS PROVIDED	ADDITIONAL
1. Reasons for Meal Planning	■ Pencils for participants
2. Nutrition Facts Label	■ Chalkboard and chalk

MATERIALS NEEDED *continued*

VISUALS PROVIDED	ADDITIONAL
3. Choosing Free Foods	■ Commercial food product containers or labels from a variety of products, including dietetic foods
Handouts (one per participant)	■ *Reading Food Labels* (booklet available from the American Diabetes Association, 800-232-6733)
1. Shopping Guide	
2. Money-Saving Shopping Tips	
3. Nutrient Claims	

METHOD OF PRESENTATION

Start by introducing yourself and telling what you do. Ask participants to introduce themselves. Explain that the purpose of this session is to provide information on how to shop for foods that fit their meal plans. It will include label reading and an update on artificial fats and sweeteners. This information may be taught as part of the *Planning Meals* session. Because recommendations for and availability of special products change often, it is necessary to stay up-to-date to provide accurate information.

Present material in a question/discussion format. Begin by asking how they did with their short-term goal and what they learned from it.

CONTENT OUTLINE

CONCEPT	DETAIL	INSTRUCTOR'S NOTES
1. Choosing food	1.1 Having the food items or ingredients available is a first step in using your meal plan.	Ask, "What is your meal plan? What is the most important reason you use your meal plan?" Use Visual #1, Reasons for Meal Planning. Ask, "What concerns or questions do you have about shopping for food? Is the food you need for your meal plan available at your home? Who does the grocery shopping?"
	1.2 Plain foods that you prepare yourself, such as fresh fruits, vegetables, meats, fat-free (skim) milk, bread, unseasoned rice, noodles, and dried beans, fit easily into meal plans used by people with diabetes.	Cooking from scratch is the least expensive way to prepare food, but many people choose to spend their time in other ways.
	1.3 Most people also use products that have been partly prepared by someone else. Prepared foods are more	Use the publication *Reading Food Labels* with participants.

CONTENT OUTLINE

CONCEPT	DETAIL	INSTRUCTOR'S NOTES
	likely to contain extra sugar, salt, and fat. The package label can help you decide if a product will help you meet your nutrition goals.	
	1.4 Including food items low in sugar, fat, sodium, and calories may also help you meet your nutrition goals.	Most new convenience foods are lower in sugar, salt, and sodium than they used to be.
2. Planning a shopping list	2.1 A shopping list can help you buy the foods you need.	Ask, "How many of you make a shopping list before you go to the grocery store?"
	2.2 Look at your meal plan and think about the foods you will need. For example, to use the food guide pyramid, you need to buy at least 14 pieces of fruit per person each week (or about 1 quart of juice and seven pieces of fruit).	Ask, "How much fruit is recommended each day? How many pieces of fruit do you need to buy to last one week?" Note that 14 pieces of fruit for one person adds up to 56 for a family of four.
	2.3 The food guide pyramid recommends 2 cups of milk per day. To follow the guide, you need to buy a gallon per person each week.	Ask, "How many servings of milk do you plan to drink each day? How much milk do you need to buy to last a week?"
	2.4 You also need to buy vegetables and meat. The food guide pyramid recommends 3–5 servings of vegetables; 6 or more servings of bread, cereal, or starches; and 4–6 oz of meat each day.	Repeat with other food groups to demonstrate the planning required for participants to purchase the food that fits their plan. Amounts needed per person per week to meet minimum serving recommendations: ■ vegetables 4 lb frozen ■ meat 2–3 lb
	2.5 This shopping guide lists foods that can help you use your meal plan. Different foods help reach different nutrition goals.	Use Handout #1, Shopping Guide. Ask, "What items on this list do you enjoy eating?"
	2.6 These items are examples of foods that are low in fat, saturated fat, calories, or added sugar or high in fiber.	The meats contain ≤3 gm of fat per ounce. Low-fat meat and dairy products are recommended because they are also low in saturated fat. Fiber is part of a balanced diet for good health.

CONTENT OUTLINE

CONCEPT	DETAIL	INSTRUCTOR'S NOTES
	2.7 No single food is "good" or "bad." All foods may be included in your meal plan. You may need to eat very small amounts of some foods if you want to reach your nutrition and blood glucose goals.	Ask, "What items would you add to the shopping guide to make it a grocery list that fits your meal plan and the way others in your family eat?"
	2.8 Many people worry that it costs more for food when you have diabetes. It may mean spending more on some items (such as low-fat meats and fresh fruits) and less on others (such as snacks and convenience foods). Eating with diabetes does not need to cost more than it does for other people.	Ask participants to brainstorm for ideas for saving money on food. Distribute Handout #2, Money-Saving Shopping Tips.
	2.9 No special products are needed to use a meal plan for diabetes, although artificial sweeteners, diet soft drinks, and low-fat margarine may make your diet more enjoyable and easier to use.	
3. Label information	3.1 Food labels give information to help you decide if a food fits into your meal plan.	Use Visual #2, Nutrition Facts Label, or distribute product containers or labels so participants can locate the information.
	3.2 The U.S. Food and Drug Administration (FDA) requires almost all foods in the United States to have a standard nutrition label.	Restaurant menus are exempt. Nutrition information is required for any food that makes nutritional claims and is voluntary on produce, fresh meat, and poultry.
	3.3 The main parts of a food label show: ■ nutrition facts ■ list of ingredients	
	3.4 The nutrition facts panel tells you: ■ serving size ■ number of servings per container ■ nutrient content	Ask, "What do you need to know about a food product before you know when and if to include it among your food choices?" List responses on the chalkboard. Ask, "Where can you find this information?"

CONTENT OUTLINE

CONCEPT	DETAIL	INSTRUCTOR'S NOTES
	3.5 The percentage of daily values is also included. This tells how a food fits into a 2000-calorie diet.	
	3.6 Compare the serving size on a food label with the amount you usually eat. may not be the same as an	The serving sizes are given in household measurements. They exchange amount.
	3.7 The following nutrients must be included on the label: ■ total fat ■ fiber ■ saturated fat ■ sugar ■ cholestrol ■ protein ■ sodium ■ iron ■ total carbohydrate ■ calcium ■ vitamins A and C	Point out the location of the amount in grams next to each nutrient. Other nutrients such as unsaturated fats or other vitamins and minerals may be added. Foods that contain only a few of these nutrients or are in a small package may use a shortened label.
	3.8 It's important to look at grams of total fat as well as saturated fat. Saturated fat is most likely to clog blood vessels because the liver makes more cholesterol when people eat a lot of saturated fat.	The percentage of total fat in a food item can be calculated by dividing the calories of fat by the total calories. It is the percentage of fat in the *total diet* that is important, and the goal varies from person to person. This material is not usually emphasized for pediatric patients. (See Outline #18, *Eating for a Healthy Heart*.)
	3.9 Look at the ingredient list to see what types of sugar are present, then look above to see the amount.	Starches are not listed separately. Dessert and snack foods high in sugar are likely to be low in nutrients.
	3.10 Total carbohydrate includes dietary fiber, sugar, and starches. The amount of carbohydrate (starch and sugar) is what affects blood glucose levels.	Because fiber is not absorbed and does not affect blood glucose, total carbohydrate minus fiber is the most accurate measure for carbohydrate counting. This is clinically relevant only when someone eats foods very high in soluble fiber, such as legumes or oat bran.

CONTENT OUTLINE

CONCEPT	DETAIL	INSTRUCTOR'S NOTES
	3.11 People who count carbohydrates as their method of meal planning use the total carbohydrate number on the nutrition facts label.	
	3.12 Some labels tell the number of calories in a gram of fat, carbohydrate, and protein.	Find this information on different labels.
4. Foods with special claims	4.1 More and more food products are reducing their sugar, fat, calorie, and sodium contents.	
	4.2 A product must be reduced by a certain amount of sugar or fat to claim that it has less sugar or is low in fat.	See Handout #3, Nutrient Claims.
	4.3 Cautions in selecting food items with special claims: ■ low-sugar items may be high in fat ■ low-fat items may be high in sugar ■ low-fat and low-sugar items may not be any lower in calories ■ low-calorie items may be a small portion of a high-fat/high-sugar product ■ products may be expensive ■ items sweetened with concentrated fruit juice may affect your blood glucose the same as table sugar	Examples: Nutrasweet-sweetened ice cream bars Fat-free coffee cake Thinly sliced bread or small frozen dinners Cookies and fruit spreads sweetened with fruit juice tend to be expensive and just as high in sugar.
5. Dietetic foods	5.1 "Dietetic" refers to a food prepared or processed for a special diet. Commercial dietetic foods are prepared for a variety of special diets—not just for use in a diabetes diet. For example, dietetic foods made for people with kidney problems may contain a lot of sugar.	Ask, "What does the word *dietetic* mean?" A particular ingredient may be: ■ Reduced—in sodium, sugar (light fruit), fat, or protein ■ Altered—corn oil substituted for milk fat in dietetic cheese ■ Eliminated—sugar in many diet soft drinks

CONTENT OUTLINE

CONCEPT	DETAIL	INSTRUCTOR'S NOTES
	5.2 Foods that contain less than 20 calories per serving and less than 5 gm carbohydrate may be used as free foods. Two to three servings spread throughout the day will probably not raise blood glucose.	Use Visual #3, Choosing Free Foods. Ask, "Which of the products shown could be a free food?"
	5.3 Recipes for dietetic foods or foods with special claims may contain a sugar or fat substitute.	Note that sugar-free products may still contain sugar alcohols.
6. Sugar substitutes	6.1 Sugar substitutes can help satisfy the inborn taste for sweetness without increasing blood glucose.	Ask, "What sugar substitutes do you use?" Discuss only relevant ones.

	6.2 *Saccharin* is 300–400 times sweeter than sugar, although some users report a bitter aftertaste. It contains no calories.
	
	For information and recipes:
	  www.sweetnlow.com
	  Sweet 'N Low Hotline
	  800-221-1763
		The FDA 1995 guidelines for saccharin safety are 500 mg (25–35 packets) per day for children and 1000 mg (50–70 packets) per day for adults. Cancer risk with moderate use has not been shown. Heavy use during pregnancy is discouraged.

	6.3 *Aspartame* (Nutrasweet or Equal) is a protein and has no bitter aftertaste. As a protein, aspartame provides 4 kcal/gm, but since it is 180–200 times sweeter than sugar, the very small amounts used do not contribute significant calories. High temperatures destroy its sweetening power and taste; thus, aspartame cannot be used for extended cooking (>15 minutes).
	
	For information and recipes:
	  www.equal.com
	  www.nutrasweet.com
	  The Equal Information Center
	  800-323-5316
		Aspartame is made of the amino acids L-phenylalanine and L-aspartic acid. The FDA has established the acceptable daily intake (ADI) at 50 mg/kg (12–17 cans diet soda or 71 packets Equal for a 50-kg adult). Optional: Have participants calculate their own ADI. *Warning:* No safe limits have been established for children less than 2 years old. Aspartame causes mental retardation among all people with PKU.

	6.4 *Acesulfame K* (Sweet One by Sunette) is advertised to taste more	Acesulfame K was FDA- approved in July 1988 after 50 studies over

101

CONTENT OUTLINE

CONCEPT	DETAIL	INSTRUCTOR'S NOTES
	like sugar. It can be used for cooking and baking. Like other artificial sweeteners, acesulfame K increases the sweetening power of other sweeteners, so it can be used with others to reduce the overall amount of sweetener needed in a product.	15 years showed no ill effects. It is 200 times sweeter than sucrose, is a derivative of vinegar, and is excreted without being metabolized. The ADI is 15 mg/kg (18 packets for a 60-kg person). Each packet contains 11 mg potassium.

	For information and recipes:
	    www.sweetone.com
	    Sweet One Hotline
	    800-544-8610	

	6.5 *Sucralose* (Splenda) is made from sugar (sucrose). The body does not recognize it as a source of sugar or carbohydrate. Sucralose passes through your body quickly after you eat it. It has no calories. It is stable at all temperatures and has a long shelf-life.	This product was approved by the FDA in 1998. It is considered safe for all population groups.

	For information and recipes:
	    www.sucralose.com
	    Sucralose McNeil Specialty
	      Products
	    800-777-5363	

	6.6 Packets of artificial sweeteners contain dextrose or lactose as a carrier and provide 4 calories of carbohydrate per package. It is recommended that use be limited to five packets per serving (20 extra calories).	Using a variety of alternative sweeteners rather than one type is recommended. New sugar substitutes are in development and may soon be available.
7. Alternative sugars	7.1 *Sorbitol* and *mannitol* are alcohols of sugar. Because they are absorbed slowly, blood glucose rises more slowly. Because these sugars are only half as sweet as table sugar, twice as many calories are used to provide the same sweetening power. These sugars may cause diarrhea and gas.	Ask, "Have you heard of sorbitol or mannitol?" Show dietetic products that contain sorbitol and mannitol, such as hard candy.

CONTENT OUTLINE

CONCEPT	DETAIL	INSTRUCTOR'S NOTES
	7.2 *Fructose* is a sugar made from cornstarch. It has as many calories as table sugar. In pure crystalline form (expensive), it raises blood glucose more slowly than table sugar, but as high-fructose corn syrup (less costly), it affects blood glucose the same as table sugar and should be limited as such.	Fructose may taste slightly sweeter than sucrose in cold or acidic foods, such as lemonade. In insulin deficiency, crystalline fructose may be used for glucose synthesis, causing an increase in blood glucose.
8. Fat substitutes	8.1 Two of the fat substitutes that have been developed are Simplesse and Olean.	The goal of a fat substitute is to provide the feel and flavor of fat with fewer calories.
	8.2 Simplesse is finely whipped milk whey and egg white. It contains 1–2 calories per gram and can only be used in cold products. The product causes gastrointestinal (GI) symptoms among some individuals. If you are allergic to egg whites or milk, you may also be allergic to Simplesse.	Simplesse is used in frozen desserts, cheese, and other dairy products, mayonnaise, and salad dressings. It is used in foods that will not be heated. Suggest to participants that they monitor their responses to any new product.
	8.3 *Olestra* (Olean) is made from soy-bean oil and table sugar. The molecule is too large to be absorbed, so it provides no calories. The product causes GI symptoms among some individuals. For more information: www.olean.com Proctor & Gamble Co. 800-543-7276	Olestra was approved by the FDA in 1996. It is used to replace part of the fat in shortenings and oils used for deep frying. Olestra is a way to cut calories from snack foods such as chips and crackers.
9. Planning for change	9.1 Activity: Examine labels from a variety of low-sugar, low-fat, and dietetic foods. If possible, taste some of these products. Monitor your blood glucose to identify your own response to foods.	Ask participants to explain why they might use a certain product (or why not).
	9.2 Make a list of foods to include on your next grocery shopping list. Write down special products or new items you want to try.	Choose a short-term goal to try before the next session.

SKILLS CHECKLIST

Each participant will be able to use food label information to evaluate carbohydrate, fat, and calorie content of a product.

EVALUATION PLAN

Knowledge will be evaluated by achievement of learning and by responses to questions during the session; skills will be evaluated by observation. The ability to apply knowledge will be evaluated by the participants' abilities to buy food that meets their meal plan goals and through program outcome measures.

DOCUMENTATION PLAN

Record class attendance and achieved objectives as appropriate.

SUGGESTED READINGS

Holzmeister LA: *The Diabetes Carbohydrate and Fat Gram Guide*. Alexandria, VA: American Diabetes Association, 1999.

O'Connell B, Hieronymus L. Are you labelable? *Diabetes Self-Management*. 2003;20(41):42–54.

O'Connell B. Sweeteners: herbal and otherwise. *Diabetes Self-Management*. 2002; 19(4):83–88.

Warshaw HS, Franz M, Powers MA, Wheeler M. Fat replacers: their use in foods and role in diabetes medical nutrition therapy. *Diabetes Care*. 1996;19:1294–1301.

Wheeler ML, Franz M, Heins J, Schafer R, Holler H, Hobannon B, Bantle JP, Barrier P. Technical review: food labeling. *Diabetes Care*. 1994;17:480–487.

➡ Reasons for Meal Planning

- Maintain blood glucose as close to your target range as possible.

- Maintain cholesterol (blood fats) as close to your target range as possible.

- Maintain blood pressure as close to your target level as possible.

- Prevent, delay, or treat diabetes-related complications.

- Improve health through food choices.

- Meet individual nutritional needs.

➔ Nutrition Facts Label

Serving size: 4 graham crackers
Servings per container: 32

Amount Per Serving
Calories: 80   Calories from fat: 18

	Percent of Daily Value*
Total Fat 2g	5%
Saturated Fat 1g	5%
Cholesterol 0mg	0%
Sodium 66mg	3%
Total Carbohydrate 14g	5%
Dietary Fiber 1g	4%
Sugars 4g	
Protein 2g	

Vitamin A ‡   ●   Vitamin C ‡

Calcium ‡   ●   Iron 3%

‡ Contains less than 2 percent of the daily value of this nutrient.

* Percent (%) Daily Values are based on a 2,000-calorie diet. Your Daily Values may be higher or lower, depending on your calorie needs:

Nutrient		2,000 Calories	2,500 Calories
Total Fat	Less than	65 g	80 g
Saturated Fat	Less than	20 g	25 g
Cholesterol	Less than	300 mg	300 mg
Sodium	Less than	2,400 mg	2,400 mg
Total Carbohydrate		300 g	375 g
Dietary Fiber		25 g	30 g

Ingredients: Wheat flour, sugars (sucrose, corn syrup, molasses), partially hydrogenated vegetable oil, lecithin, vanilla.

➡ Choosing Free Foods

READ THE LABEL!

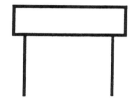

Free Foods:

- Contain less than 20 calories per serving
- Total no more than 60 calories per day

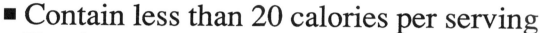

DIETETIC SALAD DRESSING

Calories: 6/Tablespoon

INGREDIENTS: Water, vinegar, corn sweetener, salt, citrate, dill, lemon juice, pectin, carrageenan, dried red pepper, guar gum

DIETETIC SALAD DRESSING

Calories: 40/Tablespoon

INGREDIENTS: Water, soybean oil, cultured low-fat buttermilk, corn syrup, monosodium glutamate, xanthan gum, onion, spices

➔ Shopping Guide

Produce Aisle

Fresh fruit

- ☐ apples
- ☐ bananas
- ☐ berries
- ☐ cantaloupe
- ☐ grapefruit
- ☐ oranges
- ☐ peaches
- ☐ pears
- ☐ strawberries
- ☐ watermelon

_____

_____

Fresh vegetables

- ☐ broccoli
- ☐ cabbage
- ☐ carrots
- ☐ celery
- ☐ corn
- ☐ cucumber
- ☐ green pepper
- ☐ greens
- ☐ kohlrabi
- ☐ lettuce
- ☐ mushrooms

- ☐ okra
- ☐ onions
- ☐ potatoes
- ☐ squash
- ☐ tomatoes

_____

_____

Frozen Food Aisle

- ☐ vegetables, plain
- ☐ entrees, low-fat or lean
- ☐ dinners, low-fat or lean
- ☐ waffles
- ☐ ice cream
- ☐ juices

_____

_____

Bakery Aisle

- ☐ bread
- ☐ rolls
- ☐ hamburger/hot dog buns
- ☐ bagels
- ☐ english muffins/muffins
- ☐ pita pockets
- ☐ tortillas
- ☐ naan

© 2004 American Diabetes Association

108

SHOPPING GUIDE *continued*

☐ angel food cake

☐ sponge cake

_____

_____

Starch Aisle

☐ whole-grain flour

☐ plain dry cereals

☐ plain cooked cereals

☐ noodles/macaroni

☐ rice (brown for more fiber)

☐ dried beans

☐ dried peas

☐ graham crackers

☐ saltine crackers

☐ low-fat crackers (whole grain for more fiber)

☐ pretzels

☐ popcorn

_____

_____

Dairy Aisle

☐ fat-free (skim) milk

☐ yogurt (plain or artificially sweetened nonfat fruit)

☐ cheese (reduced-fat)

☐ cottage cheese (low-fat)

☐ margarine

☐ eggs

☐ egg substitute

_____

_____

Meat Aisle

☐ chicken, no skin

☐ turkey, no skin

☐ fish

☐ round or sirloin steak

☐ ground round or sirloin

☐ beef round roast

☐ flank steak

☐ chipped beef

☐ leg of lamb

☐ lean lamb chops

☐ pork loin roast

☐ pork tenderloin

☐ center loin pork chop

☐ ham

☐ Canadian bacon

☐ tofu

☐ 97% fat-free lunch meat, hot dogs, or sausage

_____

_____

SHOPPING GUIDE *continued*

Canned Goods Aisle

☐ fruit

☐ fruit juice

☐ low-sodium vegetables

☐ low-sodium vegetable juice

☐ mushrooms

☐ water chestnuts

☐ tomato sauce and paste

☐ tomatoes

☐ beans (kidney, pinto, northern, garbanzo, black, black-eyed peas)

☐ broth-based soups

☐ no-fat or low-fat cream soups

☐ dried soups

☐ evaporated skim milk

☐ tuna canned in water

☐ salmon

☐ peanut butter

☐ bouillon

_____

_____

Miscellaneous

☐ spices and herbs

☐ catsup

☐ mustard

☐ mayonnaise (lite or no-fat)

☐ salad dressing (lite or no-fat)

☐ vinegar

☐ lemon juice

☐ olive oil

☐ canola oil

_____

_____

Special Products

☐ artificial sweeteners

☐ artificially sweetened jelly/jam

☐ artificially sweetened pudding

☐ artificially sweetened Jell-O

☐ artificially sweetened syrup

☐ Butter Buds

☐ nonstick cooking spray

☐ Beano

☐ salt-free seasonings

☐ diet soft drinks

_____

_____

➲ Money-Saving Shopping Tips

1. Shop only with a list.

2. Shop only once or twice a week. You'll spend more if you go more often.

3. Buy only items you really need, unless something you use often is on sale. If something you use often is on sale and can be stored, consider buying enough for a few weeks.

4. Check grocery ads for sale items and the Sunday newspaper inserts for coupons.

5. Compare discounted items with similar products at the regular price to see if you really are saving.

6. Eat before you go shopping.

7. Check unit pricing (the price per ounce or pound, usually listed on the shelf below the item). This helps you compare sizes and brands, to decide which is the least expensive.

8. Look for store brands or generic brands—they are often cheaper than national brands.

9. Prepared foods cost more than the plain ingredients from which they are made.

10. Plain cereal costs less per ounce than sugar-coated cereal.

11. Fat-free (skim) milk is less expensive than reduced-fat (2%) or whole milk.

12. Buy only the amount you will use. An item that costs less per serving will not save money if it spoils.

13. Whole, unwashed produce usually costs less than washed and cut up items.

14. Buying salad makings at the store salad bar might be less expensive than buying all the various items separately—especially for one or two people.

MONEY-SAVING SHOPPING TIPS *continued*

15. Soups, stews, and casseroles stretch a little meat to serve more people.

16. Buy plain ice cream instead of premium ice cream or sherbet.

17. Limit use of pickles, relishes, and olives. They are high in cost but low in nutrients.

18. Limit use of chips, cookies, and other snack foods. They are high in calories and cost, but low in nutrients.

Nutrient Claims

Nutrients per Serving	Free	Low	Reduced/Less	Light (Lite)
Calories	Less than 5 calories	40 calories or less	At least 25% fewer calories	At least ⅓ fewer calories
Fat	Less than 0.5 gm fat	3 gm or less fat	At least 25% less fat	At least 50% less fat
Saturated Fat	Less than 0.5 gm saturated fat	1 gm or less saturated fat and no more than 15% of calories from saturated fat	At least 25% less saturated fat	Not used
Cholesterol	Less than 2 mg cholesterol and 2 gm or less saturated fat	20 mg or less cholesterol and 2 gm or less saturated fat	At least 25% less cholesterol and 2 gm or less saturated fat	Not used
Sodium	Less than 5 mg sodium	140 mg or less sodium	At least 25% less sodium	At least 50% less sodium
Sugar	Less than 1.2 gm sugars	Not a legal claim	At least 25% less sugar	Not used

Adapted from *Label Facts for Healthful Eating*. National Food Processors Association, Washington, DC, 1993.

#7   Physical Activity and Exercise

▶ ▶ ▶ ▶ ▶

STATEMENT OF PURPOSE

This session is intended to provide information about the effects of physical activity on blood glucose and the necessary dietary adjustments for changes in activity. It also provides the opportunity to create a plan for an exercise program, if the participant desires.

PREREQUISITES

It is recommended that participants have basic knowledge about diabetes and self-care, from either personal experience or attending previous sessions.

OBJECTIVES

At the end of this session, participants will be able to:

1. list three benefits of regular activity or exercise;

2. describe the difference between aerobic and anaerobic exercise;

3. state effects of activity/exercise on blood glucose level;

4. state the benefits of a consistent exercise program;

5. determine target heart rate;

6. state possible signs and symptoms of hypoglycemia during and after exercise;

7. describe how to make adjustments in food intake or insulin doses to balance increases in physical activity;

8. develop a personal exercise plan.

CONTENT

Physical Activity.

MATERIALS NEEDED

VISUALS PROVIDED	ADDITIONAL
1. Target Heart Rates	■ Pencils for participants
	■ Chalkboard and chalk
Handouts (one per participant)	■ Information about local exercise programs
1. Treatment of Low Blood Glucose	■ Videotape of simple exercises
2. Calories Spent in Various Exercises	■ "Small Steps, Big Rewards" resource kit [available
3. Sample Activity Snacks	from the National Diabetes Education Program
4. Planning Your Exercise Program	(NDEP), www.ndep.nih.gov]
	■ Pedometers

METHOD OF PRESENTATION

Start by introducing yourself and telling what you do. Ask participants to introduce themselves and tell about their own activity programs, if any. Explain that the purposes of this session are to provide information about physical activity and, if desired, to develop a personal plan for regular exercise or increased activity level.

Present material in a question/discussion format. If possible, start the class with a walk, simple stretching, or an easy exercise videotape, using appropriate precautions for patients with diabetes complications or other health problems. Discuss only the areas that are appropriate for the participants. At the end of the class, invite participants to complete the Planning Your Exercise Program handout. Begin by asking how they did with their short-term goal and what they learned from it.

CONTENT OUTLINE

CONCEPT	DETAIL	INSTRUCTOR'S NOTES
1. Benefits of regular exercise	1.1 Exercise can lower blood pressure and cholesterol levels. Exercise strengthens your heart and circulatory system. It can decrease body fat and increase muscle tone.	Ask, "What have been your experiences with exercise? What questions do you have? What are some benefits of exercise? What are some barriers/negatives for exercise?" If not mentioned, point out that people usually look better and feel better, have more stamina, and are better able to deal with stress. Finding time to exercise, finding a place to exercise, and coming up with enjoyable activities are often barriers.
	1.2 Exercise can help you feel more relaxed. It relieves tension and stress and can be enjoyable.	Some people eat to cope with stress, but with regular exercise, they may find that they are less likely to eat when stressed.

CONTENT OUTLINE

CONCEPT	DETAIL	INSTRUCTOR'S NOTES
	1.3 While calories are burned with any exercise, regular exercise increases metabolism so more calories are burned all the time, even at rest.	Exercise supports weight loss and helps to sustain weight loss.
2. Effects on blood glucose	2.1 Generally, activity will lower your blood glucose because body cells take in glucose more efficiently.	Ask, "What effect does activity have on blood glucose?" Point out that activity lowers blood glucose only if blood glucose levels are well controlled.
	2.2 In type 2 diabetes, exercise may increase cells' sensitivity to the effects of insulin. It will also help reduce the amount of glucose released by the liver.	The duration of improvement is generally 12–72 hours. For improved control, exercise needs to be done at least every other day and preferably 5 days per week.
	2.3 Regular exercise may reduce insulin requirements.	
	2.4 Initially, exercise may make blood glucose control more difficult, because exercise needs to be balanced with your meal plan and medicines. Try not to get discouraged; planning, monitoring, and working with your health care team can help achieve this balance.	Hypoglycemia is less likely in people with type 2 diabetes and not at all likely in those treated with meal planning and exercise.
3. Choosing an exercise program	3.1 There are two types of exercise: aerobic and anaerobic. Aerobic exercise uses oxygen to help release energy from fat cells. Anaerobic exercise does not use oxygen to burn fuel.	Ask, "What kind of exercise program would you like to do?" Anaerobic exercise may not be safe or feasible for many participants.
	3.2 Choose an exercise you enjoy and will do regularly. One approach to exercise is the lifetime activity model. In this model, you accumulate a total of 30 minutes of moderately intense physical activity each day. Lower-intensity activity (e.g., light housework) can be done more often and/or for a longer period of time.	This is a good idea for everyone—even people who have an aerobic program. The goal is to use 3–4 kcal/kg/day. This level of activity provides cardiovascular benefits, but 30 minutes of continuous exercise has more effect on weight loss.

117

CONTENT OUTLINE

CONCEPT	DETAIL	INSTRUCTOR'S NOTES
	3.3 The idea is to fit 10 minutes of aerobic physical activity into your usual routine, three different times every day.	Ask, "What are ways you can increase your daily activity?" Examples: Park so you have to walk farther, take the stairs, walk the golf course. Distribute "Small Steps, Big Rewards" materials.
	3.4 Another approach is the 10,000 Steps Program; 10,000 steps is equal to 5 miles. Using a pedometer helps make walking a daily contest with yourself.	Distribute pedometers if available. Remind participants to start slowly and to gradually increase the number of steps per day.
	3.5 Another approach is a planned aerobic exercise program. Aerobic exercise is steady exercise for at least 12 minutes that increases the heart rate to at least 60% of maximum. This increases oxygen use.	Ask, "What are some aerobic exercises?" (Examples are walking, bicycling, cross-country skiing, and swimming.) If the group is fairly sedentary, point out benefits of walking programs.
	3.6 Aerobic exercise burns glucose and fat and provides the greatest benefit for blood glucose and weight management. It also helps you to cope with stress and decreases hunger.	
	3.7 Activities such as bowling and baseball are not aerobic, because long periods of inactivity occur between short spurts of activity.	Ask, "What are other examples of anaerobic exercise?" Golf is generally not aerobic unless players walk briskly and do not use a cart.
	3.8 Anaerobic exercise helps build muscle tissue. It can cause stiff and sore muscles and hunger after exercise.	Some anaerobic exercises can increase blood glucose and intraoccular pressure. Participants with diabetes complications need a medical evaluation before beginning this type of program.
4. Level and duration	4.1 Level of exercise is described as light, moderate, or strenuous. What is light exercise for one person may be moderate exercise for someone else, depending on the person's level of fitness. Your own response to exercise will change as you grow stronger.	

CONTENT OUTLINE

CONCEPT	DETAIL	INSTRUCTOR'S NOTES
	4.2 Light exercise does not make you breathe heavily, but your pulse rate may increase slightly.	Light exercise done for less than 10 minutes will not affect blood glucose; if done for longer than 10 minutes, it can lower blood glucose.
	4.3 Moderate exercise involves noticeably heavier breathing, with a pulse rate increase to more than 100 beats per minute.	Teach patients how to take their pulse rates. Count for 6 seconds and add a zero to the number to find the rate per minute.
		Moderate exercise done for less than about 10 minutes may raise blood glucose (the liver releases stored glucose); done for longer, it lowers blood glucose.
	4.4 Strenuous exercise involves rapid breathing with a pulse rate between 125 and 160 beats per minute, depending on age.	Strenuous exercise done for less than about 10 minutes may raise blood glucose. If done for longer than 10 minutes, it will lower blood glucose for a sustained period of time (if blood glucose is well controlled).
	4.5 Another way to evaluate exercise is to determine your perceived level of exertion. Perceived exertion is a method of rating how hard you are working during an activity. As you exercise, decide what you believe your rate of exertion is, using a scale of very, very light to very, very hard. Aim to work out in the somewhat-hard to hard range.	The rate of perceived exertion (RPE) scale is also known as the Borg scale. Exercise ratings range from 6 (very, very light) to 19 (very, very hard). Aim for aerobic exercise in the 12–16 range.
	4.6 If taking insulin, any level of exercise done routinely will probably require a change in your diabetes program. Ask your health care team to work with you on a plan.	
	4.7 A complete exercise program includes aerobic activity, stretching, and weight-bearing activity. Exercise continuously for 20–40 minutes.	

CONTENT OUTLINE

CONCEPT	DETAIL	INSTRUCTOR'S NOTES

	4.8 The recommended duration is 20–60 minutes. Lower-intensity exercise needs to be done for a longer period of time than higher-intensity exercise to get the most benefit.	
5. Planning your exercise program	5.1 See your health professional. Have any tests done that are recommended.	A history and physical exam are needed to look for signs of complications; a stress electro-cardiogram is recommended for people over 35 with diabetes or people over 25 with type 2 diabetes >10 years' duration or type 1 diabetes >15 years' duration; for people with an additional risk factor for coronary artery disease; or for people with macro-vascular disease, peripheral vascular disease, or autonomic neuropathy.
	5.2 Determine your target heart rate. This is the rate at which you should aim to exercise. Your target heart rate range is 60–85% of your maximum heart rate. To calculate your maximum heart rate, subtract your age from 220. Multiply by 0.60–0.85 to find your target heart rate range.	Figure an example on the chalk-board ($220 -$ age $\times$ 0.70, depending on the fitness level). Have participants calculate their own target heart rate. Point out that their health care team may recommend a different target heart rate. Use Visual #1, Target Heart Rates.
	5.3 To achieve the greatest benefit for your heart, exercise at your target heart rate for at least 20 minutes three to four times a week.	Five or six exercise sessions per week may be needed for weight loss.
	5.4 People with other medical problems, such as heart disease or hyperten-sion, or diabetes complications, such as retinopathy, need individually developed exercise programs.	For example, jogging may make retinal detachment or renal perfusion worse. Lifting weights is contraindicated in retinopathy. People with heart problems may not be able to use the target heart rate method.

CONTENT OUTLINE

CONCEPT	DETAIL	INSTRUCTOR'S NOTES
	5.5 You may need different meal plans or insulin doses for different levels of activity on different days. Seasonal changes in activity levels may also require a change in insulin dose or a snack.	For example, use one plan for exercise days, and one for rest days; or use one plan for work days and one for weekends.
	5.6 Choose footwear to protect your feet. Use of silica gels or air midsoles as well as polyester or blended socks to keep feet dry may help minimize trauma.	Remind participants to check for blisters or other injuries before and after exercise.
6. Starting to exercise	6.1 Test your blood glucose. If your blood glucose is low (below 70 mg/dl) before you begin to exercise, treat the hypoglycemia and do not exercise at that time. If your blood glucose is less than 100 mg/dl, eat additional carbohydrate. If your blood glucose is high (above 250 mg/dl), test your urine for ketones.	Wait until blood glucose is up to at least 100 mg/dl before starting to exercise.
	6.2 Do not exercise if your blood glucose is over 250 mg/dl and you have ketones in your urine. Use caution if your blood glucose is over 300 mg/dl, whether ketones are present or not. Your blood glucose levels may rise even further.	Ketones indicate insulin deficiency. Hyperglycemia due to insulin deficiency may increase with exercise.
	6.3 Gradually warm up your muscles. Do low-intensity aerobic exercise such as walking or marching in place for 5–10 minutes, then stretch for 5–10 minutes before you begin more intensive exercise. This helps prevent muscle cramps and injury.	Warm-up periods may also help to prevent postexercise hunger.
7. During aerobic exercise	7.1 Wear diabetes and personal ID, wear appropriate shoes to avoid skin breakdown, and take coins for the phone in case of emergency.	
	7.2 Take your pulse every 10–15 minutes to be sure you are working at your target heart rate.	

CONTENT OUTLINE

CONCEPT	DETAIL	INSTRUCTOR'S NOTES
	7.3 Do not overexert. You should be able to talk easily as you work out.	"No pain, no gain" is not true. If you are out of breath, you are not exercising aerobically.
	7.4 Avoid dehydration. Drink fluids every 30 minutes during your workouts.	
	7.5 Know the signs and symptoms of overexertion: increased shortness of breath, nausea or vomiting, irregular heartbeat, excessive fatigue, feeling faint or lightheaded, and pain or pressure in the chest or arm.	Stop exercising and tell your provider if you feel any of these symptoms.
8. After aerobic exercise	8.1 Gradually decrease your intensity, do low intensity aerobic activity for 5–10 min, and then finish your exercise period with about 5–10 minutes of stretching exercises. This is called a cooldown. It will help to prevent aches and muscle cramping later.	
	8.2 Test your blood to determine the effect of exercise on your blood glucose level. Everyone has his or her own response to different types of exercise.	Remind participants to monitor more frequently postexercise.
9. Hypoglycemia and exercise	9.1 Exercise uses up glucose in your blood and helps insulin work better. Because of this, exercise usually lowers your blood glucose.	Distribute Handout #1, Treatment of Low Blood Glucose.
	9.2 Know the signs and symptoms of hypoglycemia **during exercise:** undue anxiety or shakiness, as well as changes in gait, coordination, ability to think, or vision.	If possible, check your blood glucose level if you think you may be having an insulin reaction. If not possible to test, treat as a reaction.
	9.3 Carry a source of carbohydrate to treat low blood glucose.	Pin a sugar packet or package of glucose tablets to your clothes if you don't have a pocket.
	9.4 Effects of activity on your blood glucose can last for many (over 12–48) hours. It is possible to have a reaction up to 48 hours after exercising.	PEL is defined as a reaction >4 hours after exercise. It usually occurs in people with type 1 diabetes who exercise at a moderate-

CONTENT OUTLINE

CONCEPT	DETAIL	INSTRUCTOR'S NOTES
	Taking less of the insulin that is most active during/after exercise or eating a snack after exercise may help prevent postexercise late-onset hypoglycemia (PEL).	to-high intensity for more than 30 minutes. Remind participants to monitor more frequently postexercise.
	9.5 If you take insulin, you may need extra food for extra activity. Extra activity means the body is working harder and/or longer than usual. You may need extra food when you are involved in any activity that is not a usual part of your day—this includes things like raking leaves and washing windows as well as structured exercise. Just being more active in the summer may require a change in medication or meal plan.	Any activity (e.g., walking to the store) may be a usual activity (requiring no snack) for one person and an unusual activity (requiring a snack) for another. Ask the group for other examples, such as shoveling snow, painting walls, or heavy cleaning. Stress using blood glucose results for making adjustments.
	9.6 Extra food (exercise snack) is needed by people taking insulin and rarely for people taking oral agents. People who manage their diabetes with diet alone do not need extra food before exercise.	Exercising after a meal may not be enough to prevent hypoglycemia. Some participants may prefer to take a lower insulin dose rather than eat extra food. Snacks should be individualized and based on the treatment program, blood glucose levels, and response.
10. Making adjustments for activity	10.1 If you exercise regularly and take insulin, you probably need to decrease your insulin dose on exercise days or eat an exercise snack. Exercising around the same time each day will make planning insulin changes and snacks easier and more consistent.	Ask, "What questions do you have about making adjustments for exercise? What concerns do you have?"
	10.2 The decision about whether to eat additional food or adjust your medication is based on your goal for exercise. Carbohydrate replacement is most useful for unplanned exercise and/or exercise of long duration.	Ask, "What is your goal for exercise? How consistent is your exercise program?"

CONTENT OUTLINE

CONCEPT	DETAIL	INSTRUCTOR'S NOTES
Insulin Adjustments	10.3 Reducing insulin doses is particularly helpful for those who exercise routinely, as part of weight management and/or to improve control. The decision about which insulin to decrease is based on the timing and type of exercise and the insulin treatment plan.	
	10.4 The risk for hypoglycemia is less when the level of insulin in your body is lower. ■ Avoid planning your exercise program for the time when your insulin is peaking. ■ Avoid exercise for 1–2 hours after injecting rapid- or short-acting insulin. ■ Exercise before the morning insulin dose. ■ Exercise 1–3 hours after eating.	This may require insulin adjustments to accomodate the person's schedule.
	10.5 The risk for nocturnal hypoglycemia is greater when exercise is performed in the evening.	Reducing the evening insulin dose helps decrease the risk.
	10.6 Hypoglycemia is also a risk during pump therapy. Strategies for prevention include reducing the basal rate, eating an exercise snack or removing the pump during exercise.	Another option is to reduce the bolus dose for planned postmeal activity.
Carbohydrate Adjustments	10.7 The harder your body works during exercise, the more glucose it uses. The amount and timing of exercise snacks depends on the intensity of the exercise, the duration of the exercise, your pre-exercise blood glucose, and your individual response.	**Optional:** Distribute Handout #2, Calories Spent in Various Exercises. This chart is a relative measure of energy expended. It may be used to estimate the extra calories needed to replace those spent in exercise.
	10.8 Carbohydrate foods, such as fruit, juice, skim milk, and bread, turn to glucose the quickest. The harder your body works during exercise, the more carbohydrate it needs.	Distribute Handout #3, Sample Activity Snacks. Review material from Outline #4, *Food and Blood Glucose,* as needed.

CONTENT OUTLINE

CONCEPT	DETAIL	INSTRUCTOR'S NOTES
	10.9 The timing of snacks varies from person to person and with different lengths and intensities of exercise.	
	10.10 If your blood glucose is between 100–180 mg/dl, take your planned snack before you begin, and do your exercise.	This is a guideline to use as a starting point. Each individual will need to monitor and adjust accordingly.
	10.11 If your blood glucose is 180–250 mg/dl, no snack is needed before starting exercise but may be needed in 30–60 minutes or after exercise.	
	10.12 Several small carbohydrate snacks taken about every 30 minutes during exercise may be needed if exercise is very vigorous or strenuous.	
	10.13 Eat additional carbohydrate before and during exercise as needed to prevent low blood glucose.	
	10.14 It isn't always possible to stop every 30 minutes to eat during exercise. To avoid low blood glucose, eat additional carbohydrate 1–4 hours before starting, and extra carbohydrates after finishing very vigorous or strenuous exercise.	
	10.15 You may need to eat extra carbohydrates several hours after you have exercised. The longer and more intense the exercise, the longer that glucose will be lowered after exercise has stopped.	Monitoring your blood glucose after exercise will help to evaluate how well the extra food is meeting your needs.
11. Balancing food and insulin with activity	11.1 Everyone has his or her own response to exercise. Monitor blood glucose levels to determine your individual response to any adjustments that you make. You will probably need to adjust for each activity.	Encourage participants to work closely with their health care team when making adjustments.

CONTENT OUTLINE

CONCEPT	DETAIL	INSTRUCTOR'S NOTES
	11.2 The best way to know if the adjustments are adequate is to test your blood glucose before and after exercise. If the activity lasts longer than 30 minutes, check your blood glucose during the activity to monitor response.	
12. General information	12.1 Drink plenty of water before, during, and after exercise, especially if you sweat a lot. You can lose up to 2 liters of fluid per hour of exercise.	For example, drink 17 oz of fluid 2 hours before exercise.
	12.2 For long periods of strenuous exercise, such as running, drinks with 60–80 calories (15–20 gm carbohydrate) per 8 oz provide the best solution for fluid and carbohydrate absorption. Most sports drinks (such as Gatorade) meet this criterion, but juices and soft drinks may not.	Drinks with more than 25 gm carbohydrate per 8 oz are hypertonic and may cause dehydration and diarrhea. Juice and soft drinks generally need to be diluted 50:50 with water to achieve the proper fluid/carbohydrate ratio.
	12.3 Alcohol and exercise don't mix well. Less glucose is available (effect of alcohol) and more is used (effect of exercise). Alcohol consumed before, during, or after exercise can cause a low blood glucose reaction.	Because alcohol decreases the liver's ability to release glucose, and exercise enhances the muscles' ability to take up glucose, hypoglycemia can occur.
13. Tips for staying with your exercise program	13.1 Choose an exercise you enjoy and can easily do.	Ask participants to discuss exercise programs they've tried and what helped and what hindered their effort. If appropriate, work through Handout #4, Planning Your Exercise Program, as a group.
	13.2 Start slowly. Work up to more strenuous activity as you become more fit.	Walk one block the first day, and then gradually walk longer each day (e.g., add 1–2 min per session).
	13.3 If possible, exercise with your spouse or a friend.	

CONTENT OUTLINE

CONCEPT	DETAIL	INSTRUCTOR'S NOTES
	13.4 Set aside the same time each day for your exercise. Make it a habit. Choose a time that does not coincide with the peak action of your insulin.	It is easy not to exercise if you try to do it "when I get a chance."
	13.5 Take a class or join an exercise club. Many malls have walking clubs.	Give information on programs in your area.
	13.6 Choose activities that don't depend on good weather, or plan activities for good and bad weather.	For example, you can walk inside and out.
	13.7 Record your progress.	Give suggestions on how to monitor and record distance, time, and heart rate.
	13.8 Reward yourself for progress made.	Ask, "How can you reward yourself?" Examples are time for yourself, time with a friend, or going to a movie.
	13.9 Contact your health care team if you have questions, concerns, or problems. They can help you plan your activity, diet, or medication changes and solve any problems that might occur as you continue your exercise program.	Choose a short-term goal to try before the next session.

SKILLS CHECKLIST

Participants will be able to locate pulse points, count heart rates, and determine target heart rates. Select participants will be able to calculate an insulin adjustment or exercise snack.

EVALUATION PLAN

Knowledge will be evaluated by achievement of learning objectives and by responses to questions during the session. The ability to apply knowledge will be evaluated by the development of personal exercise goals, by the development and implementation of a plan to achieve those goals, and through program outcome measures.

DOCUMENTATION PLAN

Record class attendance and achieved objectives as appropriate.

SUGGESTED READINGS

Albert SG, Bernbaum M. Exercise for patients with diabetic retinopathy. *Diabetes Care*. 1995;18:130–132.

American Diabetes Association. Diabetes mellitus and exercise. *Diabetes Care*. 2004;27 (Suppl 1):S58–S62.

American Diabetes Association. *Handbook of Exercise and Diabetes*. Alexandria, VA: American Diabetes Association, 2002.

Boswell E, Davis DL, Partin L, Pichert JW: The activity activity: a tool for teaching how to adjust for exercise variations. *The Diabetes Educator* 1997;23:63–66.

Braunstein JB. Enter the high-performance zone. *Diabetes Forecast*. 2001;54(7):46–49.

Braunstein JB. Exercise made safe. *Diabetes Forecast*. 1999;52(10):35–37.

Braunstein JB. Exercise paradox: know your risk profile. *Diabetes Forecast*. 2003; 56(4):36–39.

Braunstein JB. Lifestyle activity: exercise for the masses. *Diabetes Forecast*. 2004;57(5):31.

Braunstein JB. Sports injuries. *Diabetes Forecast*. 2003;56(12):34–36.

Braunstein JB. When there are only 24 hours in a day. *Diabetes Forecast*. 2001;54(3):27–30.

Burns KJ. A new recommendation for physical activity as a means of health promotion. *The Nurse Practitioner*. 1996;21(9):18–28.

Castanaeda C, Layne JE, Munoz-Orians L, Gordon PL, Walsmith J, Foldvari M, Roubenoff R, Tucker KL, Nelson ME. A randomized controlled trial of resistance exercise training to improve glycemic control in older adults with type 2 diabetes. *Diabetes Care*. 2002;25:2335–2341.

D'Arrigo T. The wonders of walking. *Diabetes Forecast*. 2000;53(10):61–64.

Devlin JT. Exercise and the management of diabetes. *Practical Diabetology*. 2001;20(1):38–44.

Di Loreto C, Fanelli C, Lucidi P, Murdolo G, De Cicco A, Parlanti N, Santeusanio F, Brunetti P, De Feo P. Validation of a counseling strategy to promote the adoption and the maintenance of physical activity by type 2 diabetic subjects. *Diabetes Care*. 2003; 26:404–408.

Dunstan DW, Daly RM, Owen N, Jolley D, DeCourten M, Shaw J, Zimmet P. High intensity resistance training improves glycemic control in older patients with type 2 diabetes. *Diabetes Care*. 2002;25:1729–1736.

Fentress D. Simple steps to fitness. *Diabetes Forecast*. 2002;55(8):71–100.

Griffith M. Aerobic and anaerobic exercise: why you need both. *Diabetes Forecast*. 2003;56(5):64–68.

Irwin ML, Mayer-Davis CL, Addy CL, Pate RR, Durstine JL, Stolarczyk LM, Ainsworth BE: Moderate intensity physical activity and fasting insulin levels in women: The cross-cultural activity participation study. *Diabetes Care*. 2000; 23:449–454.

Jackicic JM, Leermakers EA. Commit to get fit: exercise for life. *Diabetes Spectrum*. 1996; 9:202–204.

Lorber DL. Diabetes underwater. *Practical Diabetology*. 2001;20(1):29–34.

Lynch J, Helmrich SP, Lakka TA, Kaplan GA, Cohen RD, Salonen R, Salonen JT. Moderately intense physical activities and high levels of cardiorespiratory fitness reduce the risk of non-insulin-dependent diabetes mellitus in middle-aged men. *Archives of Internal Medicine*. 1996;156:1307–1310.

Mulooly CA. Exercise. In: *A Core Curriculum for Diabetes Education*, 4th Edition, vol. 4. Franz MJ, Kwkanni K, Polonsky WH, Yarborough P, Zamudio V, eds. Chicago, IL: American Association of Diabetes Educators, 2001; 57–86.

Nies MA, Kershaw TC. Psychosocial and environmental influences on physical activity and health outcomes in sedentary women. *Image*. 2002;34:243–249.

Soo K, Furler SM, Samaras K, Jenkins AB, Campbell LV, Chisholm DJ. Glycemic responses to exercise in IDDM after simple and complex carbohydrate supplementation. *Diabetes Care*. 1996;19:575–579.

Wasserman DH, Zinman B. Exercise in individuals with IDDM: A technical review. *Diabetes Care*. 1994;17:924–937.

➲ Target Heart Rates (1 Minute)

Age (Years)	Maximum Heart Rate	Percentage of Maximum Heart Rate		
		60%	70%	85%
20	200	120	140	170
25	195	117	137	166
30	190	114	133	162
35	185	111	130	157
40	180	108	126	153
45	175	105	125	149
50	170	102	119	145
55	165	99	116	140
60	160	96	112	136
65	155	93	109	132
70	150	90	105	128
75	145	87	102	123
80	140	84	98	119

→ Treatment of Low Blood Glucose

If your blood glucose test is:	The amount of food or drink to take is:
Between 50 and 69 mg/dl	15 gm carbohydrate (1 carbohydrate serving **or** 1 cup fat-free [skim] milk)
Less than 50 mg/dl	30 gm carbohydrate (2 carbohydrate servings)

You should feel better in 10–15 minutes after you treat yourself. If your blood glucose is still less than 70 mg/dl or you don't feel better 10–15 minutes after the treatment, take 1 more carbohydrate serving. Test your blood glucose an hour after the reaction to make sure that your blood glucose has gone above 70 mg/dl and stayed there.

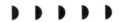

EXAMPLES OF TREATMENTS FOR LOW BLOOD GLUCOSE
(All equal about 15 gm carbohydrate or 1 fruit serving)

If your blood glucose is between 50 and 69 mg/dl, take the amount listed. If your blood glucose is less than 50 mg/dl, take twice the amount listed.

Foods	Amount
Orange or apple juice	½ cup
Grape or cranberry juice	⅓ cup
Non-diet soft drink	½ cup
Honey or corn syrup	1 Tbsp
Sugar packets	3
Life Savers	3–8 pieces
Glucose tablets	3–4 tablets

An additional carbohydrate snack may be needed at night or after exercise to keep your blood glucose above 70 mg/dl.

➲ Calories Spent in Various Exercises

	Calories/hour	Calories/minute
LIGHT ACTIVITY		
Light housework	150	2.5
Strolling, 1.0 mile/hour	150	2.5
Golf, using power cart	175	3.0
Level walking, 2.0 miles/hour	200	3.5
MODERATE ACTIVITY		
Cycling, 5.5 miles/hour	210	3.5
Gardening	220	3.5
Canoeing, 2.5 miles/hour	230	4.0
Cleaning windows, mopping, vacuuming	240	4.0
Lawn mowing, power mower	250	4.0
Lawn mowing, hand mower	270	4.5
Walking, 3.0 miles/hour	275	4.5
Bowling	300	5.0
Golf, pulling cart	300	5.0
Scrubbing floors	300	5.0
Rowboating, 2.5 miles/hour	300	5.0
Swimming, 0.25 miles/hour	300	5.0
Cycling, 8 miles/hour	325	5.5
Golf, carrying clubs	350	6.0
Badminton	350	6.0
Horseback riding, trotting	350	6.0
Square dancing	350	6.0
Volleyball	350	6.0

CALORIES SPENT IN VARIOUS ACTIVITIES *continued*

	Calories/hour	Calories/minute
Roller skating	350	6.0
Doubles tennis	360	6.0
Calisthenics and ballet exercises	360	6.0
Table tennis	360	6.0
Walking, 4.0 miles/hour	360	6.0

STRENUOUS ACTIVITY

	Calories/hour	Calories/minute
Vigorous dancing	320–500	5.5–8.5
Cycling, 10 miles/hour	400	6.5
Ice skating, 10 miles/hour	400	6.5
Ditch digging, hand shovel	400	6.5
Wood chopping or sawing	400–600	6.5–10.0
Walking, 5 miles/hour	420	7.0
Cycling, 11 miles/hour	420	7.0
Singles tennis	420	7.0
Waterskiing	480	8.0
Jogging, 5 miles/hour	480	8.0
Cycling, 12 miles/hour	480	8.0
Hill climbing, 100 feet/hour	490	8.0
Downhill skiing	550	9.0
Running, 5.5 miles/hour	600	10.0
Squash and handball	600	10.0
Cycling, 13 miles/hour	660	11.0
Running, 6–9 miles/hour	660–850	11.0–14.0
Cross-country skiing	600–1200	10.0–20.0
Running, 10 miles/hour	900	15.0

➡ Sample Activity Snacks

Intensity of activity	Examples	If blood glucose is	Then eat	Suggestions
Light	Walking a half mile or leisurely biking for less than 30 minutes	less than 100 mg/dl	10–15 gm carbohydrate per hour.	1 fruit **or** bread serving (½ cup orange juice **or** ¼ bagel)
		100 mg/dl or above	No food needed	
Moderate	Tennis, jogging, swimming, leisurely biking, gardening, golfing, vacuuming for 30 minutes to 1 hour	less than 100 mg/dl	15–30 gm carbohydrate before exercise, then 10–15 gm per 30–60 minutes of exercise	1 milk and 1 fruit serving **or** 1 milk and 1 bread (1 cup plain yogurt and ½ banana **or** cereal and 1 cup milk)
		100–180 mg/dl	10–15 gm carbohydrate per 30 minutes of exercise	1 fruit **or** 1 bread serving (½ banana **or** 8 saltine crackers)
		180–300* mg/dl	No food needed	

* Test for ketones if blood glucose is over 250 mg/dl before or after exercise.

SAMPLE ACTIVITY SNACKS *continued*

Intensity of activity	Examples	If blood glucose is	Then eat	Suggestions
Strenuous	Football, hockey, racquetball, basketball, strenuous biking or swimming, shoveling heavy snow, raking leaves	Less than 100 mg/dl	About 45 gm carbohydrate. Test blood glucose often.	2 bread servings with either 1 milk or 1 fruit (2 slices toast, with 1 cup fat-free [skim] milk or 1 small orange)
		100–180 mg/dl	30–50 gm carbohydrate (depends on intensity and duration)	1 milk and bread serving (1 slice bread and 1 cup skim milk) **or** 1 fruit and 1 bread
		180–300* mg/dl	15–30 gm carbohydrate per 30–60 minutes of exercise	

Be sure to monitor and record your blood glucose before and after exercise (and every 30 minutes during exercise). Each person responds to exercise and food differently—activity snacks need to be planned for each person with the help of a dietitian.

* Test for ketones if blood glucose is over 250 mg/dl before or after exercise.

➡ Planning Your Exercise Program

Write down the answers to the following questions:

1. What exercise programs or activities are safe and practical for you to do regularly?

2. Of these, which activities would you enjoy doing?

3. Are there any activities you plan to do?

4. Where will you do these activities?

5. What time of day will you do your program?

6. How often will you exercise?

7. How long will you exercise each time?

8. What will you do to reduce your risk for hypoglycemia?

(Please turn over)

PLANNING YOUR EXERCISE PROGRAM *continued*

9. What stretching, aerobic, and weight-bearing activities will you do?

10. What is your target heart rate?

11. What is your goal for your heart rate?

12. What is your goal for how often you will exercise once your exercise program is established?

13. How will you keep track of your exercise?

14. How will you reward yourself for your exercise program?

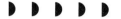

#8	Oral Medications

STATEMENT OF PURPOSE

This session is intended to provide information about the purpose, action, use, and side effects of oral diabetes medications.

PREREQUISITES

It is recommended that only people currently taking oral diabetes medications attend this session. Participants who take oral agents and insulin need information about both types of therapy.

OBJECTIVES

At the end of this session, participants will be able to:

1. define the purpose and action of oral diabetes medications (diabetes pills);

2. state that oral diabetes medications are not insulin;

3. state the name of their oral diabetes medication, the dose to take, and the time it should be taken;

4. identify one idea they will use in remembering to take the medication;

5. describe one side effect of oral diabetes medications.

CONTENT

Medications.

MATERIALS NEEDED

VISUALS PROVIDED	ADDITIONAL
1. Diabetes Pills	■ Samples of different diabetes medications ■ Sample pill bottle ■ Price information from local pharmacies ■ Compartmentalized container for medications

METHOD OF PRESENTATION

Start by introducing yourself and telling what you do. Ask participants to introduce themselves. Explain that the purpose of this session is to provide information about oral antidiabetes medications (diabetes pills) and how they work.

Present material in a question/discussion format. Discuss only the medications appropriate for the participants. Begin by asking how they did with their short-term goal and what they learned from it.

CONTENT OUTLINE

CONCEPT	DETAIL	INSTRUCTOR'S NOTES
1. Definition of oral medications	1.1 Diabetes pills are taken to lower blood glucose levels.	Ask, "What questions/concerns do you have about your diabetes medicines?"
	1.2 Diabetes pills are not insulin. Insulin cannot be taken orally—it would be destroyed by digestive enzymes.	Insulin is a protein and would be digested like other proteins. An oral medication that works like insulin is being tested.
	1.3 These pills are effective only when the pancreas still produces some insulin. Therefore, they are prescribed for people with type 2 diabetes.	
	1.4 As people get older and heavier, cells can become resistant to insulin so that the glucose remains in the bloodstream. At first, the pancreas makes more insulin; but after a time, it just isn't able to keep up. The glucose stays in the blood, and your level goes above the normal range. This is called *insulin resistance*.	
	1.5 The liver stores some glucose (sugar) to release when your blood glucose goes below normal, such as between meals and overnight. When the liver cells are resistant to insulin, the liver puts out too much glucose. This is one reason why you may have high blood glucose levels before breakfast.	Reassure participants that diabetes does not damage the liver.
	1.6 Most people with type 2 diabetes begin with meal planning and exercise and then add one pill, and then more than one, and then insulin.	Stress the use of progressive therapies to keep the blood glucose level near normal. The steps in therapy are not a sign of failure or that diabetes is worse.

CONTENT OUTLINE

CONCEPT	DETAIL	INSTRUCTOR'S NOTES
2. Types of oral medications	2.1 Currently there are five types of pills on the market. A prescription is needed for all five. These medications help your body make more insulin, help your body use insulin beter, or keep your blood glucose from going to high after meals. There are also pills that combine two types of oral medications into one pill.	Participants taking combination medications need information relevant for both agents. Combination medications are to be taken with meals and titrated gradually to reduce gastrointestinal upset, prevent hypoglycemia and determine maximum effective dose.
	2.2 Each of the five types has a different chemical structure and works differently. The types are: ■ sulfonylureas ■ biguanides ■ alpha-glucosidase inhibitors ■ thiazolidinediones ■ meglitinides	Medications that help with weight loss are also on the market, although these are not specific for diabetes. Ask, "What pills do you take?" Review those taken by participants. Use the discussion as a way to review pathophysiology. Incorporate their experiences into the discussion. Discuss synergistic effects of medications and the importance of taking all medications. Help participants correlate glucose monitoring schedules and results with medication schedule and action.
3. Types of oral medications— sulfonylureas	3.1 Sulfonylureas stimulate the pancreas to produce insulin and cause the body to respond better to the insulin it does produce. They help lower premeal blood glucose levels.	Use Visual #1, Diabetes Pills, or samples of different pills. Say each name so patients hear how it is pronounced. (Use either the brand name or generic name, not both.)
	3.2 There are seven different sulfonylureas.	The ones that were first used are called first generation. Later forms are called second generation.
	3.3 The different sulfonylurea pills work similarly but are not exactly the same and **cannot** be used interchangeably.	The action and effectiveness of older and newer sulfonylureas are similar.

CONTENT OUTLINE

CONCEPT	DETAIL	INSTRUCTOR'S NOTES
	3.4 Sulfonylureas can be used alone or in combination with other medicines. 3.5 Primary disadvantages are side effects, such as hypoglycemia, and weight gain.	Sulfonylureas, like all drugs, must be used with caution by some patients or should not be used at all by others. Review the package insert to become familiar with the risks and benefits of each drug.
4. Types of oral medications— meglitinide	4.1 Repaglinide (Prandin) and nateglinide (Starlix) cause the beta cells to release insulin. These are different than sulfonylureas in that they work more quickly and their effects are glucose-dependent. They are designed to treat post-meal hyperglycemia. 4.2 Repaglinide and nateglinide can be used with diet and exercise or with other agents, diet, and exercise. 4.3 Because they only work for a short time, take just before or up to 30 minutes before each meal or large snack. 4.4 Disadvantages include side effects, possible drug interactions, and hypoglycemia.	Repaglinide and nateglinide belong to a class of medications known as insulin secretagogues. Their effects decrease when the blood glucose is low. These are metabolized in the liver but their risk for accumulation is small because of their short half-life (1–1½ hours). Stress the importance of not taking these medications if a meal is skipped. These should not be combined with alpha-glucosidase inhibitors.
5. Types of oral medications— biguanides	5.1 Metformin (Glucophage) enhances the action of insulin on the liver and in the muscles. It works mainly by inhibiting the release of glucose from the liver. It also shows the absorption of glucose in the gut and enhances the absorption of glucose in other parts of the body. Its main effect is on fasting blood glucose 5.2 Metformin can be used with diet and exercise or with other agents, diet, and exercise.	Ask, "Is anyone taking metformin?" Ask them to describe their experiences. This medicine was approved for use in the United States in 1995 but had been used in other countries for many years. It was also tested as a drug to delay the onset of type 2 diabetes in people with impaired glucose tolerance. If sulfonylureas alone are ineffective, metformin should be added—not used in place of the sulfonylurea.

CONTENT OUTLINE

CONCEPT	DETAIL	INSTRUCTOR'S NOTES
	5.3 Metformin may also decrease cholesterol and triglycerides and does not promote weight gain, as sulfonylureas and insulin do.	Review the package insert to become familiar with the risks and benefits of the drug.
	5.4 Disadvantages include side effects, possible drug interactions, and risk for lactic acidosis. It is not appropriate for people with liver or kidney damage damage or heart failure. Side effects are primarily gastrointestinal—loss of appetite and an unpleasant metallic taste. Taking the daily dose at supper may decrease stomach upset and taking it with food may decrease the metallic taste.	Review symptoms of lactic acidosis, surgical contrast dye, and alcohol precautions. Furosemide and cimetadine may interact with metformin. Because cimetadine is available over the counter, instruct participants to use a different preparation (e.g., Pepsid AC).
6. Types of oral medications— thiazolidinediones	6.1 Rosiglitazone (Avandia) and pioglitazone (Actos) act primarily to reduce insulin resistance by improving target cell response (sensitivity) to insulin. They also decrease glucose output from the liver and increase glucose disposal in the skeletal muscles.	Ask, "Is anyone taking any of these?" Ask them to describe their experiences. Rosiglitazone and pioglitazone were approved in 1999. A related drug, troglitazone (Rezulin), was removed from the market in 2000.
	6.2 Rosiglitazone and pioglitazone may be taken with or without food.	
	6.3 These medicines are generally safe and do not cause hypoglycemia when used alone.	Edema may occur among some people.
	6.4 These medicines can take 2–12 weeks to become effective. They should be used with caution if you have liver and heart disease.	These agents may lower lipid levels. Like all drugs, these must be used with caution by some patients or should not be used at all by others.
	6.5 Watch for possible side effects, including jaundice, nausea and vomiting, stomach pain, and dark urine. Blood tests of liver function should be done before starting these drugs and periodically thereafter.	Refer to product literature for specific testing recommendations. Stress the importance of these tests for the participants' safety.

CONTENT OUTLINE

CONCEPT	DETAIL	INSTRUCTOR'S NOTES
7. Types of oral medications— alpha-glucosidase inhibitors	7.1 Acarbose (Precose) and miglitol (Glyset) block the enzymes that break down starches so that they are more slowly absorbed. This blunts the increase in blood glucose that occurs after eating.	Ask, "Is anyone taking acarbose or miglitol?" Ask them to describe their experiences. Acarbose was approved for use in the U.S. in 1996 and miglitol in 1999.
	7.2 They can be used with diet and exercise, with other oral agents, or with insulin, diet, and exercise.	These agents only affect post-prandial (not fasting) blood glucose levels. They should not be used with lispro.
	7.3 To be effective, take them with the first bite of food at all meals.	These agents, like all drugs, must be used with precaution by some people or should not be used at all by others. Obtain the package insert to become familiar with the risks and benefits of the drug.
	7.4 Primary disadvantages are side effects, such as bloating, gas, and diarrhea. The side effects generally disappear after 6 months.	
8. Side effects	8.1 As with all drugs, all oral diabetes medicines may have side effects.	
	8.2 Side effects to look for include: ■ unpleasant metallic taste ■ diarrhea ■ nausea or vomiting ■ loss of appetite ■ abdominal discomfort ■ skin rash or itching ■ dizziness ■ flushing and nausea with alcohol intake (chlorpropamide)	Assure participants that sul-fonylureas are no longer thought to cause hypertension or heart disease. Glucatrol XL is contained in a nonabsorbable shell; participants should not be concerned if they occasionally notice the shell in their stool. Second-generation agents do not cause alcohol intolerance.
	8.3 Report side effects to your provider.	
	8.4 It is a good idea to get all prescriptions filled at the same pharmacy, so the pharmacist can be alert for any drug interactions.	
9. Hypoglycemia	9.1 Hypoglycemia (low blood glucose reaction) can occur when taking sulfonylureas and glitinides.	Ask, "What are the signs and symptoms of hypoglycemia?" Refer to Outline #11, *Managing Blood Glucose.*

CONTENT OUTLINE

CONCEPT	DETAIL	INSTRUCTOR'S NOTES
	9.2 Metformin, acarbose, miglitol, and glitazones do not cause hypoglycemia if taken alone.	If taken with a sulfonylurea, a glitinide, or insulin, hypoglycemia may occur.
	9.3 Duration of action affects when hypoglycemia is likely to occur and how long it lasts.	Other medications (e.g., non-steroidal anti-inflammatory drugs) potentiate hypoglycemia.
	9.4 Hypoglycemia from oral agents may need to be treated repeatedly. If taking acarbose or miglitol, hypo-glycemia should not be treated with sucrose-containing products. Use milk or glucose tablets instead.	Ask, "How do you treat low blood glucose?" Hypoglycemia occurs less often but is more difficult to treat than for patients on insulin because of the long duration of action of the sulfonylureas. In addition, hypo-glycemia may persist beyond the standard duration of action of these drugs. Hypoglycemia may recur anytime while the patient is taking sulfonylureas.
	9.5 If your hypoglycemia does not respond to treatment, contact your health care team right away.	Glucagon is generally not an appropriate treatment for hypo-glycemia for patients with type 2 diabetes.
10. Using diabetes pills	10.1 Because the pills work differently, the choice of which pill is best for you is based on your blood glucose goals, your costs and coverage, and your levels before and after you start taking the pill. Some people take one type of pill, some take two types of pills, and others take pills plus insulin because the medicines work well together.	Ask, "How much do your dia-betes pills costs?" Provide infor-mation about lower cost options and sources.
	10.2 Blood glucose monitoring helps you to know if the medicines are working	Ask, "Do you check your blood glucose levels? Review the sched-ule and results in relation to the medications' actions and timing.
	10.3 Never take anyone else's diabetes pills (or any other kind of pill) or give anyone yours.	

CONTENT OUTLINE

CONCEPT	DETAIL	INSTRUCTOR'S NOTES
	10.4 It's important that you know: ■ the name of your pills ■ how many pills to take ■ when to take your pills ■ the shape and color of your pills	Ask participants to name their medication, dosage, and how often it should be taken. Remind patients to read the label when they get a new bottle from their pharmacy, to be sure the name, dose, and times it should be taken are correct. Show these points on sample bottles.
	10.5 Prices for prescription medicines vary, so you may want to shop around.	Have price information available from different pharmacies, or ask participants to find out and bring this information to the next session.
11. Duration of action	11.1 Duration of action refers to the length of time the pill is effective.	Use Visual #1, Diabetes Pills.
	11.2 Duration affects the dose and how often the pills need to be taken. Almost all last 6–24 hours.	Exceptions are chlorpropamide (48 hours), acarbose, miglitol, repaglinide, and nateglinide.
12. When to take diabetes pills	12.1 You may need to take your pill(s) only once per day or as many as three times per day.	Frequency depends on duration of action and how the body responds to medication.
	12.2 It is important to take these pills as prescribed, not only when you think your blood glucose is high.	
	12.3 It's helpful to take them at about the same time each day.	This helps the pancreas to establish a more consistent pattern and helps the patient to remember the medication.
	12.4 Most of these pills are taken at mealtime, usually at breakfast. Glucotrol (glipizide) will work best if taken 30 minutes before your meal. Glitinides work best if taken 1–30 minutes before your meal. Alpha-glucosidase inhibitors should be taken only at meal time, with the first bite of food. If insulin is used with sulfonylureas or biguanides, the insulin is usually taken at bedtime.	Emphasize that the timing of a medication dose can influence the medication's effectiveness and/or its side effects.

CONTENT OUTLINE

CONCEPT	DETAIL	INSTRUCTOR'S NOTES
13. Remembering to take the medication	13.1 If you forget to take your **daily** dose but remember later in the day, go ahead and take the pill.	Ask, "What happens to your blood glucose if you forget your pill? What happens if you were to take a double dose?"
	13.2 If you take one pill each day and forget one day, do **not** take two pills the next day.	If you have any questions, call your health care team.
	13.3 If you take pills two times a day and forget your morning pill, do **not** take both doses in the evening.	
	13.4 Missed doses of acarbose, miglitol, nateglinide, or repaglinide should not be made up at the next meal.	
	13.5 The following are tips for remembering to take your medicine: ■ Take it at the same time each day. ■ Take it at the same time you take other pills or do a routine activity (e.g., brushing teeth). ■ Store pills in plain sight, close to where you will take them. ■ Focus attention on times that are hard for you.	Ask, "How do you remember to take other medicines?" Coupling a new behavior with an already established behavior increases the likelihood the new behavior will be done. Example: If it's hard to remember a pill at lunchtime at work, put a note in your lunch or set an alarm.
	■ Make it easy to remember by giving yourself cues. ■ Devices are manufactured that can be set to buzz as a reminder of your pill times.	Load a compartmentalized container, either purchased or homemade, with pills for the day or week. Have one available to show.
14. Care and storage	14.1 Store medications at room temperature.	
	14.2 Do not use medicines after the expiration date.	Show a bottle and point out the expiration date.
	14.3 If pills are discolored, discard them.	
	14.4 Always keep your medicines with you when traveling (not in your suitcase). Take enough for the trip, plus extras.	A prescription and/or provider's letter is helpful for overseas travel.

CONTENT OUTLINE

CONCEPT	DETAIL	INSTRUCTOR'S NOTES
15. Meal planning and exercise	15.1 Food raises blood glucose. The more you eat, the more insulin your body needs to lower blood glucose. Even with the pills, your body can only make so much insulin.	It is a common misunderstanding that a meal plan is no longer needed once medicines are added. Medications may not be needed after weight loss.
	15.2 Your blood glucose will stay lower and more even if you divide your food into several small meals and snacks throughout the day. Too much food at once can raise blood glucose too high.	Personalize this by asking participants when they plan to eat.
	15.3 Exercise helps burn calories, improves sense of well-being, increases insulin sensitivity, and lowers blood glucose levels.	Exercise snacks are usually not necessary for patients on oral medications.
16. Other facts	16.1 Oral agents should not be taken by women who are pregnant, lactating, or planning to become pregnant. They may be harmful to the baby.	
	16.2 If you are ill and unable to eat, you still need to take your diabetes pills.	Blood glucose may actually increase because of the infectious process.
17. Research	17.1 New oral agents are being tested and may be on the market in the near future.	Insulin-like agents are areas of great research interest.
	17.2 Ask your provider if any new treatments are available that would help you.	Choose a short-term goal to try before the next session.

SKILLS CHECKLIST

None.

EVALUATION PLAN

Knowledge will be evaluated by achievement of learning objectives and by responses to questions during the session. The ability to apply knowledge will be evaluated by appropriate use of oral medications and through program outcome measures.

DOCUMENTATION PLAN

Record class attendance and achieved objectives as appropriate.

SUGGESTED READINGS

Agnew B. Dangerous combinations. *Diabetes Forecast.* 2002;55(10):89–991.

Bailey C, Path M, Turner R. Metformin. *The New England Journal of Medicine.* 1996;334:574–579.

Barzilai N. Clinical use of metformin in the United States. *Diabetes Spectrum.* 1995; 8:194–197.

Birkeland KI, Furseth K, Melander A, Mowinckel P, Vaaler S. Long-term randomized placebo-controlled double-blind therapeutic comparison of glipizide and glyburide. *Diabetes Care.* 1994;17:45–49.

Buse JB. Progressive use of medical therapies in type 2 diabetes. *Diabetes Spectrum.* 2000;13:211–220.

Carlisle BA, Kroon LA, Koda-Kimble MA. *101 Medication Tips for People with Diabetes.* Alexandria, VA: American Diabetes Association, 1999.

Clark CM Jr. Oral therapy in type 2 diabetes: pharmacological properties and clinical use of currently available agents. *Diabetes Spectrum.* 1998;11:211–221.

Cohen FJ, Neslusan CA, Conklin JE, Song. Recent antihyperglycmic prescribing trends for US privately insured patients with type 2 diabetes. *Diabetes Care.* 2003;26:1847–1831.

Funnell MM, Barlage DL. Treating diabetes with agent oral. *Nursing.* 2004;34(3).

Gordon D. Acarbose. *Diabetes Forecast.* 1997;50(2):25–28.

Grant RW, Devita NG, Singer De, Meigs JB. Polypharmacy and medication adherence in patients with type 2 diabetes. *Diabetes Care.* 2003;26:1408–1412.

Johnson MA. Medical nutrition therapy and combination medication for the treatment of type 2 diabetes. *On the Cutting Edge.* 1998;19(2):11–13.

Kanzer-Lewis G. Early combination therapy with a thiazolidinedione for the treatment of type 2 diabetes. *The Diabetes Educator.* 2003;29:954–961.

Karl DM. Sulfonylureas: new thoughts about old friends. *Practical Diabetology.* 2004; 23(1):26–29.

Kordella T. A gut response: the next generation of type 2 drugs. *Diabetes Forecast.* 2004; 57(4):39–42

Kroner BA. Common drug pathways and interactions. *Diabetes Spectrum.* 2002;15:256–261.

Leichter SB, Thomas S. Combination medications in diabetes care: an opportunity that merits more attention. *Clinical Diabetes.* 2003;21:175–178.

Marino MT. Dangerous drug combinations. *Diabetes Self-Management.* 2004;21(2):33–38.

McCarren M. Class action. *Diabetes Forecast.* 2004;57(1):R10–R13.

McCarren M. New drug for type II. *Diabetes Forecast.* 1997;50(5):26–29.

Nesto RW, Bell D, Bonow RO, Fonseca V, Grundy SM, Horton ES, Le Winter M, Porte D, Semenkovich CF, Smith S, Young LJ, Kahn R. Thiazolidinedione use, fluid retention, and congestive heart failure. *Diabetes Care.* 2004;27:256–263.

Piette JD, Heisler M, Wagner TH. Problems paying out of pocket medication costs among older adults with diabetes. *Diabetes Care.* 2004;27:384–391.

Quartetti HR. Talking points. *Diabetes Forecast.* 2002;55(10):109–112.

Rhodes KR. Prescribed medication and OTCs: interactions and timing issues. *Diabetes Spectrum.* 2002;15:256–261.

Roberts SS. Controlling costs. *Diabetes Forecast.* 2002;55(10):105–106.

Roberts SS. Diet pills for the long haul. *Diabetes Forecast.* 1996;49(7):25–30.

Roberts SS. Generic drugs. *Diabetes Forecast.* 2002;55(11):51–53.

SUGGESTED READINGS *continued*

Roberts SS. Take at the right time. *Diabetes Forecast.* 2002;55(10):99–101.

Roberts SS. The juggling act. *Diabetes Forecast.* 2002;55(10):85–86.

Sharp AR. Nutritional implications of new medicines to treat diabetes. *On the Cutting Edge.* 1998;19(2):8–10.

Sherwin R. Pill time. *Diabetes Forecast.* 1996; 49(3):36–39.

Sysowski DK, Armstrong G, Governale L. Rapid increase in the use of oral antidiabetic drugs in the United States, 1990–2001. *Diabetes Care.* 2003;26:1852–1855.

The Diabetes Prevention Program Research Group. Effects of withdrawal from metformin on the development of diabetes in the Diabetes Prevention Program. *Diabetes Care.* 2003;26:977–980.

UK Prospective Diabetes Study (UKPDS) Group. Effect of intensive blood-glucose control with metformin on complications in overweight patients with type 2 diabetes (UKPDS 34). *The Lancet.* 1998;352:854–865.

Wright A, Burden FAC, Paisey RB, Cull CA, Holman RR, UKPD Study Group. Sulfonylurea inadequacy. *Diabetes Care.* 2002;25:330–335.

➲ Diabetes Pills

Class	Name	Description	Dosage (mg)	Number of Times per Day
Sulfonylureas	Micronase (glyburide)	Round, scored tablet: White Dark pink Blue	 1.25 2.5 5.0	1–2
	Diabeta (glyburide)	Oval, scored tablet: White Pink Green	 1.25 2.5 5.0	1–2
	Glynase PresTab (glyburide)	Oval, scored tablet: White Blue Yellow	 1.5 3.0 6.0	1–2
	*Glucotrol (glipizide)	White, scored, diamond-shaped tablet	5.0 10.0	1–2
	Glucotrol XL (glipizide XL)	White, round tablet	5.0 10.0	1
	Amaryl (glimepiride)	Oval, scored tablet: White Pink Green	 1.0 2.0 4.0	1
Biguanides	Glucophage (metformin)	White, round tablet White, round tablet White, oval tablet	500 800 1000	2–3
	GlucophageXL (metformin)	White capsule		1
Insulin sensitizers	Avandia (rosiglitazone)	Five-sided tablet: Pink Orange Red/brown	 200 400 800	1–2

*Take 30 minutes before meals.

DIABETES PILLS *continued*

Class	Name	Description	Dosage (mg)	Number of Times per Day
	Actos (pioglitazone)	Tablets: White, round, convex White, round, flat White, round, flat	 15 30 45	1
Glitinides Meglitinide	***Prandin (repaglinide)	Unscored, round tablet: White Yellow Pink	 0.5 1.0 2.0	3–4
Phenylalanine derivative	***Starlix (nateglinide)	Pink, round tablet Yellow, oval tablet	60 120	3
Alpha-glucosidase inhibitors	**Precose (acarbose)	White, round, scored tablet	50	3
	**Glyset (miglitol)	White, round tablet	25 50 100	3
Sulfonylurea** and biguanide combination**	Glucovance (glyburide/ metformin)	Capsule shape: Pale yellow Pale orange Yellow	 1.25/250 2.5/500 5/500	1–2
	****Metaglip (glipizide/ metformin)	Oval Tablet Pink White Pink	 2.5–250 2.5–500 5.0–500	2
Insulin sensitizer and biguanide combination	***Avandamet (rosiglitizone/ metformin)	Oval Tablet Pale yellow Pale pink Orange Yellow Pink	 1.0/500 2.0/500 4.0/500 2.0/1000 4.0/1000	2

**Take with the first bite of meal.   ***Take 1–30 minutes before meal.   ****Take with meals.

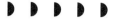

#9	All About Insulin

STATEMENT OF PURPOSE

This session is intended to provide information about what insulin is, how it works, and how it is administered; intensive insulin therapy is also discussed.

PREREQUISITES

It is recommended that only participants starting insulin therapy or currently taking insulin attend this session. Participants who take oral diabetes medications and insulin need information about both types of therapy.

OBJECTIVES

At the end of this session, participants will be able to:

1. define insulin, including where it comes from and what it does;
2. state that different kinds of insulin preparations differ as to source, strength, and length of action;
3. state how to store insulin properly;
4. state how to tell if a particular bottle of insulin is useable;
5. list the equipment needed to administer insulin;
6. state the importance of accurate measurement of insulin dosage;
7. state the importance of accurate timing of insulin dosage;
8. state how to tell if it is suitable to inject insulin at a particular site;
9. state how to treat hypoglycemia;
10. state the purpose of intensive insulin therapy;
11. define intensive insulin therapy;
12. define normal blood glucose values in pre- and postprandial states;
13. identify three circumstances that are indications for intensive insulin therapy;
14. describe treatment options available to achieve goals of intensive insulin therapy;
15. identify advantages of intensive insulin therapy;
16. identify disadvantages of intensive insulin therapy;
17. describe resources needed to implement an intensive insulin program.

CONTENT

Medications.

MATERIALS NEEDED

VISUALS PROVIDED

1. Normal Blood Glucose and Insulin Levels
2. Insulin Action Times
3. Insulin Programs
4. Timing of Regular Insulin and Meals
5. Injection Sites

Handouts (one per participant)
1. Comparison of Insulins
2. Insulin Programs
3. Intensive Programs
4. Giving an Insulin Injection
5. Treatment of Low Blood Glucose
6. How to Use Glucagon

ADDITIONAL

- Chalkboard and chalk
- Samples of all types of insulin syringes and pens
- Sample bottles of all types of insulin
- Sample boxes of insulins
- Alcohol swabs
- Price information from local pharmacies
- Samples of insulin pens and injection devices
- Information about local syringe disposal policies
- MedicAlert or other diabetes identification information
- Insulin pump and tubing
- Injection aid devices
- Glucagon kit
- Samples of glucose products

METHOD OF PRESENTATION

Start by introducing yourself and telling what you do. Ask participants to introduce themselves. Explain that the purpose of this session is to provide information about insulin and how it works and to describe different types of insulin programs. Actual injection technique is usually taught individually; however, a demonstration of the procedure may be useful as a review, at the appropriate point in the session.

Some participants attending this session will be initiating insulin for the first time. The first section of the outline provides information for these participants. It is essential to begin by addressing their fears and concerns about insulin by asking then to describe these fears. Participants who have experiences with insulin may be helpful to them as well. It is also important to reassure participants with type 2 diabetes that initiating insulin does not mean that they have failed or that their diabetes is worse. A discussion of the decision-making process they used may be a useful way to begin. It may also help alleviate fear by starting the class by having participants insert an insulin needle.

This outline provides information from initiating insulin through implementing intensive programs. Provide only the content that is appropriate for the audience. Present material in a question/discussion format. Begin by asking how they did with their short-term goal and what they learned from it.

CONTENT OUTLINE

CONCEPT	DETAIL	INSTRUCTOR'S NOTES
1. Initiating insulin therapy	1.1 Beginning insulin therapy is often difficult. Most people have questions, fears and concerns.	Ask, "What are your thoughts about insulin therapy? What questions or concerns do you have?"

CONTENT OUTLINE

CONCEPT	DETAIL	INSTRUCTOR'S NOTES
	1.2 As with every other type of treatment, there are advantages and disadvantages. What disadvantages are there for you? What advantages are there for you?	Encourage participants to voice disadvantages and advantages without offering positive or negative comments. What are advantages for some will be disadvantages for others. Common disadvantages are: Fear of needles and pain with injections; weight gain; loss of flexibility in lifestyle and independence; fear of hypoglycemia; view insulin as a personal failure or sign of worsening diabetes; fear that insulin causes complications; and fear that they will lose support of family and friends. Common advantages are: Feel better and more energetic; more flexibility in lifestyle; "not as bad as I thought;" can be more involved with care; prevent complications; better quality of life. Once the list is complete, ask participants who take insulin to address some of the concerns or provide information as appropriate. Providing emotional support through active listening is likely to be more useful than information at this point.
	1.3 Weighing the advantages and disadvantages is something that only you can do.	Ask, "What do you think is the biggest barrier for you? What supports do you have?" Remind participants with type 2 diabetes that while their health care team, family and friends can help, the final decision is up to them.
	1.4 The purpose of this class is to give you the information you need to begin insulin safely and effectively.	Ask, "What information or other help would be the most useful for you as you begin insulin therapy?"

CONTENT OUTLINE

CONCEPT	DETAIL	INSTRUCTOR'S NOTES
2. What is insulin?	2.1 Insulin is a hormone, a protein substance.	Ask, "What questions or concerns do you have about insulin? What is insulin? What insulin(s) do you take?"
	2.2 Insulin is produced in the pancreas.	Insulin is produced in the beta cells of the pancreatic islets (islets are 1% of the pancreas).
	2.3 Insulin attaches to the outside of most body cells and allows glucose to enter those cells. This lowers blood glucose (glucose leaves the blood).	Ask, "How does insulin work? How does insulin affect blood glucose?"
	2.4 In diabetes, there is not enough insulin action. Insulin injections may be needed to lower blood glucose.	Review differences in types of diabetes related to insulin production.
	2.5 At this time, insulin cannot be taken as a pill because it would be destroyed by digestive enzymes before it could act to lower blood glucose levels.	Insulin is a protein and would be digested like other proteins. Devices that would allow oral delivery of insulin are being tested.
3. Types of insulin	3.1 Insulin is made by three companies in the United States and is available worldwide under various brand names.	Show examples of each. Patients may notice some blood glucose variability with different brands.
	3.2 All insulins are classified by general types: rapid-acting, short-acting, intermediate-acting, and long-acting.	Distribute Handout #1, Comparison of Insulins. Show examples of different insulins.
	3.3 Rapid-acting: insulin lispro (Humalog) and insulin aspart (Novolog).	These insulin analogs are created when two amino acids on the human insulin chain are switched or altered. Another rapid-acting insulin analog called glulisine (Apidra) will be available in the near future.
	3.4 Short-acting: regular.	
	3.5 Intermediate-acting: NPH and lente.	NPH and lente should not be used interchangeably.
	3.6 Long-acting: glargine (Lantus) and ultralente.	Another basal insulin analog called insulin detemir (Levemir) will be available in the near future.

CONTENT OUTLINE

CONCEPT	DETAIL	INSTRUCTOR'S NOTES
	3.7 Combinations of NPH and regular are available in 70:30 and 50:50 ratios, NPH and lispro in a 75:25 ratio, and NPH and aspart in a 70:30 ratio.	
	3.8 When purchasing insulin, be sure to buy the brand, type, and strength that has been prescribed for you.	
4. Choosing an insulin program	4.1 In people who don't have diabetes, the body makes a steady amount of insulin throughout the day (basal), with an extra boost of insulin while eating (bolus).	This pattern keeps blood glucose in the normal range.
	4.2 Insulin programs attempt to provide insulin in much the same way as the body does. The goal is to maintain the glucose level in the target range.	Both bolus and basal insulin action is needed, through a combination of insulins, oral agents, and/or pancreatic function (for people with type 2 diabetes).
	4.3 Various types of insulin can be used alone or in combination to produce specific action effects. Some programs use only one type of insulin, while others use more than one type.	
	4.4 The intensity of the program is based on your blood glucose levels, meal plan, and activity. Equally important are your personal glucose and other goals, how often you are willing to inject and monitor, and how hard you are willing and able to work on caring for your diabetes.	Stress the importance of the role participants have in decision-making about the type of insulin program.
	4.5 Intensive programs are generally recommended for people with type 1 diabetes, women with diabetes who are pregnant or planning a pregnancy, or people who want to feel more in charge of their diabetes. They are also used by people with type 2 diabetes as necessary to safely and adequately manage glucose levels.	If appropriate, stress the importance of preconception care. Ask, "What advantages and disadvantages can you identify for more intensive insulin management?" Examples of disadvantages include cost, increased risk of hypoglycemia, weight gain, and more time and effort. Examples of advantages include greater flexibility in lifestyle, more even

155

CONTENT OUTLINE

CONCEPT	DETAIL	INSTRUCTOR'S NOTES
		blood glucose levels, feeling more energetic, feeling more in charge, and reduced risk for complications.
	4.6 Intensive programs usually include three or more shots per day along with frequent monitoring. Insulin pumps may also be used. Meal planning is often based on carbohydrate counting and use of insulin:carbohydrate ratios.	Clarify the difference between intensive insulin programs and optimizing control through other treatments. See Outline #20, *Carbohydrate Counting*.
5. Insulin programs	5.1 In someone without diabetes, normal preprandial blood glucose is 70–110 mg/dl. (Preprandial means before eating, usually 30 minutes premeal.)	Use Visual #1, Normal Blood Glucose and Insulin Levels.
	5.2 In someone without diabetes, a small amount of insulin is continuously released by the pancreas to maintain the blood glucose in this range. This is the basal level of insulin.	The word "fasting" is often used as a synonym for preprandial. Fasting usually means no eating for 8 or more hours, so it usually refers to the first morning blood test.
	5.3 In someone without diabetes, normal blood glucose 2 hours postprandial is less than 140 mg/dl. (Postprandial means after eating, usually 90–120 minutes postmeal.)	Timing for postprandial glucose levels is based on when the meal begins.
	5.4 An additional burst of insulin is released by the pancreas in response to the rising blood glucose levels after eating, causing the blood glucose go back to normal. This is to called a bolus of insulin.	Ask, "Do you ever check your blood glucose after meals? What have you found?"
	5.5 Insulin programs attempt to imitate the pancreas by providing insulin in a basal and bolus pattern either through oral medication to enhance insulin production or use and/or through insulin shots.	
	5.6 Each type of insulin has its own characteristic onset, peak, and length	Refer to Handout #1, Comparison of Insulins. Define *onset*,

CONTENT OUTLINE

CONCEPT	DETAIL	INSTRUCTOR'S NOTES

of action and can be combined to mimic the body's normal pattern.

peak, and *length of action*. Help participants find the insulin they take on the chart, plus its onset, peak, and length of action.

5.7 Onset, peak, and length of action of a particular insulin vary depending on injection technique, physical activity, and the way the body uses insulin.

5.8 This information is important because it helps you balance your insulin with your food and activity. It also helps you know when an insulin reaction is likely to occur.

Ask, "Based on the insulins you take, when are you most likely to have a reaction?"

5.9 The basal insulin dose can be provided by:
- intermediate-acting insulin (NPH/lente)
- long-acting insulin (glargine/ ultralente), often used because of its long duration and relatively low peak

Use Visual #2, Insulin Action Times, to show basal insulins. This mimics the constant output of insulin in people without diabetes. Rapid- or short-acting insulins are used for the basal insulin in a pump. Multiple basal rates can be given.

5.10 The onset of action of the intermediate- and long-acting insulins is gradual and their effects last longer.

Point out which insulins have the greatest effect on which blood glucose levels.

5.11 Rapid- or short-acting insulins are always used for bolus doses. Bolus doses of rapid- or short-acting insulins are given before eating, so that the insulin can get into the bloodstream and begin to work before glucose levels rise.

Use Visual #2 to illustrate. The bolus dose can be given via an insulin pump or by injection. Insulin pens and other devices make it easier to give bolus doses.

5.12 The rapid-acting and short-acting insulins begin to act very quickly after injection and last a short time. They are usually given to prevent the rise in blood glucose after meals.

Define bolus dose. Use Visual #2 to illustrate. Discuss onset, peak, length of action for each type of insulin, and the need for basal and bolus insulin availability.

CONTENT OUTLINE

CONCEPT	DETAIL	INSTRUCTOR'S NOTES

5.13 Examples of insulin programs:

- **Intermediate-acting insulin only.** One shot before breakfast or at bedtime; or two shots—one before breakfast, one before supper.
- **Oral agents plus intermediate- and long-acting insulin taken at bedtime.**
- **Intermediate-acting plus rapid-acting or short-acting insulin.** One shot before breakfast; or two shots—one before breakfast, one before supper. Sometimes a third shot of rapid- or short-acting is taken before lunch, or the rapid-acting or short-acting is taken before supper and the intermediate-acting at bedtime for a total of three shots.
- **Long-acting plus rapid-acting or short-acting insulin.** One or two shots a day of long-acting, plus two or more shots of rapid- or short-acting insulin, one before each meal.

Instructor's Notes: Use Visual #3, Insulin Programs. Point out that there are a variety of insulin programs, and that the choice of program is based on personal goals, glucose goals, and individual response.

Use of premixed 70:30, 75:25 and 50:50 provide this type of program.

Distribute Handout #2 to all participants and Handout #3 to participants using insulin: carbohydrate ratios.

5.14 Dosage is based on your individual response. Your dosage and program will probably change over time. This does not mean your diabetes is worse.

Instructor's Notes: In children, insulin dose needs to increase with growth.

5.15 Your insulin needs vary because your eating, activity, and stress levels vary. You can learn to make adjustments in your insulin doses, meal plan, and exercise level to keep your blood glucose in the target range.

Instructor's Notes: A variety of approaches for pattern management are available. Most include compensatory and anticipatory modifications. Problem-solve using participants' records or sample records and approaches used in your site.

5.16 Many people with diabetes learn to make these adjustments based on blood glucose levels. Talk with your health care team if you are interested in learning this skill.

Instructor's Notes: In a person without diabetes, the body does not make the same amount of insulin each day; the amount needed varies, based on blood glucose levels.

CONTENT OUTLINE

CONCEPT	DETAIL	INSTRUCTOR'S NOTES
6. Mixing insulins	6.1 Most commonly used mixtures are rapid-acting or short-acting plus NPH or lente; these can be given in one syringe.	See insulin package insert for specific product guidelines regarding mixing insulins.
	6.2 Draw up the rapid- or short-acting insulin first.	If intermediate- or long-acting insulin is drawn up first, traces of the retarding agent on the needle may contaminate the short-acting insulin and slow down its action time.
	6.3 When mixing lente insulins, the injection should be given within 5 minutes after mixing. The action times of the insulins may change if you wait longer. Lispro is stable when mixed with NPH. (*Note*: Most insulin manufacturers recommend giving all mixtures within 5 minutes after they are mixed.)	The excess zinc in lente binds with the regular, decreasing its potency and increasing the potency of the lente. The other option is always to wait 24 hours after mixing before injection, to allow the mixture to stabilize. Discuss sections 6.5–6.9 only if appropriate for your audience.
	6.4 Glargine insulin has a lower pH level and cannot be mixed in the same syringe with other insulins.	Some users note burning with injection. The absorption of glargine is not affected by the injection site.
	6.5 If it is necessary to have someone predraw mixed doses for later administration, combinations of NPH and regular insulins are generally recommended.	Studies suggest that predrawn NPH and regular insulins can be safely stored in syringes for 21 days.
	6.6 Store these in the refrigerator; allow the insulin to come to room temperature before injecting.	
	6.7 Store predrawn syringes for at least 24 hours before use to allow them to stabilize.	Always have an extra day's worth of syringes ready, so that you don't have to use a freshly drawn syringe, which will have a different action time.
	6.8 Store syringes horizontally. Roll gently between palms before use to remix the solution.	Storing with the needles downward can cause them to clog.

CONTENT OUTLINE

CONCEPT	DETAIL	INSTRUCTOR'S NOTES
	6.9 Various proportions of NPH and regular insulins can be mixed by a pharmacist. These are stable for 3 months when refrigerated and for 1 month at room temperature.	These are in addition to commercially prepared premixed insulins.
7. Source of insulin	7.1 You can buy synthetic human and pork insulins.	Show examples of different types of insulin. Mixtures of beef and pork insulins were discontinued in 1998.
	7.2 Most insulin is made in a laboratory. This type is called "human insulin," but it is not actually insulin from humans.	Human insulins are made using recombinant DNA technology, where bacteria are used to make parts of the human insulin molecule, which are then joined together.
	7.3 Insulin from pork acts very much like insulin made by the human body. Animal insulin is purified when it is bottled.	It is anticipated that only human insulins will be available in the near future.
8. Strength of insulin	8.1 U-100 is the strength of insulin most commonly available. U-40 and U-500 insulins are also available.	Show an example of the U-100 insulin bottle. U-500 insulin reaches peak blood levels more slowly because of its greater concentration. Insulin can be diluted to U-10 by a pharmacist.
	8.2 U-100 means 100 units of insulin per cc (cubic centimeter).	U-100 was developed in 1973 because it can be used by nearly all patients. It is compatible with the decimal system, and having a single strength of insulin helps make errors less likely.
9. Purity of insulin	9.1 All commercial preparations of insulin have small amounts of impurities.	Show examples of various insulins.
	9.2 Human insulin preparations are the most pure. Insulins made from animals have small amounts of other proteins.	*Proinsulin* is the precursor for insulin. Not all of the proinsulin can be removed from pork insulin. The amount of proinsulin is an indicator of impurities.

CONTENT OUTLINE

CONCEPT	DETAIL	INSTRUCTOR'S NOTES
	9.3 The impurities are not a problem for most people. Some people do become sensitive (allergic) to the impurities.	
10. Storing insulin	10.1 The insulin bottle in use can be kept at room temperature. Keep extra bottles in the refrigerator.	For most insulins, if the temperature is over 86°F, store in the refrigerator.
	10.2 Insulin vials generally remain stable at room temperature for 28–30 days after opening. Storage guidelines vary for cartridges and prefilled pens and range from 10 to 28 days.	Refrigerated, unopened vials can be used until the expiration date.
	10.3 Insulin can lose its potency at greater than 86°F (e.g., in a steamy bathroom) and at freezing temperatures. Do not use insulin that has been exposed to temperature extremes.	Do not store insulin in direct sunlight (e.g., a window sill). If insulin freezes, do not use it. Once frozen, it has zero potency.
	10.4 Taking insulin at room temperature is more comfortable than taking chilled insulin and may cause fewer skin irritations.	
	10.5 You do not need to refrigerate insulin when traveling unless expecting temperatures over 86°F or below freezing; then pack insulin in an insulated container.	Caution participants about leaving insulin in a hot or very cold car. They can pack insulin in a thermos or plastic foam container to keep cool.
	10.6 When traveling in airplanes, trains, or buses, pack insulin and syringes in a carry-on bag. Do **not** put in checked luggage.	Luggage can be lost on public transportation, and luggage compartments on buses and planes are often very cold.
11. Usability of insulin	11.1 Check the expiration date on the box.	Show the date on the box.
	11.2 Usability is not guaranteed by the manufacturer after that date.	
	11.3 Plan so that the amount you buy will be used up by the expiration date.	Sometimes, insulin on sale is short-dated.

CONTENT OUTLINE

CONCEPT	DETAIL	INSTRUCTOR'S NOTES
	11.4 Calculate dosages from one bottle. The number of days a bottle of a particular kind of U-100 insulin will last is calculated by determining the total number of units of that kind used in a day and dividing that number into 1000 (the number of units in a bottle of U-100).	Remember that some insulin may be lost while drawing it up. Use a participant's dosage to illustrate this activity.
	11.5 Examine insulin for change in color or for "stringiness"; do not use the insulin if it doesn't mix or if color is abnormal.	Define "stringy," or show an example.
12. Syringes and needles	12.1 Different sizes of syringes available are: ■ ⅓ cc (30 units) ■ ½ cc (50 units) ■ 1 cc (100 units) ■ 2 cc (200 units)	Mention that several companies make syringes. Show examples of different syringes. Use U-100 syringes with U-100 insulin. The 2-cc syringes may need to be specially ordered.
	12.2 Consider insulin dose, ease of reading scale, accuracy, and convenience when deciding which kind to use.	Ask, "What syringes do you use? What are your experiences with them?"
	12.3 Very fine and short needles may be less painful to use. Syringes with larger gauges have finer needles.	Short needles are not appropriate for obese patients.
	12.4 Dispose of needles and syringes carefully. A plastic detergent bottle or metal container with a screw top can be used for collecting and then capped before disposal. Dispose with the regular trash—do not recycle. Label the container as containing used syringes.	Provide information from the local health department about syringe disposal regulations. Disposal guidelines can vary. If none, use the procedures outlined in 11.4. Commercial disposal boxes are available that can be returned when full.
	12.5 Some people prefer to reuse syringes. Put the cap back on, being careful not to touch the needle. Move the plunger up and down after each use; this helps to prevent needle clogs. Needles will get dull with use.	Wiping the needle with alcohol between uses is not needed. Alcohol removes the silicone and makes the injection more painful. Reusing syringes may lead to infections for some people.

CONTENT OUTLINE

CONCEPT	DETAIL	INSTRUCTOR'S NOTES
	12.6 Various injection devices can be purchased, including simple spring-loaded devices in which the syringe is loaded, cartridge pen-type injectors, and jet-injector devices.	These may be helpful for some patients, particularly those with an aversion to needles or on intensive programs. Show examples of these products.
13. Cost of equipment	13.1 Cost of insulin and syringes varies from store to store. Shop around for the lowest prices.	Distribute a list of price information from different pharmacies in your area, or ask participants to find out and bring this information to the next session.
	13.2 Some insurance plans will cover costs with a prescription.	
14. Preparing insulin for injection	14.1 Clear insulin is already in solution and does not need to be mixed.	
	14.2 Longer-acting cloudy insulins must be mixed by rolling or shaking gently.	Show precipitate in bottle of unmixed insulin.
	14.3 Here's how to draw up one type of insulin.	Distribute Handout #4, Giving an Insulin Injection. Demonstrate drawing up of insulin, if appropriate.
	14.4 Here's how to draw up two types of insulin.	Demonstrate, if appropriate.
15. Injecting insulin	15.1 Here's how to inject insulin.	Ask, "What questions or concerns do you have about injecting?" Demonstrate proper injection technique. The angle used depends on body build and subcutaneous tissue. The deeper the injection, the faster the absorption, in general.
	15.2 Bleeding at the site may occur, caused by the needle going through the capillary.	Distinguish between bleeding at the site and blood in the syringe.

CONTENT OUTLINE

CONCEPT	DETAIL	INSTRUCTOR'S NOTES
16. Injection sites and rotation	16.1 The abdomen is the recommended site for some types of insulin.	Because absorption varies for some insulins, rotating to various parts of the body may lead to erratic blood glucose levels.
	16.2 Other parts of the body (arms, thighs, or buttocks) can be used. These areas are used because they have fewer nerves and a pad of fat underneath.	Use Visual #5, Injection Sites, to show abdominal and other sites. The abdomen is not appropriate for thin, young children or patients who cannot pinch a half an inch of fat.
	16.3 Do not use other places—there is not enough fat, and also nerve endings and blood vessels are closer to the surface.	
	16.4 Insulin is absorbed most rapidly when injected into the abdomen, followed by the arms, thighs, and buttocks for some insulins.	Ask, "What site do you prefer?" Review manufacturer guidelines for site recommendations.
	16.5 Use sites 1½ inches apart. Rotate sites within one area of your body only.	If the abdomen is not used, choose another area and rotate injections around that area.
	16.6 Rotating sites will help to prevent fat hypertrophy (a thickening at the site associated with poor insulin absorption), probably caused by overusing a site or injecting superficially.	Fewer nerve endings in hypertrophied areas mean decreased pain, but these areas should not be used for injection because insulin absorption is affected and may be unpredictable.
	16.7 Rotating sites will help to prevent fat atrophy (a depressed area with loss of subcutaneous fat).	This can be treated by injecting a pure insulin subcutaneously into the periphery of the area.
	16.8 Ask your nurse or physician to check your injection sites if you think you have fat atrophy or hypertrophy.	
	16.9 Localized skin reactions may develop. A more pure insulin may solve this problem.	

CONTENT OUTLINE

CONCEPT	DETAIL	INSTRUCTOR'S NOTES
17. Tips for taking insulin	17.1 Giving yourself an injection can be frightening. It does get easier with time.	Ask, "What makes giving injections easier for you?" Suggest taking a deep breath before injection. If others in class give insulin already, they may offer reassurance. Approach children with a matter-of-fact and confident attitude. Parents may want to practice on themselves or other adults before injecting a child.
	17.2 Timing the insulin dose with time of eating leads to more even blood glucose levels. Glucose levels begin to rise about 10 minutes after you begin to eat.	If participants are taking regular insulin, use Visual #4, Timing of Regular Insulin and Meals, to illustrate this point. Stress the importance of not taking rapid-acting insulins until the meal is prepared and ready to serve.
	17.3 Rapid-acting insulins may begin to work within 5 minutes.	
	17.4 If rapid-acting insulin is used for the bolus, give your shot 15 minutes or less before eating. If given too early, low blood glucose may result.	These insulins are given to children at meals (or just after). Glulisine can be given after eating.
	17.5 Regular insulin takes at least 15 minutes to get into the bloodstream. The standard recommendation is to take any injection containing regular insulin 30 minutes before eating. This helps prevent the rise in blood glucose that occurs after meals.	Ask, "When do you give your insulin in relation to meals?"
	17.6 If taken too early, low blood glucose may result. If taken at mealtime, food will cause the blood glucose to rise before the insulin can begin working. This may result in a postprandial blood glucose level that is above the target.	Use Visual #4, Timing of Regular Insulin and Meals, to stress the importance of timing. For more precise management, if your blood glucose is:

50–69 take a bolus dose with your meal

70–119 wait 15 minutes before eating

120–180 wait 30 minutes before eating

>180 wait 45 minutes before eating

CONTENT OUTLINE

CONCEPT	DETAIL	INSTRUCTOR'S NOTES

17.7 Take your insulin at about the same time(s) each day. This helps you to remember and will help keep your blood glucose levels more even.

17.8 Keep all supplies together near where you will give your injection.

17.9 When you first start taking insulin, you will need to plan a few extra minutes into your schedule. Take your shot at the time you do other routine activities (e.g., testing blood glucose or brushing your teeth).

17.10 Use visual cues like notes or signs, or other cues such as an alarm clock.

17.11 Putting off your shot doesn't make it easier. Sometimes you just need to set a time and stick to it.

17.12 Blood glucose monitoring provides the information you need to see how well the insulin program is working and to make adjustments for meals, activity, and as needed.

Ask, "What are reasons you check your blood glucose?" Stress the importance of this information for daily decision-making.

17.13 Some people gain weight when starting insulin. Individuals on an intensified insulin program may gain up to 8–15 lb in the first year. Work with your dietitian to create a meal plan that will help you prevent this.

Fewer calories are lost as glucose in the urine and more calories are stored as fat because of the insulin action.

17.14 Insulin therapy takes more time and effort on the part of both the person with diabetes and the health care team.

The need for family involvement and support may also increase.

17.15 At first, you will have a great deal of contact with your health care team as your program is developed and fine-tuned. You need to find a team of people who are knowledgeable, easily accessible, and with whom you can develop a collaborative relationship.

It is likely that participants will be in frequent telephone contact with their health care team members.

CONTENT OUTLINE

CONCEPT	DETAIL	INSTRUCTOR'S NOTES
	17.16 Insulin therapy gives you the opportunity and responsibility to make many daily decisions about your treatment plan. By learning how different insulins work and how exercise and specific foods affect your blood glucose, and by using information from blood testing and working closely with your health care team, you can develop an intensive insulin plan that works for you.	Point out that continuing education will help them keep abreast of new findings, treatments, and technology.
18. Miscellaneous	18.1 Accurate measurement of insulin is critical. Bubbles contain no insulin and take up space.	Show how small a unit is by squirting 5 units on the table.
	18.2 It is very important to wear identification that states you have diabetes.	Provide information about diabetes identification resources.
	18.3 In most states, a prescription is required to purchase insulin.	Clarify laws in your state. Even if available, most insurance companies require a prescription for reimbursement.
	18.4 You need a prescription when traveling overseas and a letter from your provider.	
	18.5 Take your insulin even if you are ill and cannot eat.	Illness or infection can raise blood glucose levels.
	18.6 Avoid: ■ rubbing the site ■ long, hot baths right after a shot	These both alter absorption rates.
19. Hypoglycemia	19.1 Hypoglycemia can occur when using insulin.	Ask, "What are signs and symptoms of hypoglycemia?" Refer to Outline #11, *Managing Blood Glucose.*
	19.2 It is most likely to occur at peak insulin action times.	Help participants determine when they would be most likely to have a reaction.

CONTENT OUTLINE

CONCEPT	DETAIL	INSTRUCTOR'S NOTES
	19.3 Hypoglycemia must be treated with food or drink containing sugar.	Ask, "How do you treat an insulin reaction?" Distribute and review Handout #5, Treatment of Low Blood Glucose and Handout #6, How to Use Glucagon. Remind participants who are lactose-intolerant to avoid using milk as a treatment.
20. Research	20.1 Amylin is a hormone secreted by the pancreas in response to hyperglycemia. Clinical trials are underway with synthetic versions of these hormones.	Pramlintide (Symlin) and exenatide are being tested.
	20.2 Insulin administration and new products are areas of much research.	Inhaled, nasal and oral insulins and insulin patches are both being tested.
	20.3 Choose a short-term goal to try before the next session.	

SKILLS CHECKLIST

Each insulin-taking participant will be able to:

1. draw up the correct amount of insulin;

2. inject the insulin properly; and

3. rotate injection sites appropriately.

EVALUATION PLAN

Knowledge will be evaluated by achievement of learning objectives and by responses to questions during the session; skills will be evaluated by observing return demonstration of techniques. The ability to apply knowledge will be evaluated by appropriate use of insulin or an intensive insulin therapy program and through program outcome measures.

DOCUMENTATION PLAN

Record class attendance and achieved objectives as appropriate.

SUGGESTED READINGS

Ahern JA, Mazur ML. Site rotation. *Diabetes Forecast*. 2001;54(4):66–68.

American Association of Diabetes Educators. Position Statement: Insulin self-administration instruction: use of engineered sharps injury protection devices to meet OSHA regulations. *The Diabetes Educator*. 2002;28:730–734.

American Association of Diabetes Educators. Position Statement. Intensive diabetes management: implications of the DCCT and UKPDS. *The Diabetes Educator*. 2002;28:735–740.

American Diabetes Association. *Intensive Diabetes Management*, 2nd Edition. Alexandria, VA: American Diabetes Association, 1998.

American Diabetes Association. Position statement: insulin administration. *Diabetes Care*. 2004;27(Suppl 1):S107–S109.

American Diabetes Association Resource Guide 2004. Carrying cases. *Diabetes Forecast*. 2004;57(1):RG70-RG73.

American Diabetes Association Resource Guide 2004. Insulin. *Diabetes Forecast*. 2004;57(1):RG14-RG37.

Carlisle BA, Kroon LA, Koda-Kimble MA. *101 Medication Tips for People with Diabetes*. Alexandria, VA: American Diabetes Association, 1999.

Childs B. Death to the sliding scale. *Diabetes Spectrum*. 2002;16:68–73.

Clarke, K. No needles needed. *Nursing*. 2002;32(5):49–50.

DeCosta S, Brackenridge B, Hicks D. A comparison of insulin pen use in the United States and the United Kingdom. *The Diabetes Educator*. 2002;28:52–60.

DeWitt DE, Hirsch IB. Outpatient insulin therapy in type 1 and type 2 diabetes mellitus. *JAMA*. 2003;289:2254–2264.

Fain JA. Unlocking the mysteries of insulin therapy. *Nursing*. 2004;34(3):41–45.

Fleming DR, Jacober SJ, Vandenberg MA, Fitzgerald JT, Grunberger G. The safety of injecting insulin through clothing. *Diabetes Care*. 1997;20:245–248.

Funnell MM, Kruger DF, Spencer M. Self-management support for insulin therapy in type 2 diabetes. *The Diabetes Educator*. 2004;30:274–280.

Grajower MM, Fraser CG, Holcombe JH, Daugherty ML, Harris WC, DeFelippis MR, Santiago OM, Clark NG. How long should insulin be used once a vial is started? *Diabetes Care*. 2003;26:2665–2669.

Herbst KL, Hirsch IR. Insulin strategies for primary care providers. *Clinical Diabetes*. 2002;20:11–17.

Hirsch EI, Farkas-Hirsch R. Sliding scale or sliding scare: it's all sliding nonsense. *Diabetes Spectrum*. 2001;14:84–87.

Hunt LM, Valenzuela MA, Pugh JA. NIDDM patients' fears and hopes about insulin therapy. *Diabetes Care*. 1997;20:292–298.

Jordan LS. Using the dummy tummy to teach insulin injection. *The Diabetes Educator*. 1996;22:245–246.

Kanzer-Lewis G. *Patient Education: You Can Do It!* Alexandria, VA: American Diabetes Association, 2003.

Kaufman FR, Halvorson M. New trends in managing type 1 diabetes. *Contemporary Pediatrics*. 1999;16:112–123.

Kissin A, Katzeff HL. New insulin therapies for the management of type 2 diabetes. *Practical Diabetology*. 2002;21(1):14–20.

Koerbel G, Korytkowski M. Insulin-therapy resistance. *Practical Diabetology*. 2003; 22(2):36–40.

Kordella T. Overcoming the fear. *Diabetes Forecast*. 2004;57(3):52–58.

Kordella T. The future of insulin. *Diabetes Forecast*. 2003;56(3):63–69.

Korytkowski M. When oral agents fail: practical barriers to starting insulin. *International Journal of Obesity*. 2002;26(suppl 3):S18–S24.

McCarthy JA, Covarrubias BM, Sink P. Is the traditional alcohol wipe necessary before an insulin injection? *Diabetes Care*. 1993; 16:402.

Meece JD, Campbell RK. Insulin lispro update. *The Diabetes Educator*. 2002;28:269–277.

Nath C, Ponte CD. Lessons about insulin therapy. *Nursing*. 2000;30(11):34–39.

SUGGESTED READINGS *continued*

Peragallo-Dittko V. Aspiration of the subcutaneous insulin injection: clinical evaluation of needle size and amount of subcutaneous fat. *The Diabetes Educator.* 1995;21:291–296.

Pearson J, Bergenstal R. Fine-turning control: pattern management versus supplementation. *Diabetes Spectrum.* 2001;14:75–82.

Ratner RE. Insulin-delivery systems in the management of diabetes. *Practical Diabetology.* 2004;23(1):14–24.

Riddle MC, Rosenstock J, Gerich J, on behalf of the Insulin Glargine 4002 Study Investigators. The Treat to Target Trial. *Diabetes Care.* 2003;26:3080–3086.

Rizor HM, Richards S. All our patients need to know about intensified diabetes management they learned in fourth grade. *The Diabetes Educator.* 2000;26:392–404.

Roberts SS. Diabetes essentials: insulin administration. *Diabetes Forecast.* 2004; 57(3):44–46.

Rosenstock J, Schwartz SL, Clark, CM, Jr., Park GD, Donley DW, Edwards MB. Basal insulin therapy in type 2 diabetes. *Diabetes Care.* 2001;24:631–636.

Silva SR, Clark L, Goodman SN, Plotnick LP. Can caretakers of children with IDDM accurately measure small insulin doses and dose changes? *Diabetes Care.* 1996;19:56–59.

Snoek F. Psychological insulin resistance: what do patients and providers fear most. *Diabetes Voice.* 2001;30(3):26–28.

Spollett GR. Basal-bolus insulin therapy. *Practical Diabetology.* 2002;21(1);33–36.

Springer J. Basal insulin in combination with oral hypoglycemic agents in the management of type 2 diabetes. *The Diabetes Educator.* 2004;30:68–70.

Stephens EA, Ryan-Turek T, Frias JP. New directions in diabetes management: Pramlintide as an adjunct to insulin therapy in type 1 and type 2 diabetes. *Practical Diabetology.* 2004;23(1):7–13.

Tsui E, Barnie A, Ross S, Parkes, R, Zinman B: Intensive insulin therapy with insulin lispro: a randomized trial of continuous subcutaneous insulin infusion versus multiple daily insulin injection. *Diabetes Care.* 2001;24:1722–1725.

Whitlock WL, Brown A, Moore K, Pavliscak H, Dingbaum A, Lacefield D, Buker K, Xenakis S, Reichard P, Toomingas B, Rosenqvist U. Changes in conceptions and attitudes during five years of intensified conventional insulin treatment in the Stockholm Diabetes Intervention Study (SDIS). *The Diabetes Educator.* 1994;20:503–508.

Wulffele MG, Kooy A, Lehert P, Betes D, Ogterop JC, van der Burg BB, Donker AJM, Stehouwer CDA. Combination of insulin and metformin in the treatment of type 2 diabetes. *Diabetes Care.* 2002;25:2133–2140.

➔ Normal Blood Glucose and Insulin Levels

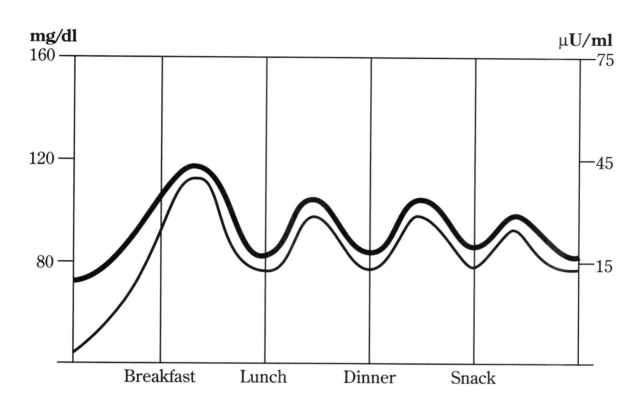

Blood Glucose Level

Plasma Insulin Level

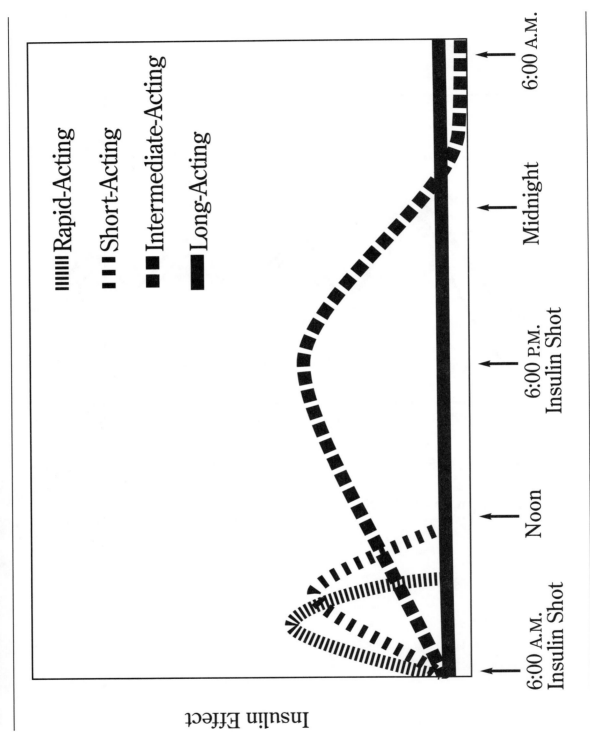

Insulin Action Times

Rapid-Acting
Short-Acting
Intermediate-Acting
Long-Acting

Insulin Effect

6:00 A.M.
Insulin Shot

Noon

6:00 P.M.
Insulin Shot

Midnight

6:00 A.M.

Insulin Programs

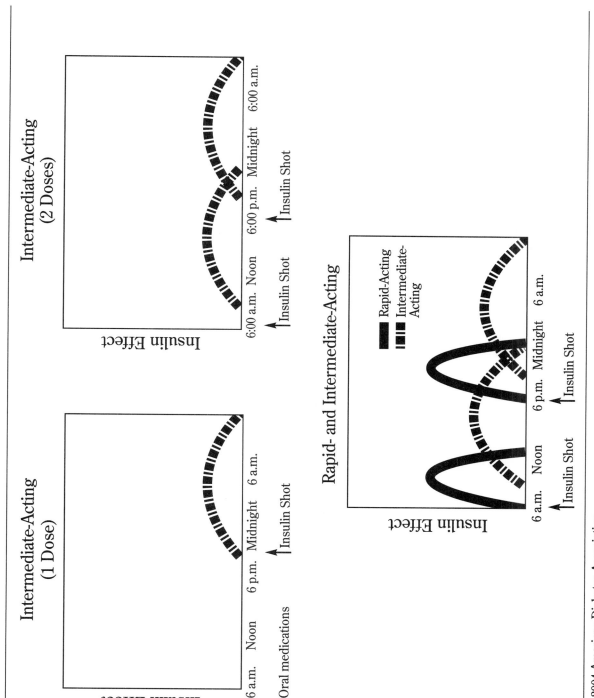

Intermediate-Acting
(1 Dose)

Intermediate-Acting
(2 Doses)

Rapid- and Intermediate-Acting

Insulin Effect

Insulin Effect

Insulin Effect

6 a.m.   Noon   6 p.m.   Midnight   6 a.m.

Oral medications

Insulin Shot

6:00 a.m.   Noon   6:00 p.m.   Midnight   6:00 a.m.

Insulin Shot

Insulin Shot

Rapid-Acting

Intermediate-
Acting

6 a.m.   Noon   6 p.m.   Midnight   6 a.m.

Insulin Shot

Insulin Shot

173

INSULIN PROGRAMS *continued*

Insulin Programs

Short- and Intermediate-Acting

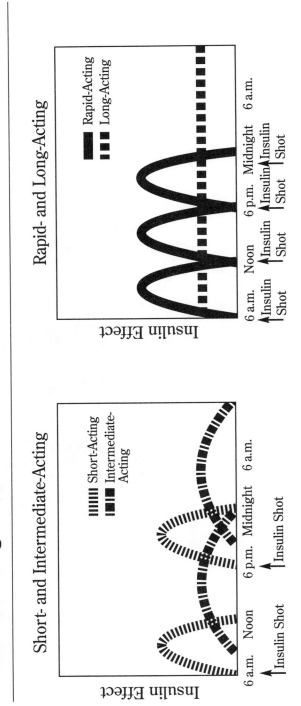

Rapid- and Long-Acting

Short- and Long-Acting

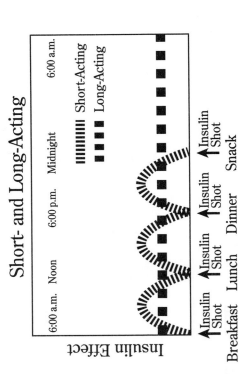

INSULIN PROGRAMS *continued*

Insulin Programs

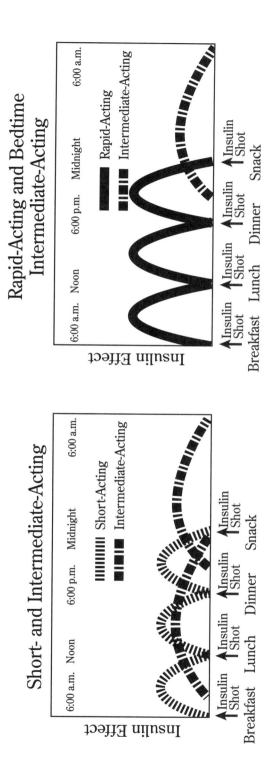

Short- and Intermediate-Acting

Insulin Effect

6:00 a.m. Noon   Midnight   6:00 p.m.   6:00 a.m.

Short-Acting
Intermediate-Acting

Insulin Shot   Insulin Shot   Insulin Shot

Breakfast   Lunch   Dinner   Snack

Rapid-Acting and Bedtime Intermediate-Acting

Insulin Effect

6:00 a.m. Noon   Midnight   6:00 p.m.   6:00 a.m.

Rapid-Acting
Intermediate-Acting

Insulin Shot   Insulin Shot   Insulin Shot

Breakfast   Lunch   Dinner   Snack

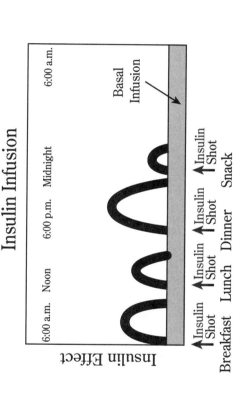

Continuous Subcutaneous Insulin Infusion

Insulin Effect

6:00 a.m. Noon   Midnight   6:00 p.m.   6:00 a.m.

Basal Infusion

Insulin Shot   Insulin Shot

Breakfast   Lunch   Dinner   Snack

175

Timing of Regular Insulin and Meals

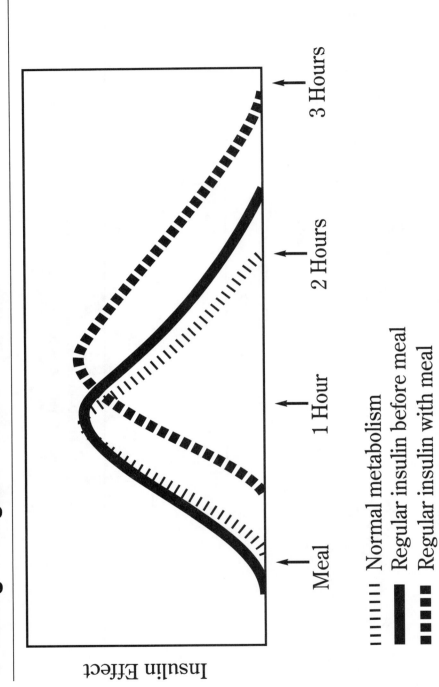

Insulin Effect

Meal   1 Hour   2 Hours   3 Hours

||||||| Normal metabolism

Regular insulin before meal

Regular insulin with meal

➔ Injection Sites

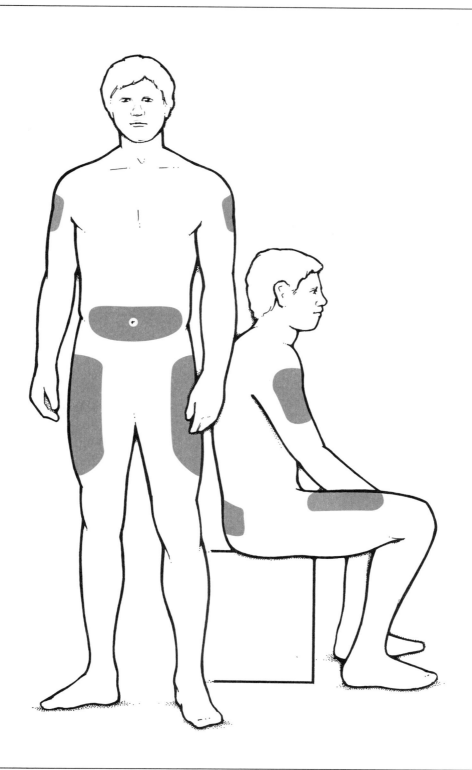

➡ Comparison of Insulins

Type	Source	Color	Approximate Length of Action (Hours)		
			Onset	**Peak**	**End**
Rapid-acting Lispro Aspart	Human	Clear	5 minutes	1	2–4
Short-acting Regular	Human Pork	Clear	½–1	2–5	6–16
Intermediate-acting NPH	Human Pork	Milky-white when mixed	1–1½	4–12	24+
Lente	Human	Milky-white when mixed	1–2½	6–15	22+
Long-acting Ultralente	Human	Milky-white when mixed	4–6	8–30	24–36+
Glargine	Human	Clear	5	—	24+
Mixtures NPL 75: H 25	Human	Milky-white when mixed	15	½–4	24
NPH 70: R 30	Human	Milky-white when mixed	½	2–12	24
NPH 50: R 50	Human	Milky-white when mixed	½	1–6	14+

H, human; R, regular.

➊ Insulin Programs

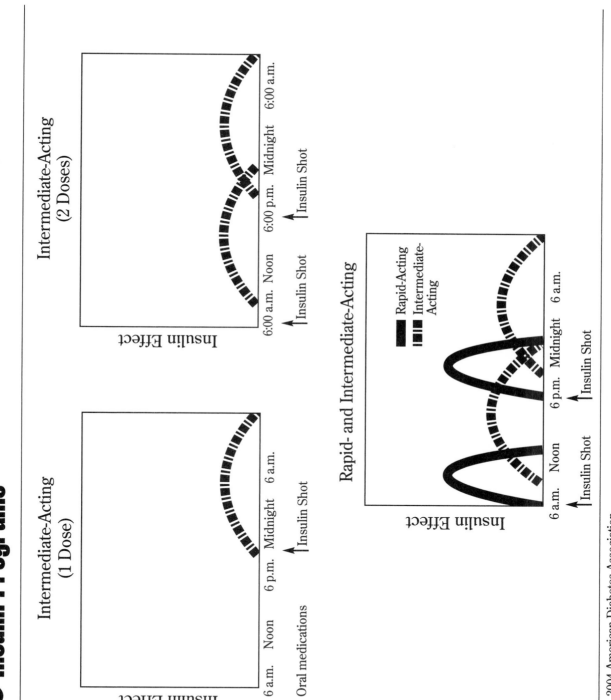

Intermediate-Acting
(1 Dose)

Insulin Effect

6 a.m.   Noon   6 p.m.   Midnight   6 a.m.

Oral medications   ↑ Insulin Shot

Intermediate-Acting
(2 Doses)

Insulin Effect

6:00 a.m. Noon   6:00 p.m. Midnight   6:00 a.m.

↑ Insulin Shot   ↑ Insulin Shot

Rapid- and Intermediate-Acting

▮ Rapid-Acting
▮▮▮ Intermediate-Acting

Insulin Effect

6 a.m.   Noon   6 p.m.   Midnight   6 a.m.

↑ Insulin Shot   ↑ Insulin Shot

INSULIN PROGRAMS *continued*

Insulin Programs

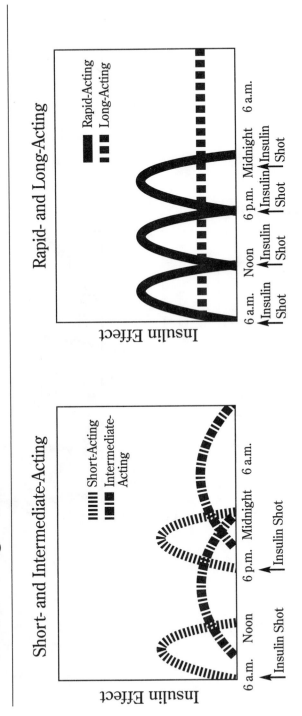

Short- and Intermediate-Acting

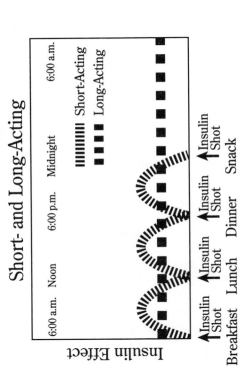

Rapid- and Long-Acting

Short- and Long-Acting

INSULIN PROGRAMS *continued*

Insulin Programs

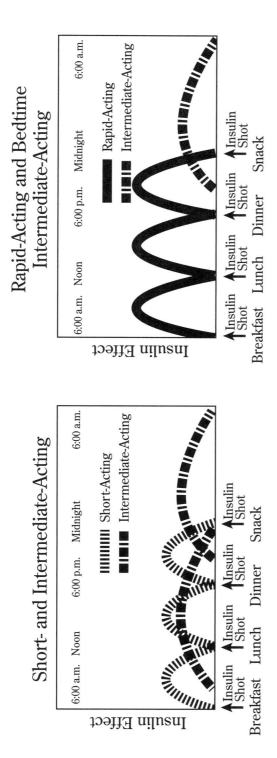

Short- and Intermediate-Acting

6:00 a.m. Noon 6:00 p.m. Midnight 6:00 a.m.

||||||| Short-Acting

▬▬▬ Intermediate-Acting

Insulin Effect

↑Insulin Shot ↑Insulin Shot ↑Insulin Shot

Breakfast Lunch Dinner Snack

Rapid-Acting and Bedtime Intermediate-Acting

6:00 a.m. Noon 6:00 p.m. Midnight 6:00 a.m.

▬ Rapid-Acting

▬▬▬ Intermediate-Acting

Insulin Effect

↑Insulin Shot ↑Insulin Shot ↑Insulin Shot

Breakfast Lunch Dinner Snack

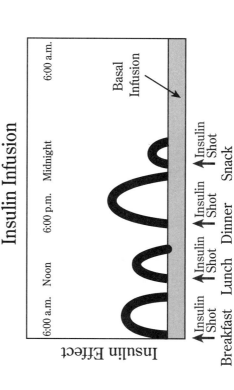

Continuous Subcutaneous Insulin Infusion

6:00 a.m. Noon 6:00 p.m. Midnight 6:00 a.m.

Basal Infusion

Insulin Effect

↑Insulin Shot ↑Insulin Shot

Breakfast Lunch Dinner Snack

181

➔ Intensive Programs

Name_____ Date _____

BASAL INSULIN
The brand name and type of your basal insulin is:

_____

Please take the designated units of this insulin at the following times:

Breakfast	Lunch	Dinner	Bedtime Snack

BOLUS INSULIN
The brand name of your bolus insulin is:

_____

Please take the designated units of this insulin at the following times:

Breakfast	Lunch	Dinner	Bedtime Snack

INTENSIVE INSULIN THERAPY PROGRAM *continued*

Blood Glucose Ranges (mg/dl)	Breakfast	Lunch	Dinner	Bedtime Snack

Please use the scale below to give your premeal insulin, according to your blood glucose levels.

For each 15 grams of additional carbohydrate eaten, add _____ unit(s) to the designated dose.

For each 15 grams of carbohydrate not eaten, subtract _____ unit(s) from the designated dose.

For exercise, subtract _____ unit(s) from the pre-exercise dose.

For stress, add _____ unit(s) to the designated dose.

➜ Giving an Insulin Injection

ONE KIND OF INSULIN

1. Gather your equipment:
   - syringe
   - insulin

2. Wash your hands.

3. Roll the bottle of insulin between the palms of your hands or shake gently to mix the insulin well. Do not shake vigorously. This can leave air bubbles that can get into the syringe.

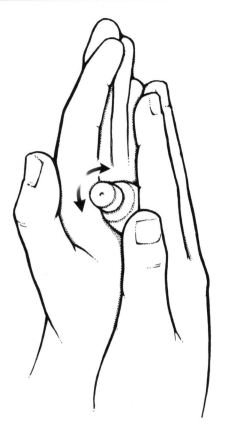

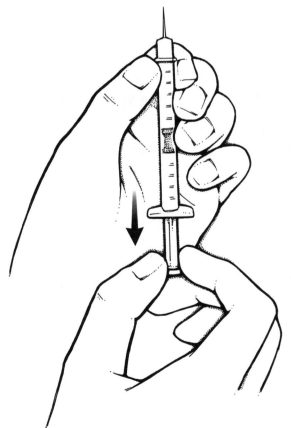

4. Take the needle cap off the syringe.

5. Hold the syringe with the needle pointing toward the ceiling. Keep the syringe at eye level, so you can easily see the markings on the barrel.

6. You must put air into the insulin bottle before you can get the insulin out of the bottle. First, pull the syringe plunger down until the top of the black tip crosses the mark of the dose to be taken. This draws air into the syringe.

   For example: If you take 40 units of insulin, draw about 40 units of air into the syringe.

GIVING AN INSULIN INJECTION *continued*

7. Now turn the syringe tip down. Put the needle through the rubber stopper of the insulin bottle. Push down all the way on the plunger, and hold the plunger in. This puts air into the bottle.

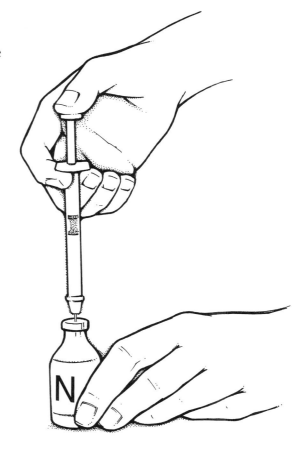

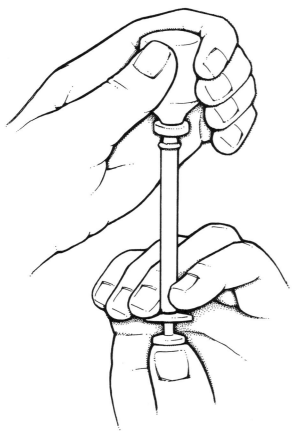

8. Turn the bottle and syringe upside down, so the bottle is on the top and the syringe is on the bottom. Leave the needle in the bottle with the plunger pushed all the way in.

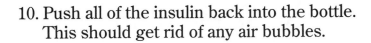

GIVING AN INSULIN INJECTION *continued*

9. Make sure the tip of the needle is in the insulin. Pull down slowly on the plunger. This brings insulin into the syringe. Pull it down until the black tip is 2 or 3 units past your dose.

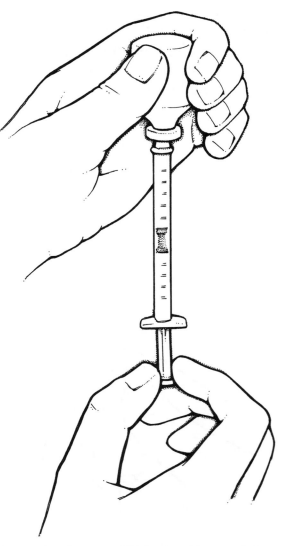

10. Push all of the insulin back into the bottle. This should get rid of any air bubbles.

11. Pull down slowly on the plunger to the exact line of your insulin dose. The right amount of insulin should now be in your syringe.

12. Look in the syringe for air bubbles. If you see air bubbles, push the insulin back into the bottle. Then pull the plunger back to the exact line of your insulin dose. If bubbles are still in the syringe, repeat the process until they are gone.

13. When all the bubbles are out and you have the right dose, pull the bottle straight up and off the needle. Put the needle cap back on the syringe over the needle. Put the syringe down. Check to be sure that you have the right dose. You'll know that it's right if the top of the plunger crosses the right mark on the syringe and there are no air bubbles.

14. Now you are ready to give yourself your shot. Take a deep breath and let it out slowly to help you relax.

GIVING AN INSULIN INJECTION *continued*

TWO KINDS OF INSULIN IN THE SAME SYRINGE

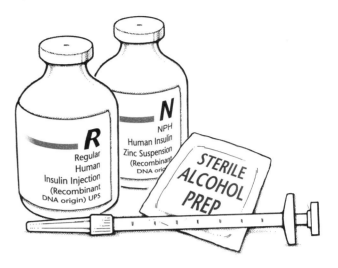

_____insulin (cloudy) _____ units

_____insulin (clear) _____ units

Total _____ units

1. Get your insulin bottles and syringe ready. Wash hands with soap and water.

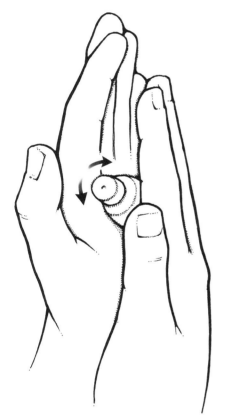

2. Roll _____ insulin between your hands or shake gently. This insulin looks cloudy.

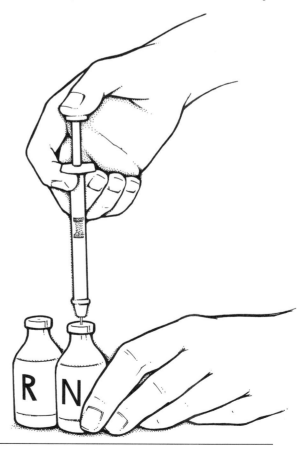

3. Take the needle cap off of the syringe.

4. Pull _____ units of air into the empty syringe. Put the needle through the rubber stopper of the bottle of cloudy insulin. Push air into the bottle. Remove the needle.

© 2004 American Diabetes Association

GIVING AN INSULIN INJECTION *continued*

5. Pull _____ units of air into the same empty syringe. Put the needle into your rapid- or short-acting insulin bottle. This insulin is clear. Push air into the bottle.

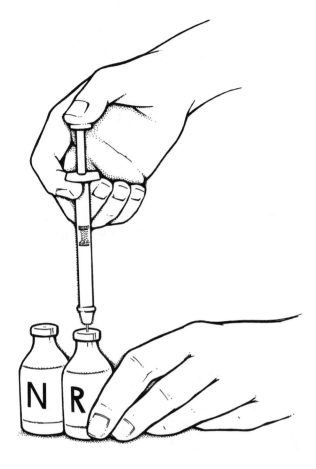

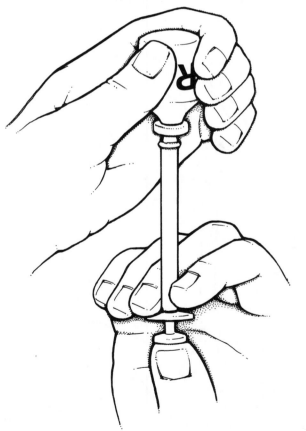

6. With the needle still in the regular insulin bottle, turn the bottle upside down. Pull the plunger halfway down the syringe. This brings insulin into the syringe. Push the insulin back into the bottle to get rid of the air bubbles. Now pull your dose of insulin into the syringe. Carefully measure _____ units of clear insulin. Pull the syringe out of the bottle.

GIVING AN INSULIN INJECTION *continued*

7. Turn the cloudy _____ insulin bottle
   upside down. Put the needle into the bottle.
   Pull the plunger back slowly to total _____
   units. Pull the bottle off the needle.

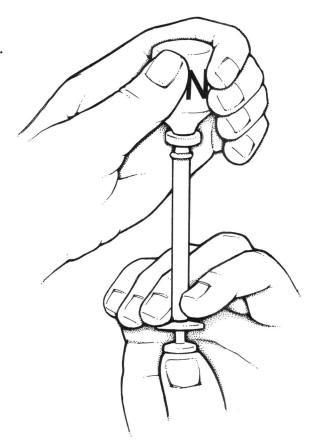

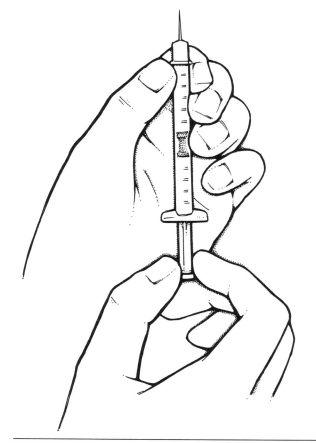

8. Check the total dosage. The dose should
   be:

   _____ (cloudy) ____ units.

   _____insulin (clear) ____ units.

   Total of _____ units now in the syringe.

GIVING AN INSULIN INJECTION *continued*

GIVING THE INJECTION

1. You will inject yourself in your abdomen. Insulin is absorbed most evenly from this site. Your abdomen also has fewer nerves than other places and a pad of fat underneath. Pick a spot from the chart and then find this spot on yourself. Pick a spot at least 1 inch from the place you gave your last shot.

2. If desired, clean the spot with alcohol. Let dry.

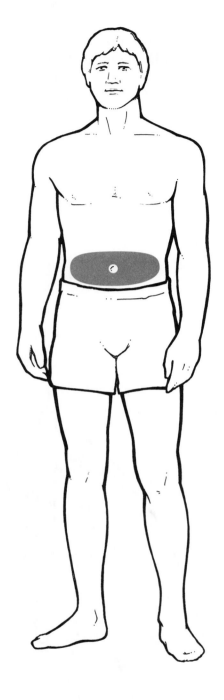

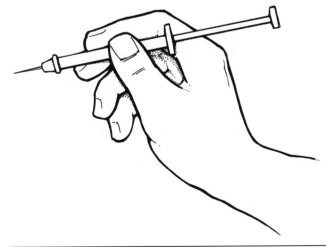

3. Remove the top from the needle. Hold the syringe in one hand as you would hold a pencil.

GIVING AN INSULIN INJECTION *continued*

4. With your other hand, pinch up a couple of inches of skin.

5. Stick the needle straight into the pinched skin. Put the needle all the way in through the skin with one smooth motion.

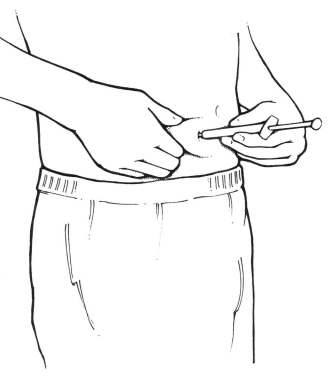

6. Relax the pinch, and slowly push the plunger all the way down. Be sure the insulin is in, then remove the needle.

7. Lightly press down on the site. Don't rub the spot. Don't worry if a drop of blood appears where the needle was.

8. When you are ready to discard your used needles and syringes, put them into a hard plastic or metal container with a screw-on lid. Label and discard according to local regulations.

9. Record the insulin dose you just gave yourself in your diabetes diary.

It may be hard to give yourself a shot the first time, but with practice it will become much easier.

© 2004 American Diabetes Association

➲ Treatment of Low Blood Glucose

If your blood glucose test is:	The amount of food or drink to take is:
Between 50 and 69 mg/dl	15 gm carbohydrate (1 carbohydrate serving **or** 1 cup fat-free [skim] milk)
Less than 50 mg/dl	30 gm carbohydrate (2 carbohydrate servings)

You should feel better in 10–15 minutes after you treat yourself. If your blood glucose is still less than 70 mg/dl or you don't feel better 10–15 minutes after the treatment, take 1 more carbohydrate serving. Test your blood glucose an hour after the reaction to make sure that your blood glucose has gone above 70 mg/dl and stayed there.

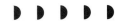

EXAMPLES OF TREATMENTS FOR LOW BLOOD GLUCOSE

(All equal about 15 gm carbohydrate or 1 fruit serving)

If your blood glucose is between 50 and 69 mg/dl, take the amount listed. If your blood glucose is less than 50 mg/dl, take twice the amount listed.

Foods	Amount
Orange or apple juice	½ cup
Grape or cranberry juice	⅓ cup
Non-diet soft drink	½ cup
Honey or corn syrup	1 Tbsp
Sugar packets	3
Life Savers	3–8 pieces
Glucose tablets	3–4 tablets

An additional carbohydrate snack may be needed at night or after exercise to keep your blood glucose above 70 mg/dl.

➡ How to Use Glucagon

Glucagon is an emergency drug that is given as a shot to raise the blood glucose level. It should be given when the person is not able to swallow or is at risk for choking, or in case of a severe insulin reaction or coma.

A prescription is needed to buy glucagon. It comes in two ways: in a kit or in a box to be mixed. If you use the kit, follow the package instructions.

To prepare glucagon for injection if you do not use a kit:

1. Remove the flip-off seals on bottles 1 and 2. Bottle 1 holds a diluting liquid and bottle 2 holds a white powder.

2. Draw the plunger of an insulin syringe (U-100) back to the 50-unit mark.

3. Steady the smaller bottle with the liquid in it (bottle 1) on the table. Push the needle through the stopper.

4. Inject the air from the syringe into the bottle and then turn the bottle upside down.

5. Withdraw as much of the liquid as possible into the syringe.

6. Remove the needle and syringe from bottle 1 and insert this same needle into bottle 2, the bottle with the powder. Inject all of the liquid from the syringe into bottle 2.

7. Remove the needle and syringe. Shake the bottle **gently** until the glucagon powder dissolves and the liquid becomes clear.

8. Withdraw the entire contents of bottle 2 (the mixed glucagon) into the syringe.

9. Inject the glucagon in the same way you would insulin, using the buttock, thigh, or arm.

10. Turn the person onto one side or stomach. (Vomiting is common after glucagon.)

11. As soon as the person is alert and not feeling sick, he or she should eat something, because glucagon acts for only a short period of time. First, give some juice or a non-diet soft drink, and then additional carbohydrate.

HOW TO USE GLUCAGON *continued*

12. If the person does not wake up within 15 minutes, the dose may be repeated. Call an ambulance.

13. Always call the doctor after an insulin reaction when coma or seizure occurs.

14. Check the package of glucagon periodically to be sure that it hasn't passed the expiration date. It's a good idea to keep an insulin syringe taped to the box so it will be ready.

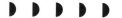

#10	Monitoring Your Diabetes

STATEMENT OF PURPOSE

This session is intended to provide information about the purpose of regular blood testing for glucose and urine testing for ketones and how to record and use the results.

PREREQUISITES

It is recommended that participants bring their meters, as well as blood glucose and urine test records.

OBJECTIVES

At the end of this session, participants will be able to:

1. explain that blood is tested to determine the actual level of glucose in the blood;

2. state the importance of A1C tests;

3. state when to test blood glucose and urine ketones;

4. explain the importance of keeping a complete diabetes record;

5. test blood and urine and record results accurately;

6. define the usefulness of these tests in blood glucose regulation;

7. list personal benefits of monitoring blood glucose levels;

8. list at least four factors that can affect the results of blood tests;

9. name four factors that can affect test results;

10. define personal glucose goals.

CONTENT

Monitoring.

MATERIALS NEEDED

VISUALS PROVIDED	ADDITIONAL

VISUALS PROVIDED

1. Relationship of A1C to Risk of Complications
2. Normal Blood Glucose and Insulin Levels
3. Target Levels
4. Sample Diabetes Record

Handouts (one per participant)
1. Relationship of A1C Levels and Blood Glucose
2. Target Levels
3. Diabetes Record

ADDITIONAL

- Chalkboard and chalk
- Samples of blood glucose and ketone meters and test strips
- Samples of lancets and lancet devices
- Samples of urine ketone test strips
- Samples of records and log books
- Samples of stickers to use for children

METHOD OF PRESENTATION

Start by introducing yourself and telling what you do. Ask participants to introduce themselves. Explain that the purpose of this session is to provide information about the value and use of monitoring.

Present material in a question/discussion format. Begin by asking how they did with their short-term goal and what they learned from it. Conclude the session by presenting examples of records and helping participants make recommendations from data presented. If parents of children or adolescents are in the class, you will need to adapt blood glucose goals and include testing at school, grandparents' homes, child-care facilities, etc.

Monitoring procedures are best taught on a one-on-one basis; however, you may want to demonstrate a blood glucose test to begin the session if any participants are unfamiliar with the procedure.

CONTENT OUTLINE

CONCEPT	DETAIL	INSTRUCTOR'S NOTES
1. Introduction	1.1 Monitoring your diabetes gives you information about your blood glucose level and the effects of meal timing, food intake, medication, activity, and stress.	Ask, "What questions do you have about blood glucose monitoring?" Ask participants how they currently monitor their diabetes. Many participants dislike the use of the word "test" and prefer "check" or "monitor."
	1.2 Your diabetes record helps you keep track so you can use this information more easily.	Stress the importance of monitoring data for use by participants in daily self-care.
2. Methods used to monitor blood glucose levels	2.1 Home blood glucose monitoring is a direct method that tells you what your blood glucose level is at that time.	Ask, "How can you find out your blood glucose level? Your blood glucose patterns?"

CONTENT OUTLINE

CONCEPT	DETAIL	INSTRUCTOR'S NOTES

2.2 An additional test is the A1C test. This is a measure of your blood glucose levels over the previous 3–4 months. It can be done in a laboratory or with a fingerstick drop of blood.

Ask, "Do you know your A1C? What does this number mean to you?" Provide to participants if available. Distribute Handout #1, Relationship of A1C Levels and Blood Glucose. Fructosamine is a less frequently used measure of short-term control, generally a 2–3 week average.

Less than 6% is generally considered the normal value. Use Handout #1, Relationship of A1C Levels and Blood Glucose. A1C results are not directly affected by food or activity on the day of the test. Remind participants to request this test if not done at least every 6 months.

2.3 Your red blood cells carry the memory of all your blood glucose levels. Glucose attaches itself to the hemoglobin in the red blood cell, forming glycated hemoglobin. (This is different from the test done for iron or anemia and used to be called glycosylated hemoglobin or hemoglobin A1C.)

2.4 Measuring A1C gives you the big picture of your glucose level, while a blood glucose check gives you a snapshot of that moment.

Remind participants that blood glucose levels change frequently during the day. Use Visual #2, Normal Blood Glucose and Insulin Levels.

2.5 If your readings and your A1C levels don't match, it may mean that your blood glucose levels are high or low at times when you are not checking— for example, after meals.

2.6 Your A1C reading is not a simple average, but a weighted average. You never have a complete turnover of red blood cells all at once. About half were formed within the last month. So your glucose levels in the last month count for about half of your A1C level, and cells from the previous 2–3 months make up the other half of the measure.

CONTENT OUTLINE

CONCEPT	DETAIL	INSTRUCTOR'S NOTES

2.7 This number tells you about your risk for complications. Research has shown that keeping A1C levels at 7% or lower helps to prevent or delay the long-term complications of diabetes. Every time you lower your A1C level, you lower your risk.

Use Visual #1, Relationship of A1C to Risk of Complications. Ask, "Where is your A1C level now? Where would you like your A1C to be?" Stress the importance of this number for their long-term outcomes.

2.8 Your A1C is important for you because it helps you know how your blood glucose levels are affecting your body and how your treatment plan and hard work are paying off.

Use Visual #1 to illustrate that every decrease in A1C helps lower their risk for complications.

2.9 The Diabetes Control and Complications Trial (DCCT) was a large study of people with type 1 diabetes that showed that people in the group using intensive insulin therapy significantly reduced their risks for some of the long-term complications of diabetes compared with people using standard therapy. Participants in the intensive group had significantly lower blood glucose and A1C levels than those in the standard group.

Ask, "How many of you have heard about the DCCT?" This was a multicenter 10-year trial with 1441 participants. It ended in 1993.

2.10 The risk for diabetic retinopathy was decreased by 76%, neuropathy by 60%, and nephropathy by 35–56%.

Retinopathy = eye disease.
Neuropathy = nerve disease.
Nephropathy = kidney disease.

2.11 The United Kingdom Prospective Diabetes Study (UKPDS) was a large study conducted among people with type 2 diabetes. The results showed that the risk for retinopathy, nephropathy, and perhaps neuropathy was reduced by lowering glucose levels. The overall complication rate was reduced by 25%. For every percentage point decrease in A1C, there was a 35% decrease in risk of complications.

This study was conducted among 5102 patients with newly diagnosed type 2 diabetes. Participants were followed for an average of 10 years.

There is no evidence for reduced risk at below-normal levels (<6.2%). A 16% reduction (which was not statistically significant) in the risk of combined fatal or nonfatal myocardial infarction and sudden death was observed with lower blood glucose levels.

CONTENT OUTLINE

CONCEPT	DETAIL	INSTRUCTOR'S NOTES
	2.12 The UKPDS also showed that reducing blood pressure significantly reduced strokes, diabetes-related deaths, heart failure, microvascular complications, and visual loss.	
3. Home blood glucose monitoring	3.1 Level of glucose in the blood results from interaction of: ■ meal plan ■ medicines for diabetes ■ exercise ■ stress	Ask, "What questions do you have about home blood glucose monitoring? How does glucose get into your blood? What factors affect blood glucose?" Write the list on the board.
	3.2 Glucose levels change throughout the day and night.	Refer to the list on the board. Use Visual #2, Normal Blood Glucose and Insulin Levels. Ask, "What would you expect your glucose to do 1 hour after you eat? When your insulin is peaking?"
4. Blood glucose testing methods	4.1 All blood glucose meters require a drop of blood. Noninvasive meters are being developed.	Ask, "What ways have you found to make testing less painful?" Examples: Use sides of fingers, use lancet devices, wash with warm, soapy water, and use a different finger for each test. Show examples of various lancets and lancet devices. Review disposal procedure.
	4.2 The meter reads the blood glucose value from a test strip. The different meters vary in features, readability, portability, site of testing, and cost.	Show examples of various meters. Specific techniques for the chosen method will be taught on a one-on-one basis by the health care team.
	4.3 Choice of meter is based on personal preference, cost, features (e.g., memory), and ease of use.	Demonstrate alternative site meters if available and visual strips if appropriate.
	4.4 Computer programs are available to you and your health care team that can download the results from your meter's memory.	Point out that this does not replace recording the numbers for pattern management.

CONTENT OUTLINE

CONCEPT	DETAIL	INSTRUCTOR'S NOTES
5. When to check your blood	5.1 When to check is based on the information you need, your blood glucose goals, and your treatment plan.	Ask, "How often do you monitor? How do you use the results?" Schools and workplaces may have policies about blood glucose testing.
	5.2 Checking blood glucose at various times of the day gives a better picture of control than testing only in the morning. Some options are: ■ 1–8 times per day ■ before each meal and at bedtime ■ fasting and 2 hours after the start of each meal ■ before and after each meal ■ once a day, but at different times each day (e.g., Monday before breakfast, Tuesday before lunch) ■ fasting and once more at different times of the day (as above) ■ each day before breakfast	Ask, "How often do you need to check to get the information you need?" Postprandial testing is especially useful for people using rapid-acting insulins or a carbohydrate uptake inhibitor, people who are counting carbohydrate, people with disparate A1C and blood glucose levels, and people with type 2 diabetes or IGT.
	5.3 Test every 2–4 hours when ill.	Ask, "How do you handle monitoring at work? At school? Away from home? How do you respond to people who ask about it?"
6. Factors that affect blood glucose test results	6.1 Factors that affect your blood glucose level: ■ food and beverages ■ medicine for diabetes ■ other medicines ■ exercise ■ stress ■ timing of food and diabetes medication ■ time of day the test is performed	Ask, "What have you noticed that affects your blood glucose level?"
	6.2 Outdated strips: check expiration date.	Ask, "What other factors can affect your test results?"
	6.3 Technique errors: ■ collection methods (e.g., inadequate blood sample) ■ meter not correctly calibrated to strips ■ meter needs to be cleaned	Most meters are now calibrated to plasma glucose values. Plasma values are 10–15% higher than whole blood values.

CONTENT OUTLINE

CONCEPT	DETAIL	INSTRUCTOR'S NOTES
	6.4 Spoiled materials: do not use test materials if there is a color change on the test pad.	Store in a cool dry place. Do not store test materials in direct sunlight, or on or near a stove, radiator or window sill. Heat and dampness can affect test materials.
	6.5 Meter malfunction.	Check the directions for the meter. If it still doesn't work, contact the manufacturer's toll-free hot line or your health care team.
	6.6 If your blood glucose results do not seem right to you, ask yourself if any of these factors might have caused the problem.	Multiple factors affect blood glucose values and participants do not have control over many of them.
7. Use of monitoring information	7.1 Monitoring gives you the information you need to make decisions as you care for your diabetes each day. Without this information, you aren't able to make informed choices.	Ask, "What do you learn by monitoring?"
	7.2 You can determine if you are hypoglycemic by testing your blood glucose. Sometimes you feel as if you are having a reaction, but you are not certain.	A blood glucose level below 70 mg/dl generally indicates hypoglycemia.
	7.3 You can help detect and prevent nightime hypoglycemic reactions by checking your blood glucose before bedtime. This is especially important if your blood glucose was lower than usual or you exercised more than usual that day.	If your blood glucose is low, eat a larger-than-usual bedtime snack. A change in your insulin dose is needed if the finding is consistent.
	7.4 You can determine the effects of a particular activity or food on your blood glucose by checking before and after you do the activity or eat the food.	Monitoring can provide flexibility by increasing the ability to make adjustments and decisions.
	7.5 You can determine if your insulin dose was adequate for the amount of carbohydrate eaten.	

CONTENT OUTLINE

CONCEPT	DETAIL	INSTRUCTOR'S NOTES

8. Blood glucose goals

8.1 Selecting your personal blood glucose goal is one of the most important decisions you can make for about your health. It is the basis your treatment plan and for developing a collaborative relationship with your health care team.

Stress the importance of setting blood glucose goals as a needed first step in choosing treatment options. Clarity in goals establishes collaboration with providers and decreases frustration on both sides.

8.2 It helps to know where you want your glucose levels to be most of the time. Set personal blood glucose goals with your health care team. Setting a range rather than an exact number is more realistic. These goals may change from time to time. You'll use these goals as a guide for using your monitoring data.

Ask, "What is normal blood glucose?" Use Visual #3, Target Levels. These goals are based on whole blood values. Plasma values and goals are 10–15% higher than whole blood values.

	People Without Diabetes (mg/dl)	People with Diabetes (mg/dl)
Before meals	80–125	90–130
After meals	80–130	<180

Remind participants that multiple factors affect blood glucose levels. Because they do not have control over many of these, it is often unrealistic to expect (and to set as a goal) blood glucose levels always in the normal or even the target range.

8.3 Fasting blood glucose tells what your blood glucose is before breakfast. The other levels take into account the effect of food. Blood glucose levels are highest just after a meal.

Point out that if participants have a lower fasting blood glucose level, blood glucose levels are generally lower for the rest of the day. After-meal values are 1–2 hours after the start of the meal.

8.4 These are suggested blood glucose levels. However, you need to choose personal blood glucose goals based on your health, lifestyle, diabetes care goals, and other events in your life. Talk with your health care team about these goals, so you can work together to achieve them.

Ask, "Where would you like your blood glucose to be most of the time? How often do you need to test so that you have the information you need to help keep your blood glucose there?" Encourage participants to set and record personal goals. Ask,

CONTENT OUTLINE

CONCEPT	DETAIL	INSTRUCTOR'S NOTES
		"How do you feel emotionally when your results are in range? Out of range? How does this affect how you manage your diabetes? What are some ideas for ways to handle these times?"
	8.5 Your blood glucose goals may change over time. It is important to remember that every improvement in metabolic control decreases your risks for the long-term complications. Factors to consider are: ■ what is reasonable for you to do ■ what you are able to do ■ your personal risks, barriers, and benefits to various treatment options	Stress the importance of decreasing blood glucose levels slowly.
	8.6 Costs and barriers for optimizing glucose control may include increased risk for low blood glucose, weight gain, expense, and effort involved.	Ask, "What costs and barriers do you see for yourself?" The meal plan may need to be changed to prevent weight gain with improved glucose control.
	8.7 Benefits may include prevention of complications, feeling more energetic, decreased symptoms.	Ask, "What benefits do you see for yourself?" Listing these on a board can help participants consider their options (see Outline #15, *Changing Behavior*).
	8.8 If your blood glucose levels aren't in your goal range, think about what might have caused the problem, such as: ■ more (or less) food, activity, or medicine ■ illness ■ stress	Ask, "What is it like for you when your blood glucose is out of range? How do you handle your feelings? How does it affect how you care for yourself?"

CONTENT OUTLINE

CONCEPT	DETAIL	INSTRUCTOR'S NOTES
	8.9 Try not to get discouraged or dwell on what went wrong. Think about what you can do differently tomorrow. Many people find it more helpful to look for patterns in their blood glucose levels. Look at your record for the past 1–2 weeks. Were there times of the day when your blood glucose levels were too high or too low most days? If so, you may need a change in your medicines or meal plan.	Review participants' records for patterns, use Visual #4, Sample Diabetes Record, or develop an example with the group. Point out that it's often less frustrating to look at patterns. It is where the blood glucose level is most of the time that matters.
9. Tips for blood glucose monitoring	9.1 Blood glucose monitoring may seem hard to do at first. As you learn to use the results to understand your body better and manage your treatment, it will become easier.	Ask, "What barriers have you encountered to monitoring? What strategies have you used to overcome the barriers?" Brainstorm a list of ideas.
	9.2 Before you do a test, gather all test materials and get them in order. You may want to keep your testing equipment in a small box or bag so that all materials are stored together.	Keeping all materials in a pouch or bag helps you be ready to take them with you.
	9.3 Keep your testing equipment near the place you usually test so it will take less time. Keep your diabetes record and a pen in the same place.	Some people own more than one meter to keep in different places. Humidity in a bathroom may damage strips.
	9.4 If you have trouble remembering, put a reminder where you'll be sure to see it (if you test in the morning, put your equipment by your alarm clock). Plan ways to make testing part of your daily routine.	
	9.5 To obtain an adequate drop of blood: ■ wash your hands in warm water before the finger prick ■ dangle fingers at your side for 30 seconds before the finger prick ■ squeeze below the place on your finger you are going to prick until it turns red ■ prick the sides of your fingertips, not the fatty middle part	Laser lancet devices are now on the market, as are devices that allow you to obtain blood from areas other than the fingertips.

CONTENT OUTLINE

CONCEPT	DETAIL	INSTRUCTOR'S NOTES
	■ keep your hand below the level of your heart while you wait for the drop to reach an adequate size ■ gently milk your finger ■ try your thumb or fourth finger—they have a rich blood supply	
	9.6 Do not use monitoring equipment that belongs to another person, and avoid sharing your equipment with others.	Point out the need for precautions to prevent blood-borne infections.
	9.7 Learn to use the results to adjust your medications, diet, or activity.	Teach pattern management here, if appropriate. Refer to Outline #19, *Carbohydrate Counting,* and Outline #9, *All About Insulin.*
10. Recording and use of test results	10.1 Write down test results and bring to your appointments. Bring your meter also, so it can be downloaded.	Use Visual #4, Sample Diabetes Record. Be sure to include comments on the record—note any symptoms or deviations from your usual program.
	10.2 You need to understand personal benefits and barriers for monitoring.	Ask, "What are benefits of blood glucose monitoring for you?" List on the chalkboard. Ask, "What are some barriers you face? What can you do about these barriers?"
	10.3 Monitoring alone will not control your blood glucose. You can learn to use the results of your tests to adjust your diet, medicine, and exercise.	Ask, "What do you need to be able to do with the results to make monitoring worthwhile for you?" List on the chalkboard.
	10.4 Look for patterns in your blood glucose levels. Think about possible causes for your blood glucose patterns or changes from your usual pattern. This is the first step in using the results.	Ask, "Is your blood glucose often high or low at a certain time of day?" Put sample situations on a record form and ask questions about them. Distribute Handout #3, Diabetes Record, if desired.

CONTENT OUTLINE

CONCEPT	DETAIL	INSTRUCTOR'S NOTES
	10.5 Call your doctor or nurse if any problems arise between visits or if there are major changes in your results. Also call if you have low blood glucose reactions for reasons you don't understand, or if your blood glucose tests change suddenly and you don't know why or what to do.	All participants should have individual blood glucose parameters and know when to contact their health care teams. Remind participants to ask for these parameters.
	10.6 It is important to keep careful records.	Demonstrate the record-keeping process and discuss results and potential actions to take. Use of monitoring results is discussed in more detail in Outline #11, *Managing Blood Glucose.*

SKILLS CHECKLIST

Each participant will be able to do a blood glucose test using the appropriate technique and record the results. Select participants will be able to do a urine ketone test using the appropriate technique and record the results.

EVALUATION PLAN

Knowledge will be evaluated by achievement of learning objectives and by responses to questions during the session. Skills will be evaluated by observing a return demonstration of techniques. The ability to apply knowledge will be evaluated by development and implementation of a personal monitoring plan and through program outcome measures.

DOCUMENTATION PLAN

Record class attendance and achieved objectives as appropriate.

SUGGESTED READINGS

AADE Position Statement. Educating providers and persons with diabetes to prevent the transmission of blood-borne infections and avoid injuries from sharps. *The Diabetes Educator.* 1997;23:401–403.

American Diabetes Association. Bedside blood glucose monitoring in hospitals. *Diabetes Care.* 2004;27(Suppl 1):S104.

American Diabetes Association. Consensus Statement: Postprandial blood glucose *Diabetes Care.* 2001; 24;775–778.

American Diabetes Association. Concensus statement: self-monitoring of blood glucose. *Diabetes Care.* 1996;18(Suppl 1): 62–66.

American Diabetes Association. Resource Guide 2004. Blood glucose monitors and data

SUGGESTED READINGS *continued*

management systems. *Diabetes Forecast.* 2004;57(1):RG39–RG58.

American Diabetes Association. Tests of glycemia in diabetes. *Diabetes Care.* 2004;27(Suppl 1):S91–S93.

Carroll MF, Burge MR. Compliance with home blood glucose monitoring among patients with diabetes mellitus. *Practical Diabetology.* 2001;20(4):16–19.

Carter JK, Houston CA, Gilliland SS, Perez GE, Owen CL, Pathak DR, Little RR. Rapid HbA$_{1c}$ testing in a community setting. *Diabetes Care.* 1996;19:764–767.

Chase HP, Pearson JA, Wightman C, Roberts MD, Oderberg AD, Garg SK. Modem transmission of glucose values reduces the costs and need for clinic visits. *Diabetes Care.* 2003;26:1475–1479.

DeCherney GS. Time for a tune-up? *Diabetes Forecast.* 1997;4:23–24.

Deitz PW. Be proactive with patterns. *Diabetes Forecast.* 2000;53(7):54–60.

Derr R, Garrett E, Stacy GA, Saudek CD. Is HbA$_{1c}$ affected by glycemic instability. *Diabetes Care.* 2003;26:2728–2733.

Goldstein DE, Little RR, Lorenz RA, Malone JI, Nathan D, Peterson CM. Tests of glycemia in diabetes: a technical review. *Diabetes Care.* 1995;18:896–909.

Gottlieb SH. Know your ABC's. *Diabetes Forecast.* 2002;55(10):34–36.

Griffin C. Using A1C to gauge blood glucose control. *Nursing.* 2003;33(12):72.

Harris MI. Frequency of blood glucose monitoring in relation to glycemic control in patients with type 2 diabetes. *Diabetes Care.* 2001;24:979–982.

Hoffman RM, Shah JH, Wendel CS, Duckworth WC, Adam KD, Bokhari SU, Dalton C,

Murata GH. Evaluating once-and twice-daily self-monitored blood glucose testing strategies for stable insulin-treated patients with type 2 diabetes. *Diabetes Care.* 2002;25:1744–48.

Park J-Y. Daly JM. Evaluation of diabetes management software. *The Diabetes Educator.* 2003;29:255–267.

Parkin CG, Brooks N. Is postprandial glucose control important? Is it practical in primary care settings? *Clinical Diabetes.* 2002;20:71–74.

Peragallo-Dittko V. Alternative site testing: *Practical Diabetology.* 2002;21(4):48.

Polonsky WH. Ten good reasons to hate blood glucose monitoring. *Diabetes Self-Management.* 2000;17(3):24–30.

Sacks DB, Bruns DE, Goldstein DE, Maclaren NK, McDonald JM, Parrott M. Guidelines and recommendations for laboratory analysis in the diagnosis and management of diabetes mellitus. *Diabetes Care.* 2002;25:750–786.

Scheiner G. Analyze this: interpreting your monitoring log. *Diabetes Self-Management.* 2002;19(2):39–49.

Schwedes U, Siebolds M, Mertes G, the DMBG Study Group. Meal-related structured self-monitoring of blood glucose. *Diabetes Care.* 2002;25:1928–1932.

Sokol-McKay D, Buskirk K, Whittaker P. Adaptive low-vision and blindness techniques for blood glucose monitoring. *The Diabetes Educator.* 2003;29:614–630.

Spollett G. Choosing a meter for home glucose monitoring. *Practical Diabetology.* 2003; 22(1):40–47.

Vincze G, Barner JC, Lopez D. Factors associated with adherence to self-monitoring of blood glucose among persons with diabetes. *The Diabetes Educator.* 2004;30:112–125.

➔ Relationship of A1C to Risk of Complications

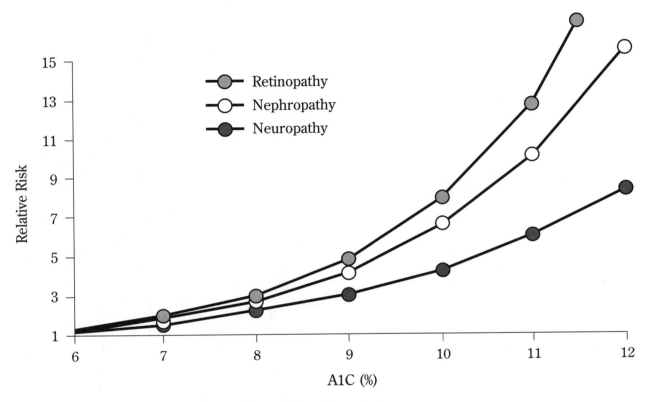

Source: Skyler. *Endocrinol Metab Clin*. 1996;25:243–254, with permission.

➡ Normal Blood Glucose and Insulin Levels

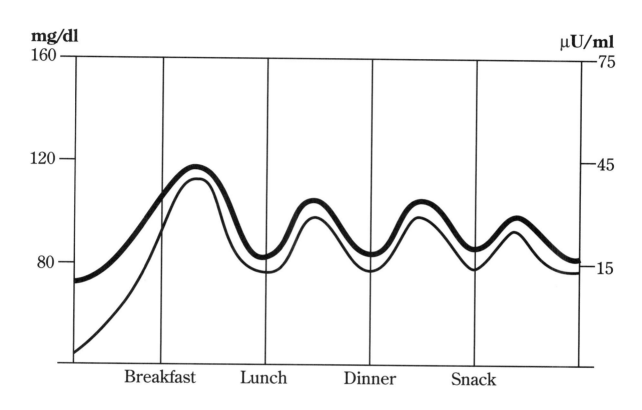

Blood Glucose Level

Plasma Insulin Level

➲ Target Levels

	People Without Diabetes	**People with Diabetes**
Blood glucose (plasma)		
Before meals	80–125 mg/dl	90–130 mg/dl
After meals	80–130 mg/dl	Less than 180 mg/dl
A1C	Less than 6%	Less than 7%
Blood pressure	Less than 130/80	Less than 130/80

➡ Sample Diabetes Record

	Breakfast		Lunch		Supper		Bedtime		Other		Ketones	Comments
	Dose	Blood Glucose	Dose	Blood Glucose	Dose	Blood Glucose	Dose	Blood Glucose	Dose	Blood Glucose		
Sun	18L 6R	220			10L 4R			100			7 A.M. SM	Ate at 10 A.M.
Mon	18L 4R	80		120	12L 4R	170		140		30	7 A.M. Neg	Reaction 3 A.M.
Tues	18L 4R	240		180	12L 4R	240		110		70	7 A.M. SM	Walk 7-8 P.M.
Wed	18L 4R	90			10L 4R	120		80		90	10 P.M. Neg	Walk 7-8 P.M.
Thur	18L 4R	100			10L 4R	180					7 A.M. Neg	Walk 7-8 P.M.
Fri	18L 4R	120		150	10L 4R	160		120			6 P.M. Neg	
Sat	18L 4R	90		70	10L 4R	180		240			10 P.M. Neg	Ate 9 A.M. Tennis 10-12 Reaction 3 P.M.
Number of measurements		7		4		6		6		3		
Total of blood glucose values		940		520		1050		790		190		
Average of blood glucose values		134		130		175		132		64		

➥ Relationship of A1C Levels and Blood Glucose

The A1C blood test tells you your blood glucose levels over the past 3–4 months. This test, along with your home blood glucose checks, can give you a more complete picture of your blood glucose. It also helps you know your risk for long-term complications. The closer your A1C level is to normal, the lower your risk.

Hemoglobin is one part of a red blood cell. It carries oxygen throughout your body. The glucose (sugar) in your blood attaches to the hemoglobin, where it stays for the life of the red blood cell. The combined hemoglobin and glucose unit is called A1C. This test measures the percentage of total hemoglobin that has glucose attached to it. Because red blood cells live for about 120 days, these tests reflect your glucose levels for the previous 3–4 months. The results are not affected much by what you did the day before the test. This is not the same as the test for anemia or iron levels in your blood.

This chart shows how the A1C results compare with average blood glucose levels. The relationship between A1C and plasma glucose levels is shown.

A1C (%)	Average Plasma Glucose	
	(mg/dl)	(mmol/l)
6	135	7.5
7	170	9.5
8	205	11.5
9	240	13.5
10	275	15.5
11	310	17.5
12	345	19.5

4–6 Normal

Your A1C level should be measured every 3–6 months so that you and your health care team can assess your overall diabetes care plan.

➡ Target Levels

	People Without Diabetes	**People with Diabetes**
Blood glucose (plasma)		
Before meals	80–125 mg/dl	90–130 mg/dl
After meals	80–130 mg/dl	Less than 180 mg/dl
A1C	Less than 6%	Less than 7%
Blood pressure	Less than 130/80	Less than 130/80

➡ Diabetes Record

	Breakfast		Lunch		Supper		Bedtime		Other		
	Dose	Blood Glucose	Dose	Blood Glucose	Dose	Blood Glucose	Dose	Blood Glucose	Dose	Blood Glucose	Ketones	Comments
Sun											
Mon											
Tues											
Wed											
Thur											
Fri											
Sat											

Number of measurements _____

Total of blood glucose values _____

Average of blood glucose values _____

214

| #11 | **Managing Blood Glucose** |

▶ ▶ ▶ ▶ ▶

STATEMENT OF PURPOSE

This session is intended to identify and define the factors that influence blood glucose levels, show how these factors interrelate, and discuss the short-term complications of diabetes. Instructions for sick-day management and recognizing and treating hypoglycemia and hyperglycemia are included.

PREREQUISITES

It is recommended that participants have basic knowledge about the pathophysiology of diabetes. It is also suggested that participants bring their diabetes monitoring records.

OBJECTIVES

At the end of this session, participants will be able to:

1. define normal fasting blood glucose levels;

2. state benefits of near-normal blood glucose levels;

3. identify the three treatment components that affect regulation of blood glucose;

4. define hypoglycemia and hyperglycemia and list two causes of each;

5. define ketones and ketosis;

6. identify and discriminate between symptoms of hypoglycemia and hyperglycemia;

7. state actions to take that differ between hypoglycemia and hyperglycemia;

8. state action to treat hypoglycemia that is appropriate for the severity and the time of the reaction;

9. state appropriate ways to manage blood glucose when ill, and state when to seek medical care;

10. identify food and drink choices to help with sick-day management.

CONTENT

Monitoring; Acute Complications.

MATERIALS NEEDED

VISUALS PROVIDED

1. Normal Blood Glucose and Insulin Levels
2. Insulin Action Times
3. Target Levels

Handouts (one per participant):
1. Treatment of Low Blood Glucose
2. How to Use Glucagon
3. Sick-Day Guidelines
4. Sick-Day Record

ADDITIONAL

- Chalkboard and chalk
- MedicAlert or other diabetes identification information
- Glucagon kit
- Samples of glucose products

METHOD OF PRESENTATION

Start by introducing yourself and telling what you do. Ask participants to introduce themselves and say how long they have had diabetes and how it is being treated. Explain that the purposes of this session are to define factors that affect blood glucose levels and provide ways to use this information in the participants' own self-care. The first section is a review of factors that influence glucose levels. The second reviews acute problems related to blood glucose values.

Present material in a question/discussion format. Use the participants' own experiences as case studies, asking others for ideas about ways to handle the situation. Use monitoring records or develop examples that participants can use for problem-solving.

CONTENT OUTLINE

CONCEPT	DETAIL	INSTRUCTOR'S NOTES
1. Managing blood glucose	1.1 This means keeping the factors that raise your blood glucose balanced with the factors that lower it. The body maintains this balance.	Ask, "What questions or concerns do you have about your blood glucose levels? What is your target blood glucose?"
	1.2 In people who don't have diabetes, blood glucose rises promptly after food is eaten, insulin is released by the pancreas in response to the increased blood glucose levels, and blood insulin levels rise. Usually, serum blood glucose goes no higher than 140 mg/dl and returns to the pre-meal level 2 hours after beginning to eat.	Use Visual #1, Normal Blood Glucose and Insulin Levels. Insulin production increases 40 times within 5–15 minutes after starting a meal. Within 30 minutes, the pancreas releases a uniform stream of insulin for as long as it takes to digest the meal.
	1.3 In people with diabetes, very little or no insulin is made, or the insulin	Ask, "How does glucose get into the blood? Where does it come

CONTENT OUTLINE

CONCEPT	DETAIL	INSTRUCTOR'S NOTES
	doesn't work to lower blood glucose levels. You need to compensate for this lack of insulin action. You need to do what your body once did for you.	from?" Injected insulin works more slowly than insulin made by the pancreas, and its effects last longer (even rapid-acting and short-acting insulins).
	1.4 Keeping the balance will help to prevent both the short-term (acute) and long-term (chronic) problems of diabetes.	Many people with diabetes object to the word "control" in relation to diabetes. Manage or regulate are more acceptable.
	1.5 The basic factors involved in blood glucose management are food, exercise, and diabetes medicines (insulin or pills). Meal planning and exercise are part of all diabetes treatment plans.	Ask, "How does food affect your blood glucose? Diabetes medicine? Exercise?" Type 1 diabetes must be treated with insulin. In type 2 diabetes, oral medicines and/or insulin are included as needed.
	1.6 Knowing how these factors interact, your test results, and your personal blood glucose goals are the basis for decisions you and your health care team make about your plan.	
	1.7 One of the most frustrating aspects of diabetes is the difficulty of keeping all of these factors in balance.	Ask, "What do you do when your blood glucose goes off track?" Acknowledge the frustration of this and the inadequacy of current therapy. Review the following material only if appropriate based on audience interest.
2. Meal plan	2.1 There are four basic purposes of a diabetes meal plan: ■ to provide appropriate food in amounts and at intervals that will balance with insulin or oral medication to maintain target blood glucose levels ■ to achieve and maintain a reasonable body weight ■ to provide nutritional needs ■ to normalize blood fats, which minimizes risks for cardiovascular disease	Ask, "What is your main purpose for using a meal plan?" The insulin may be secreted by the individual's pancreas or administered by injection. Remind patients with type 2 diabetes that weight loss may increase the body's sensitivity to the insulin still being made by the pancreas, so they may not need to keep taking diabetes pills or insulin injections.

217

CONTENT OUTLINE

CONCEPT	DETAIL	INSTRUCTOR'S NOTES
3. Exercise	3.1 Exercise has the same beneficial effects for the person with diabetes as for those without diabetes.	Ask participants if they exercise and what their exercise program is, including type and schedule.
	3.2 Exercise usually will lower blood glucose in well-regulated diabetes.	Lower glucose levels can occur 24–48 hours after exercise.
	3.3 Consistent exercise at a comfortable level is the aim.	
	3.4 Aerobic exercise also helps reduce body fat.	
4. Medications to lower blood glucose	4.1 Oral agents stimulate the pancreas to produce more insulin, increase sensitivity to insulin, or alter your ability to absorb carbohydrates.	See Outline #8, *Oral Medications*.
	4.2 Insulin works to lower blood glucose. Combinations of insulins and multiple injections are used to provide more even blood glucose levels throughout the day and to provide peak action when meals are eaten.	Ask, "Why might it be desirable to combine two kinds of insulin? Why do some people take two or more shots a day?" Use Visual #2, Insulin Action Times. See Outline #9, *All About Insulin*.
5. Monitoring	5.1 Monitoring does not regulate your blood glucose. It gives you information about how well your meal plan, exercise, and medicines are balanced.	Ask, "What do you learn from monitoring? What are ways you use monitoring information?" See Outline #10, *Monitoring Your Diabetes*.
	5.2 Monitoring tells you if you are meeting the blood glucose goals you set for yourself.	
	5.3 You can learn to use the information from your tests to adjust your treatment plan.	
	5.4 You can use the information to find your usual pattern of blood glucose.	
	5.5 You can use the information to determine how certain foods, activities, or weight loss affect your diabetes.	Problem-solve using participants' records or sample records.
	5.6 You can use the information to determine if your blood glucose is too high or too low.	Define these as the acute or short-term complications of diabetes.

CONTENT OUTLINE

CONCEPT	DETAIL	INSTRUCTOR'S NOTES
6. Hypoglycemia	6.1 Regulating blood glucose helps to prevent the acute complications of diabetes. One of these is hypoglycemia or low blood glucose, sometimes called an insulin reaction.	Ask, "What questions or concerns do you have about hypoglycemia?" Hypo = low; Glyc = glucose (sugar); Emia = blood
	6.2 Hypoglycemia is caused by too much effect of things that lower blood glucose (insulin, sulfonylureas, exercise) and/or too little food. Physical or emotional stress can also cause low blood glucose. Hypoglycemia is not likely to occur in diabetes managed with only diet and exercise.	For each type of insulin, ask participants when before-breakfast and evening doses would lower blood glucose levels the most.
	6.3 The signs and symptoms of hypoglycemia are: blood glucose level below 70 mg/dl, sweating, weakness, hunger, anxiety, trembling, fast heartbeat, irritability, inability to think clearly, headache, drowsiness, numbness or tingling around lips, confusion, coma, and convulsions.	Ask, "What symptoms of hypoglycemia do you have?" Write these on the board. Nightmares or restlessness may be noted by others if hypoglycemia is nocturnal.
	6.4 Some people feel symptoms at higher levels and others cannot detect early symptoms at all. Some people do not have any of the listed symptoms; however, most people have the same symptoms each time they are hypoglycemic.	As blood glucose levels come into the target range, patients who have been hyperglycemic for some time and have felt low blood glucose symptoms at higher levels will notice that they don't feel symptoms until they drop close to 70 mg/dl.
	6.5 Hypoglycemia has a rapid onset (few minutes).	
	6.6 Driving with low blood glucose levels is extremely dangerous. Always carry a source of glucose in your car. Have diabetes identification clearly visible. Keep a diabetes wallet card next to your driver's license.	Stress the need for those with hypoglycemia unawareness to test their blood before driving. A small card on the dashboard will inform helpers more quickly than a necklace or bracelet that may not be seen.

CONTENT OUTLINE

CONCEPT	DETAIL	INSTRUCTOR'S NOTES
7. Treatment of hypoglycemia	7.1 Use a carbohydrate, such as sugar cubes, juice, or glucose tablets. You need to carry something with you to treat hypoglycemia at all times. Do not go off by yourself or lie down and wait for it to go away.	Distribute Handout #1, Treatment of Low Blood Glucose, and discuss. Show types of glucose products. Point out that participants who are lactose intolerant should not use milk for treatment.
	7.2 Wait 10–15 minutes. Test blood glucose again, and repeat treatment if blood glucose remains below 70 mg/dl, or if there is no relief of symptoms.	Tell participants to keep a can of juice near the bed for nightime reactions.
	7.3 At night or after exercise, you may need to follow the initial treatment with a snack to keep your blood glucose level above 70 mg/dl.	
	7.4 Glucagon is a hormone that helps the liver release its store of glucose into the bloodstream.	
	7.5 Glucagon can be given if a person is comatose or unable to eat. Call for emergency help if no glucagon is available. Glucagon may be less effective if administered in close succession, because the amount of stored glucose is less available.	Ask, "Do you have someone who knows what to do if you have a reaction?" Glucagon injection technique should be taught to families of patients prone to severe hypoglycemia, who have asymptomatic hypoglycemia, or who are using intensive insulin therapy. Glucagon is not appropriate for people with type 2 diabetes. Distribute Handout #2, How to Use Glucagon, if appropriate. Demonstrate kit.
	7.6 Record the time of day, blood glucose level, and any precipitating causes.	
	7.6 If you have more than one unexplained reaction a week, consult your health care team.	
	7.7 It is very important to wear identification that states you have diabetes.	Distribute forms from the Medic Alert Foundation (800-633-3130) or others.

CONTENT OUTLINE

CONCEPT	DETAIL	INSTRUCTOR'S NOTES
8. Hyperglycemia	8.1 Hyperglycemia (blood glucose levels above the normal range) is another acute complication.	Ask, "What questions or concerns do you have about hyperglycemia? What is hyperglycemia?" Hyper = high Glyc = glucose Emia = blood
	8.2 If your glucose reading is often higher than 130 mg/dl before meals and 180 mg/dl after meals or your A1C is 7% or higher, it is too high and needs to be treated.	
	8.3 Hyperglycemia is caused by too little effect of things that lower blood glucose (insulin, oral medication, exercise), and/or too much effect of things that raise blood glucose (insulin that has expired or "gone bad," overeating, weight gain, infection, physical or emotional stress).	Hyperglycemia for no apparent reason may be caused by illness, infection, or emotional stress.
	8.4 The signs and symptoms of hyperglycemia are: higher blood glucose than usual, increased urine output, increased thirst, dry skin and mouth, fatigue and visual blurring, and, in the extreme, marked dehydration, lethargy, confusion, coma, and sometimes stroke. Hyperglycemia usually has a gradual onset.	Ask, "What are the symptoms of hyperglycemia?" Write these on the board. Point out that there may not be any symptoms.
9. Acute consequences of hyperglycemia	9.1 In type 1 diabetes during hyperglycemia, breakdown of fats caused by lack of insulin results in ketones appearing in the blood. Ketones are acids.	Discuss ketoacidosis only if appropriate for the audience. Mild ketosis can also occur during a weight-reduction diet.
	9.2 When hyperglycemia progresses, the excess ketones appear in the urine. This is a warning sign of impending ketoacidosis.	Blood or urine can be tested for ketones. Trace urinary ketones in the morning may indicate a nocturnal insulin reaction.

CONTENT OUTLINE

CONCEPT	DETAIL	INSTRUCTOR'S NOTES
10. Ketone monitoring	10.1 Ketones appear in the blood and urine when the body cells don't have enough glucose to use for energy because there is: ■ not enough insulin activity because of inadequate dose or illness ■ not enough carbohydrate, as in a weight loss diet or with hypoglycemia	Present this section only if participants will test ketones. Ask, "What are ketones?" Blood glucose tests do not provide information about ketones. Urine or blood tests are needed for ketone results.
	10.2 The body burns fat and protein for energy when glucose is not available. Ketones are a waste product of this metabolism.	An analogy is ashes left in a fireplace when logs are burned.
	10.3 Ketones are acid. A buildup of ketones upsets the body's balance, and ketoacidosis results.	Ketoacidosis is acidosis due to ketones in the blood.
	10.4 Several products are on the market to test for urine ketones.	Show examples of various strips and meters that measure blood ketones.
	10.5 Urine tests reflect the amount of ketones in the blood during the time the urine was made by the kidneys. Blood tests show current levels.	Urine reflects ketones in the blood since the time of last voiding.
11. When to check for ketones	11.1 If you have type 1 diabetes: ■ check whenever your blood glucose is over 300 mg/dl ■ check whenever you feel ill ■ early-morning tests can tell you if you had a reaction during the night	Present information specific for participants.
	11.2 If you have type 2 diabetes: ■ check whenever you feel ill ■ check whenever your blood glucose is running high most of the time	Ketoacidosis is rare in type 2 diabetes.
12. Results of ketone tests	12.1 If ketone results are positive, drink water or other sugar-free drinks. Extra insulin and fluids may help to prevent ketoacidosis.	This helps to flush ketones from the body. Provide information about insulin coverage if appropriate.

CONTENT OUTLINE

CONCEPT	DETAIL	INSTRUCTOR'S NOTES
	12.2 Test blood glucose and urine ketones every 2 hours until normal.	
	12.3 Call your health care team if tests remain elevated or you feel sick.	
	12.4 Symptoms of ketoacidosis are those of hyperglycemia (see 8.4) plus fruity breath; loss of appetite; nausea; vomiting; abdominal pain; faster, deeper breathing; confusion; and coma. If untreated, death may occur.	Encourage patients to seek help from their health care team or go to an emergency room. Drinking sugar-free fluids and taking regular insulin may be used as an early treatment.
	12.5 If you have stomach pain, nausea, vomiting, rapid breathing, or sweet, fruity-smelling breath, call your health care team or emergency room.	These are early signs of diabetic ketoacidosis (DKA).
	12.6 In type 2 diabetes, symptoms of severe fatigue, dehydration, abdominal pain, nausea, vomiting, and confusion without ketones are serious and should be reported right away. A coma can occur if these symptoms are not treated.	These are early symptoms of hyperglycemic hyperosmolar nonketotic syndrome. Encourage patients to seek help from the health care team or go to an emergency room.
13. Treatment of hyperglycemia	13.1 Treatment is based on cause.	
	13.2 Take your usual medicines, eat planned meals, drink plenty of sugar-free fluids, and test your blood glucose and ketones (if >300 mg/dl) every 4 hours until back to the usual range.	Remind participants to try to determine possible cause. Fluids may help flush ketones from the body in early stages.
	13.3 Contact your health care team if you have any of the following: ■ blood glucose greater than 170 mg/dl for more than a week ■ any symptoms of hyperglycemia ■ presence of ketones ■ two consecutive blood glucose readings of more than 300 mg/dl ■ vomiting, confusion, or symptoms of severe dehydration	Give appropriate guidelines for your setting or patient population. Look for moderate to large ketones in the urine.

CONTENT OUTLINE

CONCEPT	DETAIL	INSTRUCTOR'S NOTES
14. Difference between hypo- and hyper-glycemia	14.1 Measure blood glucose as soon as either high or low blood glucose is suspected. If hyperglycemia is found, measure urine ketones.	Generally, blood glucose must be 70 mg/dl or less to confirm hypoglycemia.
	14.2 Hypoglycemia occurs rapidly, within minutes. Hyperglycemia develops slowly, over hours or days.	
	14.3 If unable to test, treat with glucose as though hypoglycemia were present, and test blood glucose as soon as possible.	If symptoms are relieved by treatment with glucose, they were likely due to low blood glucose levels.
15. Sick-day management	15.1 An illness or infection can affect your blood glucose control. Make a sick-day plan with your health care team before illness occurs.	Ask, "What questions or concerns do you have about sick-day care?" Distribute and review Handouts #3, Sick-Day Guidelines, and #4, Sick-Day Record.
	15.2 Take your diabetes medicine as usual. Monitor your blood glucose at least every 4 hours. Test urine ketones every time you go to the bathroom if hyperglycemic.	Illness increases insulin resistance. More frequent monitoring is needed when blood glucose levels are elevated.
	15.3 If possible, eat as usual. You may want to choose more soft or liquid foods. If you are unable to eat everything, try to have at least the carbohydrate foods. If you can't eat, drink high-carbohydrate liquids.	Ask, "What foods appeal to you when you are sick? What foods are you able to eat?" See Handout #3, Sick-Day Guidelines, page 2. Make sure all participants have a plan that includes carbohydrate and medication adjustments, fever reduction information, monitoring information, and when to contact a health care professional.
	15.4 If your blood glucose is high, you are vomiting, or you have urine ketones, call your health care team.	
	15.5 You need to tell all health professionals (doctors, podiatrists, and dentists) that you have diabetes.	This is particularly important before any type of surgery.

CONTENT OUTLINE

CONCEPT	DETAIL	INSTRUCTOR'S NOTES
16. Hints and tips	16.1 Everyone's blood glucose goes out of range now and then. This is often hard to cope with, especially when the results are unexpected.	Ask, "How do you handle these frustrations?" Some people have symptoms of low blood glucose as levels move nearer to the target range. If blood glucose is 70 mg/dl or higher, advise patients to try to wait for symptoms to decrease. If unable to tolerate symptoms, treat minimally (e.g., one saltine cracker).
	16.2 Contact your health care team if your blood glucose is out of your goal range nearly every day.	Close class by asking participants to identify their personal blood glucose goal (health outcome) and one step they will take this week to work toward this goal (behavior-change goal).

SKILLS CHECKLIST

None.

EVALUATION PLAN

Knowledge will be evaluated by achievement of learning objectives and by responses to questions during the session. The ability to apply knowledge will be evaluated by development of personal blood glucose goals, by development and implementation of a plan to achieve those goals, and through program outcome measures.

DOCUMENTATION PLAN

Record class attendance and achieved objectives as appropriate.

SUGGESTED READINGS## Overview

American Diabetes Association. *Diabetes Education Goals*. 3rd Edition. Alexandria, VA: American Diabetes Association; 2002.

Funnell MM, Kruger DF. Type 2 diabetes: treating to target. *Nurse Practitioner*. 2004; 29:11–25.

Riddle MC, Rosenstock J, Gerich J, on behalf of the insulin glargine 4002 study investigators. The treat to target trial. *Diabetes Care*. 2003;26:3080–3086.

Testa MA, Simonson DC. Health economic benefits and quality of life during improved glycemic control in patients with type 2 diabetes mellitus: A randomized, controlled, double-blind trial. *JAMA*. 1998; 280:1490–1496.

University of New Mexico Diabetes Team. *101 Tips for Improving Your Blood Sugar*. 2nd Edition. Alexandria, VA: American Diabetes Association, 1999.

Acute Complications

Bloomgarden Z. Heading off the diabetic crisis. *Emergency Medicine*. 1996;96:12–31.

Draelos MTT, Jacobson AM, Weinger K, Widom B, Ryan CM, Finkelstein DM, Simonson DC. Cognitive function in patients with insulin-dependent diabetes mellitus during hyperglycemia and hypoglycemia. *American Journal of Medicine*. 1995; 98:135–143.

Hyperglycemia

American Diabetes Association. Hyperglycemic crises in diabetes. *Diabetes Care*. 2004; 27(Suppl 1):S94–S102.

American Diabetes Association Resource Guide 2004. Urine Testing. *Diabetes Forecast*. 2004;57(1):RG64–RG69.

D'Arrrigo T. Acidosis: the snake in the grass. *Diabetes Forecast*. 2001;54:70–74.

Fain JA. Lowering the boom on hyperglycemia. *Nursing*. 2001;31(8):48–51.

Hardman L, Young FT. Combating hyperosmolar hyperglycemic nonketotic syndrome. *Nursing*. 2001;31(3):32–34.

Kitabchi AE, Umpierrez G, Murphy MB, Barrett EJ, Bokhari SU, Dalton C, Murata GH. Management of hyperglycemic crises in patients with diabetes: a technical review. *Diabetes Care*. 2001;24:131–153.

Weil RM. Getting to know ketones. *Diabetes Self-Management*. 2004;20(6):100–104.

Hypoglycemia

American Diabetes Association. Position statement: Hypoglycemia and employment/licensure. *Diabetes Care*. 2004;27 (Suppl 1):S134.

American Diabetes Association. Resource Guide 2004. Medical identification products. *Diabetes Forecast*. 2004;57(1):RG74–RG77.

American Diabetes Association. Resource Guide 2004. Products for treating low blood glucose. *Diabetes Forecast*. 2004;57(1):RG59–RG62.

Boyle PJ, Kempers SF, O'Connor AM, Nagy RJ. Brain glucose uptake and unawareness of hypoglycemia in patients with insulin-dependent diabetes mellitus. *The New England Journal of Medicine*. 1996;334:292–295.

Clark DJ, Gonder-Frederick L, Polonsky W, Schlundt D, Kovatchev B, Clarke, W. Blood glucose awareness training. *Diabetes Care*. 2001;24:637–642.

Cox DL, Gonder-Frederick LA, Kovatcher BP, Sulian DM, Clarke WL. Progressive hypoglycemia's impact on driving simulation performance: occurrence, awareness, and correction. *Diabetes Care*. 2000;23:163–170.

Cryer PE, Davis SN, Shamoon H. Hypoglycemia in diabetes: a technical review. *Diabetes Care*. 2003;26:1902–1912.

Cryer PE, Fisher JN, Shamoon H. Hypoglycemia: a technical review. *Diabetes Care*. 1994; 17:734–755.

Dailey GE. Hypoglycemia in elderly patients treated with oral agents. *Practical Diabetology*. 2002;21(2):7–14.

Dey J, Misra A, Desai NG, Mahapatra AK, Padma MV. Cognitive function in younger type II diabetes. *Diabetes Care*. 1997;20: 32–35.

Managing Blood Glucose

SUGGESTED READINGS *continued*

Drass JA, Feldman RHL. Knowledge about hypoglycemia in young women with type I diabetes and their supportive others. *The Diabetes Educator.* 1996;22:34–38.

Franz MJ. Treatment of hypoglycemia. *Practical Diabetology.* 2003;22(3):40–41.

Gonder-Fredrick L, Cox D, Kovatchev B, Schlundt D, Clarke W. A biopsychobehavioral model of risk of severe hypoglycemia. *Diabetes Care.* 1997;20:661–669.

Herter CD. Differential diagnosis of reactive hypoglycemia. *Practical Diabetology.* 2002;21(4):22–28.

Kalergis M, Schiffrin A, Gougeon R, Jones PJH, Yale J-F. Impact of bedtime snack composition on prevention of nocturnal hypoglycemia in adults with type 1 diabetes undergoing intensive insulin management using lispro insulin before meals. *Diabetes Care.* 2003;26:9–15.

Leese GP, Wang J, Broomhall J, Kelly P, Marsden A, Morrison W, Frier BM, Morris AD. Frequency of severe hypoglycemia requiring emergency treatment in type 1 and type 2 diabetes. *Diabetes Care.* 2003; 26:1176–1180.

Lincoln NB, Faleiro RM, Kelly C, Kirk BA, Jeffcoate WJ. Effect of long-term glycemic control on cognitive function. *Diabetes Care.* 1996;19:656–658.

Marrero DG, Guare JC, Vandagriff JL, Fineberg NS. Fear of hypoglycemia in the parents of children and adolescents with diabetes: maladaptive or healthy response? *The Diabetes Educator.* 1997;23:281–286.

McCall A. IDDM, countregulation, and the brain. *Diabetes Care.* 1997;20:1228–1229.

Rovner JF: Diabetes and the brain: a complex relationship. *Diabetes Spectrum.* 1997;10:23–70.

Watts SA, Anselmo JM, Smith JA. Combating hypoglycemia in the hospital and at home. *Nursing.* 2003;33(3):32.

Sick Days

Agnew B. What ails you? *Diabetes Forecast.* 2003;56(2): 67–69.

American Diabetes Association. Position statement: Immunization and prevention of influenza and pneumococcal disease in people with diabetes. *Diabetes Care.* 2004; 27(Suppl 1):S111–S113.

Centers for Disease Control. Cold and flu survivor guide. *The Diabetes Educator.* 2004;30:80–90.

Chipkin SR, Lazar H. Perioperative and postoperative glucose control. *Practical Diabetology.* 2002;21(2):33–39.

Diabetes Medicine Chest. *Diabetes Forecast.* 2001;54(2):67–86.

Geerlings SE, Stolk RP, Camps MJL, Netten PM, Collet TH, Hoepelman AI. Risk factors for symptomatic urinary tract infection in women with diabetes. *Diabetes Care.* 2000;23:1737–1741.

Gori M, Campbell RK. Sugar-free medications. *The Diabetes Educator.* 1997;23:269–270, 272, 277–278, 256.

Jacober SJ, Sowers JR. Management of diabetes in patients undergoing surgery. *Practical Diabetology.* 2001;20(4):7–15.

Legget-Frazier N, Mazur ML. Creating a diabetes sick-day plan. *Diabetes Forecast.* 2001;54(8):90–93.

Quartetti HR. FAQs on OTCs. *Diabetes Forecast.* 2004;57(2):68–71.

Smith SA, Poland GA. Use of influenza and pneumococcal vaccines in people with diabetes: a technical review. *Diabetes Care.* 2000;23:95–108

Surgery/Hospitalization

American Diabetes Association. Position statement: Concurrent care. *Diabetes Care.* 2004;27(Suppl 1):S132.

American Diabetes Association: Position statement: Hospital admission guidelines for diabetes mellitus. *Diabetes Care* 2004;27 (Suppl 1):S103.

Bejerkness SD. What to expect in the emergency room. *Diabetes Self-Management.* 2001; 18(4):8–12.

Boord JB, Graber AL, Christmas JW, Powers AC. Practical management of diabetes in critically

SUGGESTED READINGS *continued*

ill patients. *Am J Respir Crit Care Med.* 2001; 164:1763–1767.

Clement S, Braithwaite SS, Magee MF, Ahmann A, Smith EP, Schafer RG, Hirsch IB, on behalf of the Diabetes in Hospitals Writing Committee. Management of diabetes and hyperglycemia in hospitals: a technical review. *Diabetes Care.* 2004;27:553–591.

Cousineau MK, Merkin S, Cohen A, Zonszein J. Total parenteral nutrition and the management of a patient with diabetes mellitus. *Diabetes Spectrum.* 1996;9:73–75.

Finney SJ, Zekveld C, Alia A, Evans T. Glucose control and mortality in critically ill patients. *JAMA.* 2003;290:2041–2047.

Golden SH, Peart-Vigilance C, Kao WHL, Brancati FL. Perioperative glycemic control and the risk of infectious complications in a cohort of adults with diabetes. *Diabetes Care.* 1999;22:1408–1414.

Joshi N, Caputo GM, Weitekamp MR, Karchmer AW. Infections in patients with diabetes mellitus. *The New England Journal of Medicine.* 1999;341:1906–1912.

Kitabchi AE. From research to practice: acute care of patients with diabetes. *Diabetes Spectrum.* 2002;15:17–53.

Levetan C. Controlling hyperglycemia in the hospital: a matter of life and death. *Clinical Diabetes.* 2000;18(1):38–93.

Metchick L, Petit W, Inzucci S. Inpatient management of diabetes mellitus. *Am J Med.* 2002; 113(4):317–323.

Montori VM, Bistrian BR, McMahon MM. Hyperglycemia in acutely ill patients. *JAMA.* 2002;288:2167–2169.

UKPDS

American Diabetes Association. Position statement: Implications of the United Kingdom Prospective Diabetes Study. *Diabetes Care.* 2000;23(Suppl 1):S27–S31.

UK Prospective Diabetes Study (UKPDS) Group: Intensive blood-glucose control with sulfonylureas or insulin compared with conventional treatment and risk of complications in patients with type 2 diabetes (UKPDS 33). *The Lancet.* 1998;352:837–853.

DCCT

American Diabetes Association. Position statement: Implications of the Diabetes Control and Complications Trial. *Diabetes Care.* 2000;23(Suppl 1):S24–S26.

The DCCT Research Group. Influence of intensive diabetes treatment on quality-of-life outcomes in the Diabetes Control and Complications Trial. *Diabetes Care.* 1996; 19:195–203.

The DCCT Research Group. Adverse events and their association with treatment regimens in the Diabetes Control and Complications Trial. *Diabetes Care.* 1995; 18:1415–1427.

The DCCT Research Group. Resource utilization and costs of care in the Diabetes Control and Complications Trial. *Diabetes Care.* 1995; 18:1468–1478.

The DCCT Research Group. The effect of intensive treatment of diabetes on the development and progression of long-term complications in insulin-dependent diabetes mellitus. *The New England Journal of Medicine.* 1993;329:977–986.

The DCCT Research Group. Implementation of treatment protocols in the Diabetes Control and Complications Trial. *Diabetes Care.* 1995;18:361–376.

Thompson CJ, Cummings JFR, Chalmers J, Gould C, Newton RW. How have patients reacted to the implications of the DCCT? *Diabetes Care.* 1996;19:876–879.

➡ Normal Blood Glucose and Insulin Levels

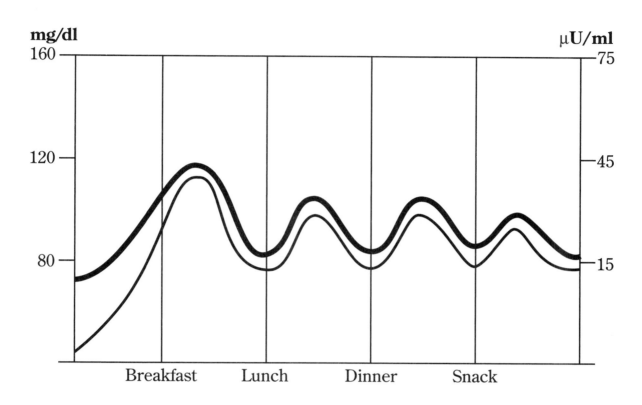

─── Blood Glucose Level

── Plasma Insulin Level

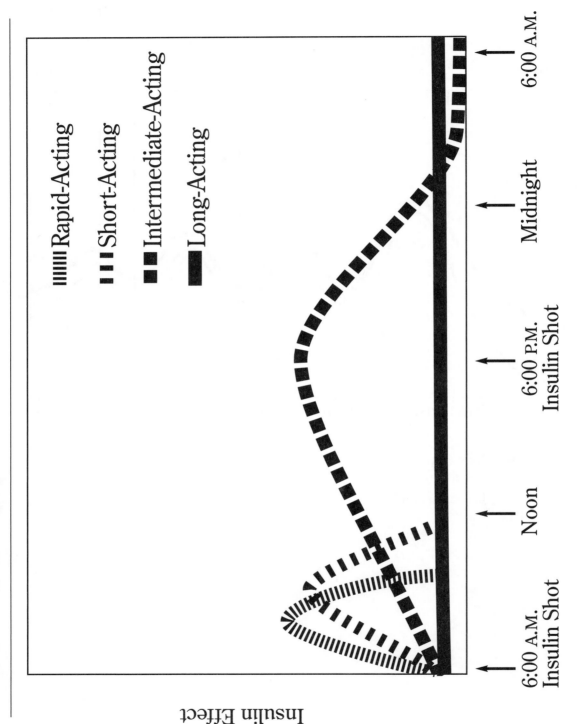

Insulin Action Times

Rapid-Acting

Short-Acting

Intermediate-Acting

Long-Acting

Insulin Effect

6:00 A.M.
Insulin Shot

Noon

6:00 P.M.
Insulin Shot

Midnight

6:00 A.M.

© 2004 American Diabetes Association

➲ Target Levels

	People Without Diabetes	People with Diabetes
Blood glucose (plasma)		
Before meals	80–125 mg/dl	90–130 mg/dl
After meals	80–130 mg/dl	Less than 180 mg/dl
A1C	Less than 6%	Less than 7%
Blood pressure	Less than 130/80	Less than 130/80

➲ Treatment of Low Blood Glucose

If your blood glucose test is:	The amount of food or drink to take is:
Between 50 and 69 mg/dl	15 gm carbohydrate (1 carbohydrate serving **or** 1 cup fat-free [skim] milk)
Less than 50 mg/dl	30 gm carbohydrate (2 carbohydrate servings)

You should feel better in 10–15 minutes after you treat yourself. If your blood glucose is still less than 70 mg/dl or you don't feel better 10–15 minutes after the treatment, take 1 more carbohydrate serving. Test your blood glucose an hour after the reaction to make sure that your blood glucose has gone above 70 mg/dl and stayed there.

EXAMPLES OF TREATMENTS FOR LOW BLOOD GLUCOSE
(All equal about 15 gm carbohydrate or 1 fruit serving)

If your blood glucose is between 50 and 69 mg/dl, take the amount listed. If your blood glucose is less than 50 mg/dl, take twice the amount listed.

Foods	Amount
Orange or apple juice	½ cup
Grape or cranberry juice	⅓ cup
Non-diet soft drink	½ cup
Honey or corn syrup	1 Tbsp
Sugar packets	3
Life Savers	3–8 pieces
Glucose tablets	3–4 tablets

An additional carbohydrate snack may be needed at night or after exercise to keep your blood glucose above 70 mg/dl.

➜ How to Use Glucagon

Glucagon is an emergency drug that is given as a shot to raise the blood glucose level. It should be given when someone is unable to swallow or is at risk for choking, or in case of a severe insulin reaction or coma.

A prescription is needed to buy glucagon. It comes in two ways: in a kit or in a box to be mixed. If you use the kit, follow the package instructions.

To prepare glucagon for injection if you do not use a kit:

1. Remove the flip-off seals on bottles 1 and 2. Bottle 1 holds a diluting liquid and bottle 2 holds a white powder.

2. Draw the plunger of an insulin syringe (U-100) back to the 50-unit mark.

3. Steady the smaller bottle with the liquid in it (bottle 1) on the table. Push the needle through the stopper.

4. Inject the air from the syringe into the bottle and then turn the bottle upside down.

5. Withdraw as much of the liquid as possible into the syringe.

6. Remove the needle and syringe from bottle 1 and insert this same needle into bottle 2, the bottle with the powder. Inject all of the liquid from the syringe into bottle 2.

7. Remove needle and syringe. Shake bottle **gently** until the glucagon powder dissolves and the liquid becomes clear.

8. Withdraw the entire contents of bottle 2 (the mixed glucagon) into the syringe.

9. Inject the glucagon in the same way you would insulin, using the buttock, thigh, or arm.

10. Turn the person onto one side or stomach. (Vomiting is common after glucagon.)

11. As soon as the person is alert and not feeling sick, he or she should eat something, because glucagon acts for only a short period of time. First, give some juice or a non-diet soft drink, and then additional carbohydrate.

12. If the person does not wake up within 15 minutes, the dose may be repeated. Call an ambulance.

13. Always call the doctor after an insulin reaction when coma or seizure occurs.

14. Check the package of glucagon periodically to be sure that it hasn't passed the expiration date. It's a good idea to keep an insulin syringe taped to the box so it will be ready.

➡ Sick-Day Guidelines

These guidelines are for you to use when you have a minor illness, such as a cold, the flu, or an upset stomach. You may also use these guidelines when you have a dental procedure such as a tooth extraction and cannot chew. You will need to talk about sick days with your doctor, nurse, or dietitian—they may have specific guidelines for you.

You will need to test and keep a record of both your blood glucose every 2–4 hours and ketones every 4 hours. Check your temperature about every 4 hours, and keep a record of it, too. If you have a fever, drink some liquid at least once every half hour. If you notice any changes from your usual blood glucose pattern or changes in the way you feel, follow any special guidelines you may have been given.

Call your doctor if you have any of the following:

- rising ketone levels
- ketones for more than 12 hours
- blood glucose levels of greater than 250 mg/dl
- vomiting and/or other unusual symptoms
- high (101.5°F) or rising fever or fever for more than 24 hours

When you call your provider, have your sick-day record nearby so you can report your blood glucose and ketone levels, your insulin dose, and your temperature. (See Handout #4, Sick-Day Record.) If you are unable to reach your doctor quickly, go to the nearest emergency room. Call for help if you are alone and are unable to care for yourself.

If you take insulin, take your usual dose. **Do not omit your insulin.** The stress of being sick can raise your blood glucose level, even if you don't eat. If you take diabetes pills (oral hypoglycemic agents) to control your blood glucose, take your usual dose.

When you are ill, it is important to eat the same amount of carbohydrate that you normally do. If possible, follow your regular diet. If you are having a hard time swallowing, eat soft foods with the same amount of carbohydrate content as your regular diet (see list on page 3). If you can't eat everything, choose carbohydrate foods. If you are sick to your stomach or vomiting, take enough liquids to equal the amount of carbohydrates that you would normally eat. You can space the liquids out over the day. Taking a small sip every 10–15 minutes (for example, during every TV commercial) will help you keep the food or liquid down. The list of liquids and their carbohydrate content on page 3 can help you plan your sick-day diet.

© 2004 American Diabetes Association

If your blood glucose is higher than 240 mg/dl, you need to drink sugar-free liquids, and you may need extra regular insulin. Your health care team will give you instructions when you call.

Even after you start to feel better, you will still need to test your blood glucose and ketones every 4 hours until you are back to your usual pattern. You may want to keep eating soft and liquid carbohydrates until your appetite is back to normal. If you've been very sick to your stomach, start by having clear liquids (things you can see through, such as broth, tea, regular soft drinks, Jell-O, apple or grape juice, and popsicles). When you can keep these down, move on to full liquids (orange or tomato juice, ice cream, and soup), and then to soft foods (oatmeal, toast, plain cooked vegetables, applesauce, rice, noodles, and crackers).

These guidelines are meant to give you the information you need to take care of yourself when you have a minor illness. Feel free to ask your nurse, doctor, or dietitian any questions you might have about this information.

SICK-DAY GUIDELINES *continued*

CARBOHYDRATE CONTENT OF LIQUIDS AND SOFT FOODS

Food Item	Amount	Grams of Carbohydrate
Non-diet soft drink	½ cup	15
Orange juice	½ cup	15
Apple or pineapple juice	½ cup	15
Grape or prune juice	⅓ cup	15
Milk	1 cup	12
Ice cream, vanilla	½ cup	15
Cereal, cooked	½ cup	15
Gelatin, regular	½ cup	20
Sherbet	½ cup	30
Popsicle	1	24
Sugar	1 tsp	4
Coffee, tea, bouillon, broth	1 cup	0
Soup, thin creamy	1 cup	15
Soup, thick chunky	1 cup	20
Cream soup, made with water	1 cup	15
Cream soup, made with milk	1 cup	27
Pudding, regular	½ cup	30
Pudding, sugar-free	½ cup	15
Yogurt, plain or artificially sweetened	1 cup	17
Yogurt, fruit flavored	1 cup	40–60

EXAMPLE: LIQUID REPLACEMENT OF CARBOHYDRATES

Food Item	Amount	Grams of Carbohydrate
Broth	1 cup	0
Jell-O, regular	½ cup	20
7-Up, regular	1 cup (8 oz)	30
Ice cream	½ cup	10
Tea	1 cup	0
Total		**60**

Managing Blood Glucose

➔ Sick-Day Record

Physician Phone _____

Pharmacy Phone _____

Time	Food/Liquids	Insulin/ Medication	Blood Glucose	Urine Ketones	Symptoms (Fever, Nausea, Vomiting, Dizziness, etc.)

| #12 | **Stress and Coping** |

STATEMENT OF PURPOSE

This session is intended to provide information about stress, how it affects glucose levels, and coping strategies. It is also intended to help participants recognize stressful situations in their lives and develop methods for coping with them.

PREREQUISITES

None.

OBJECTIVES

At the end of this session, participants will be able to:

1. define stress;

2. explain that what is stressful for one person may or may not be stressful for another;

3. explain the body's response to stress;

4. list the effects that stress may have on blood glucose;

5. identify and evaluate personally stressful situations;

6. list the ways in which they currently respond to stress;

7. identify one way to cope with a personally stressful situation.

CONTENT

Psychosocial Adjustment.

MATERIALS NEEDED

VISUALS PROVIDED	ADDITIONAL
None.	■ Chalkboard and chalk ■ Information about local diabetes and stress-management support groups and other local resources ■ Information about books on coping with diabetes or stress ■ Video or audiotape about stress or relaxation techniques.

METHOD OF PRESENTATION

Start by introducing yourself and telling what you do. Ask participants to introduce themselves and say how long they have had diabetes. Explain that the purposes of this session are to encourage expression of feelings about stress, to provide information about stress and coping, and to practice relaxation techniques.

A comfortable environment conducive to relaxation is recommended. Present materials in a question/discussion format. Begin by asking how they did with their short-term goal and what they learned from it. Show a videotape, describe a stressful situation, or ask participants to describe stressful experiences to introduce the topic, if desired. End with one of the relaxation exercises or use a relaxation audio- or videotape.

CONTENT OUTLINE

CONCEPT	DETAIL	INSTRUCTOR'S NOTES
1. Definition of stress	1.1 Stress can occur when: ■ an event produces a strain on a person ■ a person thinks of a situation as challenging or threatening, and physiological responses follow ("fight or flight")	Ask, "What questions or concerns do you have regarding stress? What is stress?" Using the chalkboard, list participants' definitions of stress.
	1.2 Stress is influenced by both the individual and the environment. Each of us defines what situations we see as stressful.	Ask, "What is stressful for you?" Stress is defined by our perceptions of a situation, not necessarily the reality.
	1.3 Positive as well as negative situations can be stressful, such as marriage, a new job, or retirement.	Point out that life would be pretty dull without stress. We all need challenges to keep life interesting. Ask, "Have you had situations that you viewed at the time as very stressful that you now see as valuable learning experiences?"
	1.4 We all experience stress from time to time. Too many stresses or a long, intense, physical response to stress can lead to health problems and will affect your diabetes control. Limiting stressful events or positively coping with them is important for your health.	Ask, "What health problems are related to stress?"
2. Evaluating stress-ful situations	2.1 When something happens to people, they size up the situation and make a	Ask, "How do you determine what is stressful to you?" Ask for

CONTENT OUTLINE

CONCEPT	DETAIL	INSTRUCTOR'S NOTES
	judgment about whether the situation could be good or harmful.	examples of situations people may or may not perceive to be stressful (e.g., traffic jam, delayed flight).
	2.2 How stressful an event is depends on how good or harmful we think it is. Other things going on in our lives can change our perception of stress. A particular event may feel very stressful one day and not stressful another day.	
	2.3 Also, our beliefs, values, and goals affect the way we feel about events.	
	2.4 Change of any kind is almost always stressful.	
	2.5 Major life stresses (events such as illness or death in the family) are stressful for almost everyone. Some major life events, such as graduating from school, marriage, the birth of a child, a new job, or retirement, are positive and challenging situations that can cause a stress response.	Have participants identify major stressors in their lives.
	2.5 Minor life stresses are the irritating, frustrating, and distressing demands of daily life, such as being in a traffic jam, arguing with a coworker, tests, phone calls, or doctor visits. Events such as holidays or vacations can also be stresses.	Have participants list or name their minor stressors. Point out that what are major stressors for some are minor for others.
3. How the body responds to stress	3.1 This is sometimes called the fight or flight response.	Ask, "How do you feel when you are in a stressful situation?" (nervous, sweaty, pounding heart, or queasy stomach). List on the board.
	3.2 The body prepares itself for stress by sending out stress hormones (catecholamines, glucagon, cortisol, and growth hormone). These hormones cause symptoms you can feel and changes in your behavior.	

CONTENT OUTLINE

CONCEPT	DETAIL	INSTRUCTOR'S NOTES
	3.3 These stress hormones increase your heart rate and blood pressure, make your breathing rapid and shallow, and may cause your blood glucose to rise.	Ask, "How do you tell the difference between a response to stress and a low blood glucose reaction?" Sometimes the symptoms of stress and hypoglycemia are similar.
	3.4 The levels of glucose and ketones in the blood rise to provide the brain and muscles with important sources of energy. This energy is needed to either fight off stress or run away from it—the fight or flight response.	Ask, "Have you noticed that your blood glucose level is affected by stress?"
	3.5 If this extra energy is not used to fight or run away, it can leave you feeling tense and tired or cause a headache.	
4. Effects of stress on blood glucose	4.1 Stress makes control of diabetes more difficult. In an individual who does not have diabetes, insulin made by the pancreas prevents the blood glucose from rising too high.	
	4.2 In a person with diabetes, the pancreas may not make enough insulin to keep the blood glucose and ketone levels from going too high.	
	4.3 In spite of this, research studies have shown that some individuals actually have a drop in blood glucose as an immediate response to stress.	
	4.4 High or fluctuating blood glucose and ketone levels may result. If stress is short-lived and repetitive, levels of blood glucose and ketones may "bounce" considerably.	
5. Effects of diabetes on stress	5.1 Some people find that they feel less able to deal with stress when they learn they have diabetes. Their energy for coping with other stressors is being used up on diabetes.	Ask, "Have you noticed any changes in the way you handle stress since you learned you have diabetes?"

CONTENT OUTLINE

CONCEPT	DETAIL	INSTRUCTOR'S NOTES
	5.2 Some people find that they feel less able to deal with stress when their blood glucose level is uneven or too high.	Ask, "Have you noticed any change in the way you handle stress when your blood glucose is high or low?"
6. Coping	6.1 One way to deal with a stressor is to eliminate it. If we can't eliminate the stress, we need to find a way to deal with it. This is called coping.	Ask, "What are ways you cope with stress?" List on the board. Diabetes is a stressor that we cannot eliminate so we need ways to cope with it.
	6.2 Everyone needs a variety of coping skills to use in different situations.	Remind participants of the many different styles and ways of coping.
	6.3 Each person deals with stress in his or her own way. We usually behave in ways that are familiar to us.	Ask, "How do you usually act before, during, and after a stressful situation?"
	6.4 Some of these strategies work and some leave us feeling tense, tired, angry, or sick. Some, such as smoking, drinking too much, and drug abuse, cause other problems.	Many people eat more or differently when they feel stressed. There is nothing wrong with that as a strategy, except most of us make choices that have other negative consequences.
	6.5 Other techniques and ways of dealing with stress can help us to feel more in control, relaxed, and less tense after a stressful event.	
	6.6 To determine if a strategy is effective, ask yourself, "Did it work? Did I feel better both temporarily and later? Is this an effective strategy to use in the future?"	People who learn to use varied coping skills and who are flexible in their approach to tough situations deal with stress more easily.
7. Tips for managing stress	7.1 There are three important factors in coping: ■ having enough information ■ feeling in control ■ having the support of others	Ask, "What helps you cope with stress? What hinders you?" Different coping devices are effective in different situations.

CONTENT OUTLINE

CONCEPT	DETAIL	INSTRUCTOR'S NOTES
	7.2 To evaluate your response to stress, you need to recognize your present behavior in a stressful situation. Sometimes it helps to keep a stress diary for 3–4 days. Jot down stresses, how you react or cope, and how you feel during and after stressful situations. You may also want to write down your blood glucose level or use your monitoring record to note stress. This can help you predict or avoid stressful events, solve the problem causing the stress, or learn other ways to cope with things you can't change.	Encourage the group to brainstorm strategies for coping with stress. List them on the chalkboard.
	7.3 Do fewer things and do them better. One technique for managing stress is to reduce the demands on your time. Are you doing too much at work, at home, in the community, with friends? Carefully look at your typical day or week. Are there activities that you can give up? Set priorities for what you need to do. Save some time for yourself every day.	
	7.4 Identify your thoughts about your diabetes or other stress factors in your life. Thoughts can affect feelings and behavior. For example, some people view diabetes as a disaster, and some see it more as a challenge.	Ask, "What are some thoughts you've had about diabetes? How did your thoughts affect your feelings or your behavior?"
	7.5 Sometimes it is healthy to avoid stressful situations until you have time to think about how you might handle them positively.	
	7.6 Redirect your reaction to stress. Use the energy in some way. Exercise (walking, biking, jogging, or aerobics) as a way to release tension. Spend energy on hobbies, keeping a journal, talking with a friend, or joining a support group.	Exercise is a form of controlled stress on the body. Exercise helps use up the stress hormones. With regular exercise, the body is better able to handle all types of stress. Exercise also increases overall stamina, which helps with long-term stress.

CONTENT OUTLINE

CONCEPT	DETAIL	INSTRUCTOR'S NOTES

7.7 Many different relaxation techniques can be used to relieve stress: meditation, yoga, biofeedback, deep breathing, visual imagery. They relieve tension by relaxing muscles. These techniques are usually done in a quiet, comfortable place where you will not be interrupted by the phone or other people. After you practice them there, you can use the same techniques anywhere you are experiencing stress.

7.8 Keep your sense of humor. Laughter releases endorphins and helps you decrease stress.

Ask, "Have you had experiences that were stressful at the time but were humorous later?"

7.9 Sometimes being with people who have similar problems helps to reduce stress. Talking about problems can help you to solve them. The American Diabetes Association may have a group in your area.

Provide information about local support groups, stress management groups, or other local resources.

7.10 Books are available that discuss coping with diabetes and other stresses.

Provide information about books or other resources that are available.

7.11 If you want help to handle stress, or feel unable to cope, ask for professional help. Your health care team can tell you about resources. It is helpful to find a mental health specialist (social worker, psychologist, psychiatrist, or nurse) who is experienced in working with people with diabetes.

7.12 Stress is something we all experience. Learning how to deal with stress effectively can help improve your quality of life.

Choose a short-term goal to try before the next session.

CONTENT OUTLINE

CONCEPT	DETAIL	INSTRUCTOR'S NOTES
8. Relaxation techniques	8.1 Deep breathing, sometimes called diaphragmatic breathing, can be relaxing. When we are tense, we tend to breathe high in our chests in a rapid and shallow fashion. You can use the deep-breathing technique in a variety of stressful situations.	Practice deep breathing and relaxation for 5–10 minutes.

Deep Breathing Exercise

Have participants assume a comfortable position. Have the room quiet, without distractions.

Ask participants to breathe in slowly through the nose for 4 counts and breathe out slowly through the nose for 8 counts.

Ask participants to close their eyes and continue to breathe deeply and slowly.

Say the following in a clear, slow, calm voice: "Now relax all the muscles in your head and neck. You can feel all the tension leaving your face, neck, shoulders, arms, and hands. You are limp and relaxed like a rag doll. Continue to breathe deeply. Now relax your back, abdomen, buttocks, thighs, legs, feet, and toes. You are totally relaxed. Breathe deeply in for 4 counts and out for 8 counts."

CONCEPT	DETAIL	INSTRUCTOR'S NOTES
	8.2 Another method of handling stress is to use visual images to relax the mind and body. Sometimes called a "mental vacation," this technique can leave you refreshed and recharged.	Practice the visual imagery to end the session for 5–10 minutes. Speak slowly and in a relaxing manner as you go through the exercise, pausing between requests.

Visual Imagery Exercise

Ask participants to close their eyes and travel in their minds to a place in their lives that was beautiful and peaceful.

"It can be any place where you feel happy, relaxed, and at peace.

"What do you smell?
"What do you hear?
"What do you feel?
"What do you see?

"Continue relaxing for a few minutes. Let go of these images. Stretch. Open your eyes."

SKILLS CHECKLIST

None.

EVALUATION PLAN

Knowledge will be evaluated by achievement of learning objectives and by responses to questions during the session. The ability to apply knowledge will be evaluated through the identification of coping strategies and program outcome measures.

DOCUMENTATION PLAN

Record class attendance and achieved objectives as appropriate.

SUGGESTED READINGS

Braunstein JB. Getting the stress monkey off your back. *Diabetes Forecast*. 2002;55(6):55–57.

Dossey B. Using imagery to help your patients heal. *American Journal of Nursing*. 1995; 95(6):41–47.

Polonsky WH. *Diabetes Burnout*. Alexandria, VA: American Diabetes Association, 1999.

Surwit RS, van Tilburg MAL, Zucker N, McCaskill CC, Parekh P, Feinglos MN,

Edwards CL, Williams P, Lane JD. Stress management improves long-term glycemic control in diabetes. *Diabetes Care*. 2002; 25:30–42.

Welch GW, Jacobon AM, Polonsky WH: The problem areas in diabetes scale. *Diabetes Care*. 1997;20:760–766.

Williamson L. Chill out. *Diabetes Forecast*. 2003;56(11):77–79.

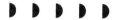

| #13 | **Personal Health Habits** |

STATEMENT OF PURPOSE

This session is intended to provide information about personal health habits that are important for people with diabetes and to suggest ways to incorporate them into daily life. Foot care, skin care, infections, and dental care are included.

PREREQUISITES

None.

OBJECTIVES

At the end of this session, participants will be able to:

1. state why it is important for people with diabetes to be particularly attentive to their personal health habits;

2. recognize early signs and symptoms of infection;

3. list two components of dental care;

4. list four preventive foot care practices;

5. list three components of daily skin and foot care;

6. describe how to cut toenails properly;

7. state how to treat minor cuts and bruises;

8. state ways to improve circulation;

9. list symptoms of urogenital infections;

10. state reasons for need of increased frequency of health monitoring.

CONTENT

Risk Reduction.

MATERIALS NEEDED

VISUALS PROVIDED

1. Foot Inspection
2. Cutting Your Toenails
3. Urogenital System

Handouts (one per participant)
1. Foot Care Guidelines

ADDITIONAL

- Pencils for participants
- Information about local resources for stopping smoking and foot and dental care
- Mirror, samples of foot lotions, foot care instruments, wound care products, other foot care products
- Monofilament to test sensation

METHOD OF PRESENTATION

Start by introducing yourself and telling what you do. Ask participants to introduce themselves. Explain that the purposes of this session are to provide information about health habits and to develop a personal foot care plan.

Present material in a question/discussion format with demonstrations. Begin by asking how they did with their short-term goal and what they learned from it. One approach for teaching foot care is to have participants remove their shoes so that they can practice the skills they need to care for their feet.

CONTENT OUTLINE

CONCEPT	DETAIL	INSTRUCTOR'S NOTES
1. Health habits	1.1 Health habits are very important for *everyone,* with or without diabetes.	Ask, "What questions or concerns do you have about your general health or health habits and diabetes?"
	1.2 Health habits include taking care of yourself physically and emotionally, such as getting adequate sleep, nutrition, and exercise. Other health habits include foot, skin, and dental care.	Ask, "What are some health habits you already have?"
	1.3 It is important to obtain medical care at appropriate intervals. Don't neglect the other areas of your health.	Tell all health care providers that you have diabetes.
2. Special care when you have diabetes	2.1 Having diabetes means paying special attention to some health habits.	
	2.2 Smoking is particularly harmful because you have diabetes. The combination of diabetes and smoking	Ask, "Are any of you interested in quitting at this time?" Provide a list of smoking cessation

CONTENT OUTLINE

CONCEPT	DETAIL	INSTRUCTOR'S NOTES
	greatly increases the risk for cardio-vascular disease and other problems.	programs in your area and offer information on available over-the-counter or prescription aids.
	2.3 Alcohol can affect blood glucose and blood fat (triglyceride) levels.	Refer to Outline #5, *Planning Meals,* for more information.
3. Infections	3.1 Infections are more common and more serious in people who have diabetes.	Ask, "What questions or concerns do you have about infections?"
	3.2 The signs of infection are pain, redness, warmth of area, swelling, discharge, and fever.	Ask, "What are the signs of infection?"
	3.3 The first sign may be elevated blood glucose levels.	Infections raise blood glucose levels; they also occur more often when blood glucose levels are high.
	3.4 Infections can occur without open cuts or injuries.	
	3.5 Call your health care team right away if you see any signs of infection.	
4. Importance of dental care	4.1 When blood glucose is high, gum and mouth infections are more common.	Ask, "What questions do you have about dental care? How do you care for your teeth?" Elevated glucose levels support bacterial growth.
	4.2 Brush your teeth at least twice a day using toothbrush and techniques that your dentist recommends. Note any bleeding or sores on gums.	Infected teeth can raise glucose levels. People with diabetes are prone to gum disease.
	4.3 Have regular dental exams. Be sure to tell your dentist that you have diabetes. Schedule your appointments after meals to decrease the risk of an insulin reaction.	See a dentist at least twice yearly or at recommended intervals.
	4.4 If you can't eat your regular meals because of dental work or tooth problems, follow your sick-day plan for a soft or liquid diet.	

CONTENT OUTLINE

CONCEPT	DETAIL	INSTRUCTOR'S NOTES
5. Importance of foot care	5.1 Decreased circulation causes slow healing of injuries.	Ask, "What questions or concerns do you have about caring for your feet? What do you do to take care of your feet?"
	5.2 Peripheral neuropathy (diabetic nerve disease in the leg and foot) causes decreased sensation and puts the foot at risk for undetected trauma.	Some people with diabetes have little or no feeling in their feet. They can injure or burn their feet without noticing it.
	5.3 Early discovery and treatment of foot injuries or other problems can prevent serious complications. Untreated problems may lead to infection and potentially to amputation. Most amputations from diabetes are preventable with appropriate care.	Two of the most important things participants can do is to get into the habit of looking at their feet each day and to seek prompt treatment for problems or changes.
6. Prevention of foot problems	6.1 Wear shoes and socks that fit. Poorly fitting shoes are the most common cause of foot trauma. Shoes and socks made of natural fibers are recommended because they allow feet to breathe. Change your shoes at least once during the day.	Ask, "What questions do you have about choosing shoes and socks."
	6.2 Shop for shoes in the afternoon when feet are larger. Buy shoes that have room for your toes to wiggle. Avoid shoes that are too tight. Try on both shoes and buy for the bigger foot. Shoes that don't fit well can lead to sores, blisters, and calluses. Break in new shoes slowly by wearing them for 1–2 hours a day at first.	Poorly fitting shoes are the most common cause of foot trauma.
	6.3 When taking shoes off, look for areas of redness. These are most often caused by improper fit.	Ask participants to remove shoes and socks. The instructor should also.
	6.4 Shake out or feel inside your shoes for foreign objects before putting them on.	Demonstrate. Ask participants to check their shoes.
	6.5 Avoid heating pads, hot water bottles, and microwavable warmers. These can cause burns.	

CONTENT OUTLINE

CONCEPT	DETAIL	INSTRUCTOR'S NOTES
	6.6 Avoid going barefoot indoors and outdoors.	Shoes help prevent injury. Hard-soled slippers are recommended.
	6.7 Wear wool socks to keep feet warm and warm, waterproof shoes or boots for outdoor winter activities.	
	6.8 At the beach, avoid walking barefoot on hot sand or shells. Put sunscreen on tops of feet.	Beach sandals and swim shoes (e.g., Aquasocks) are available at stores that stock beach supplies.
	6.9 Take your shoes off when you see your provider as a reminder to check your feet.	Ask, "When did you last have your feet examined?"
	6.10 Your provider can test for sensation using a small device called a monofilament. This should be done at least once a year. You can also do this test at home.	Encourage participants to ask for monofilament testing annually. Demonstrate the test with a monofilament. Monofilaments are available for home use from several sources.
7. Daily care of feet	7.1 Wash daily with mild soap and warm water and dry completely.	Ask, "What can you do to care for your feet each day?" Suggest times for foot care (during bath or dressing).
	7.2 Look at tops and bottoms of your feet for fissures, cracks, calluses, red spots, cuts, bruises, etc. Treat appropriately.	Demonstrate. Pass mirror for participants to use if they can't see bottoms of feet. Use Visual #1, Foot Inspection.
	7.3 If skin is dry, use lanolin-based lotion to keep feet soft. If feet sweat a lot, use powder.	Show products. Care is most important if cracks or fissures are present. Soaking feet is drying for skin.
	7.4 Corns and calluses may be related to shoe fit. Remove calluses by gently rubbing with an emery board or pumice stone. Work on callused areas over time.	Point out corns, calluses, and other abnormalities during the demonstration.
	7.5 Treat corns or bunions by padding. Do not use caustic corn removers or sharp instruments.	These chemicals can burn your skin. Show appropriate products.

CONTENT OUTLINE

CONCEPT	DETAIL	INSTRUCTOR'S NOTES
	7.6 Trim toenails to follow the curve of your toe and be even with the end of the toe. Nails are softer and easier to cut after a bath.	Show tools for cutting nails. Nails that have fungal infections or are ingrown should be cut by a podiatrist. Use Visual #2, Cutting Your Toenails.
	7.7 If toes overlap, sheepskin or cotton placed between can prevent blisters.	
8. Other foot care	8.1 Treat small cuts by washing, rinsing well, drying, and covering with sterile dressing held in place with nonallergenic tape.	Show examples of tape, dressings, ointment, and antiseptics.
	8.2 Avoid iodine, merthiolate, mercurochrome, or liniment. These can burn skin, and their colors hide signs of infection.	
	8.3 If cuts do not show signs of healing within 2 days, contact your provider.	
	8.4 See a foot care specialist for continuing care of foot problems.	Refer as needed.
9. Decreased circulation to extremities	9.1 The signs and symptoms of decreased circulation are decreased hair growth, change in color (blue or red when standing, blanched when elevated), cold feet, and swollen feet and ankles.	
	9.2 Some clothing can further decrease circulation. Avoid tight clothing such as girdles. Make sure knee-high stockings do not cut off blood flow. The type with wide elastic tops generally allows more circulation. If you wear support stockings, make sure they fit without wrinkles. Avoid crossing your legs at the knee.	Distribute Handout #1, Foot Care Guidelines. Help participants complete the Foot Care Plan portion. Ask, "When will you be able to do your foot care?"
	9.3 Circulation (blood flow) can be improved (stop smoking or begin an exercise program including walking and foot exercises).	Demonstrate some foot exercises and have participants perform them.

CONTENT OUTLINE

CONCEPT	DETAIL	INSTRUCTOR'S NOTES
10. Urogenital infections	10.1 Symptoms include vulvovaginal itching and burning, urethral or penile discharge, frequent urination with urgency and pain, difficulty in initiating stream, fever, bloody urine, and suprapubic and back pain.	Use Visual #3, Urogenital System, to show the relationship between the kidneys, ureters, bladder, and urethra. Use words participants understand.
	10.2 Cultures are needed to determine appropriate treatment.	
	10.3 Prevent bladder infections by urinating often, drinking lots of water, and keeping blood glucose levels in your target range.	Empty the bladder every 2 hours while awake.
	10.4 Do not ignore small problems; they may become big problems.	
11. Regular examinations	11.1 Diabetes exams and tests: ■ every visit—foot and blood pressure check ■ every 3–6 months—A1C test ■ yearly—foot examination, tests for lipids, and microalbuminuria as appropriate.	Emphasize that a diabetes checkup may not assess total physical health.
	11.2 Dilated eye exam: ■ adults and adolescents with type 1—within 3–5 years of diagnosis and annually thereafter ■ people with type 2—at diagnosis and annually thereafter	This can prevent blindness from retinopathy. Stress this point and that the pupils must be dilated by an eye specialist. It is not sufficient for your provider or an optician to examine the eyes during an office visit.
	11.3 **Before** becoming pregnant, have an exam by a diabetes doctor and obstetrician. Tight blood glucose management is necessary **before** and during pregnancy.	Tight glucose regulation before conception and in early weeks of pregnancy will decrease risk of birth defects.
	11.4 Write down questions and problems before the visit, and bring the list with you.	
	11.5 Be sure to tell each of your providers that you have diabetes.	Choose a short-term goal to try before the next session.

SKILLS CHECKLIST

Each participant will be able to inspect feet, cut toenails, treat small cuts and mild injuries, and demonstrate foot exercises.

EVALUATION PLAN

Knowledge will be evaluated by achievement of learning objectives and by responses to questions during the session. Skills will be evaluated by observing a demonstration of techniques. The ability to apply knowledge will be evaluated by the development and implementation of a personal foot care plan and through program outcome measures.

DOCUMENTATION PLAN

Record class attendance and achieved objectives as appropriate.

SUGGESTED READINGS

Foot and Skin Care

Adler AI, Boyko EJ, Ahroni JH, Smith DG. Lower-extremity amputation in diabetes. *Diabetes Care.* 1999;22:1029–1035.

American Diabetes Association. Position statement: Preventive foot care in patients with diabetes mellitus. *Diabetes Care.* 2004;27(Suppl 1):S63–S64.

American Diabetes Association. Resource Guide 2004. Wound gels and prescription lotions. *Diabetes Forecast.* 2004;57(1):RG63.

Barry PJ. Using human skin equivalents to heal chronic wounds. *Nursing.* 2003;33(3):68–69.

Bonham P. A critical review of the literature: part II-antibiotic treatment of osteomyelitis in patients with diabetes and foot ulcers. *J Wound Ostomy Continence.* 2001;28:141–149.

Booth J, Young MJ. Differences in the performance of commercially available 20-g monofilaments. *Diabetes Care.* 2000;23:984–988.

Corbett CF. A randomized pilot study of improving foot care in home health patients with diabetes. *The Diabetes Educator.* 2003;29:273–282.

Dahmen R, Haspels R, Koomen, B, Hoeksma AF. Therapeutic footwear for the neuropathic foot. *Diabetes Care.* 2001;24:705–709.

DeBeradis G, Pellegrini F, Fanciosi M, Belfiglio M, Di Nardo B, Greenfield S, Kaplan SH, Rossi MCE, Sacco M, Tognoni G, Valentini M, Nicolucci A. Physician attitudes toward foot care education and foot examination and their correlation with patient practice. *Diabetes Care.* 2004;27:286–287.

Dunlap C. All about amputation. *Diabetes Forecast.* 2003;56(8):68–71.

Frykberg RG, Armstrong DG, Giurini J, Edwards A, Kravette M, Kravitz S, Ross C, Stavosky J, Stuck R, Vanore J. Diabetic foot disorders: a clinical practice guideline. *J Foot and Ankle Surg.* 2000;39(5):S1–S60.

Gottlieb SH. From heart to sole. *Diabetes Forecast.* 2002;55(9):37–39.

Haas LB. Lower extremity amputations: strategies for prevention. *Diabetes Spectrum.* 1995;8:205–231.

Ledda MA, Walker EA, Basch CE. Development and formative evaluation of a foot self-care program for African Americans with diabetes. *The Diabetes Educator.* 1997;23:48–51.

Manam RK, Edelson GW. Lower extremity edema in diabetes mellitus. *Practical Diabetology.* 1997;16(2):6–7.

SUGGESTED READINGS *continued*

Margolis DJ, Allen-Taylor L, Hoffstad O, Verlin JA. Diabetic neuropathic foot ulcers. *Diabetes Care.* 2002;25:1835–1839.

Mayfield JA, Rieber GE, Sanders LJ, Janisse D, Pogach LM. Preventive foot care in people with diabetes: a technical review. *Diabetes Care.* 1998;21:2161–2177.

McCarren M. Simple test saves feet. *Diabetes Forecast.* 1996;49(4):28–31.

Patout CA, JR., Birke JA, Horswell R, Williams D, Cerise FP. Effectiveness of a comprehensive diabetes lower extremity amputation prevention program in a predominately low-income African American population. *Diabetes Care.* 2000;23:1339–1342.

Pham H, Armstrong DG, Harvey C, Harlesss LB, Giurini JM, Veves A. Screening techniques to identify people at high risk for diabetic foot ulceration. *Diabetes Care.* 2000;23:606–611.

Scheffler NM. All about socks. *Diabetes Forecast.* 2001;54(9):78–82.

Scheffler NM. How to shop for shoes. *Diabetes Forecast.* 2004;57(3):70–73.

Scheffler NM. The ins and outs of Charcot foot. *Diabetes Forecast.* 2000;53(7):68–70.

Sumpio BE. Foot ulcers. *New England Journal of Medicine.* 2000;343:797–793.

Tannenberg RJ, Pfeifer MA. Fend off foot ulcers. *Diabetes Forecast.* 2001;54(8):86–89.

Valk GD, Kriegsman DMW, Assendelft WJJ. Patient education for preventing diabetic foot ulceration (Cochrane Review). In: The Cochrane Library, Issue 3, 2002.

Dental Care

Gutkowski S. Disease treatment and oral health. *Diabetes Self-Management.* 2002; 19(3):83–85.

Gutkowski S. All about toothpastes, toothbrushes, and mouthwashes. *Diabetes Self-Management.* 2002;19(6):98–103.

Gutkowski S. Beyond brushing. *Diabetes Self-Management.* 2002;19(5):98–105.

Gutkowski S. Choosing dental care. *Diabetes Self-Management.* 2003;20(1):51–55.

Gutkowski S. Power cleaning your teeth. *Diabetes Self-Management.* 2002;19(2):56–61.

Mealey B, Varon F. Under the gums. *Diabetes Forecast.* 1998;51(10):54–58.

Roberts SS. Top ways to prevent dental problems. *Diabetes Forecast.* 2001;54(4):71–72.

Stillman N, Genco RJ. Periodontal disease and diabetes: interdependent conditions. *Practical Diabetetology.* 2002;19(4):19–27.

Tomar SL, Lester A. Dental and other health care visits among US adults with diabetes. *Diabetes Care.* 2000;23:1505–1510.

➔ Foot Inspection

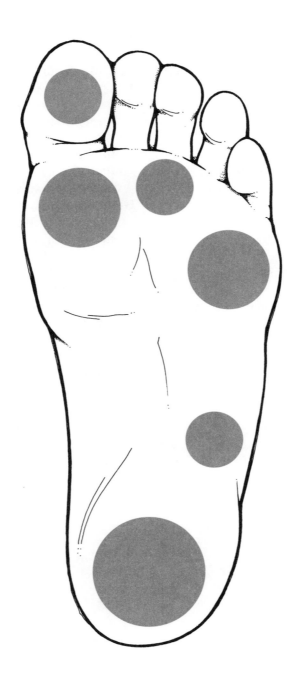

➔ Cutting Your Toenails

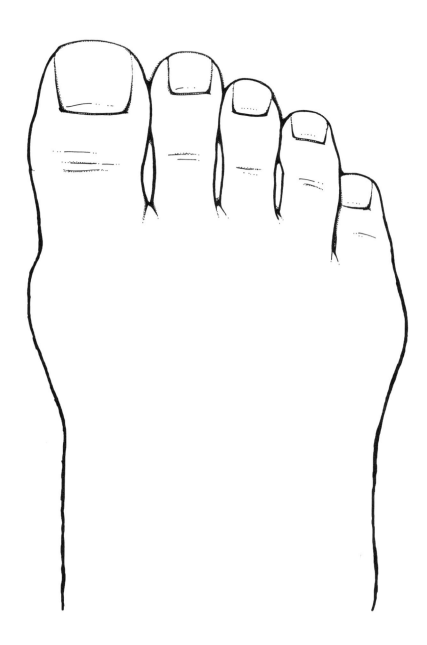

Urogenital System

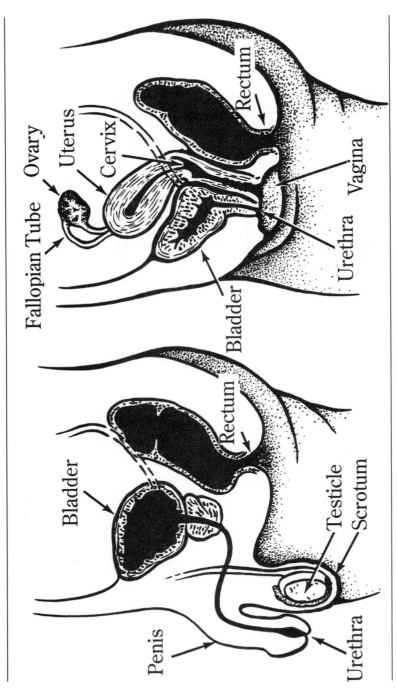

Fallopian Tube
Ovary
Uterus
Cervix
Rectum
Vagina
Urethra
Bladder

Bladder
Rectum
Penis
Urethra
Testicle
Scrotum

➲ Foot Care Guidelines

INSPECTION

- Look at your feet each day in a place with good light. Use a mirror if you can't bend over to see the bottoms of your feet. If looking at your feet is hard for you, ask a family member to help.
- Look for dry places and cracks in the skin, especially between the toes and around the heel.
- Check for ingrown toenails, corns, calluses, swelling, sores, or places that are red or pale. If corns, calluses, or other problems persist, see a foot doctor (podiatrist).

BATHING

- Wash your feet daily in warm—not hot—water. Before you put your feet into the water, test the temperature with your wrist or elbow to prevent burning your feet.
- Do not soak your feet, because soaking will dry your skin.
- Use a mild soap and rinse well. Gently dry your feet with a soft towel, making sure to dry between the toes.
- Cracks in the skin are places where infection can enter. To soften dry feet and keep the skin from cracking, use a mild cream or lotion, except between your toes where athlete's foot often occurs.
- If your feet sweat a lot, lightly dust with foot powder. Wear socks that are mostly cotton, and change them if they become damp.

TOENAILS

- Cut your toenails after bathing, when they are soft and easy to trim.
- Cut or file nails to follow the natural curve of your toe. Avoid cutting nails shorter than the ends of your toes. Sharp corners and rough edges of toenails need to be filed with an emery board so they don't cut the toes next to them.
- Don't use sharp objects to poke or dig under the toenail or around the cuticle.
- Ingrown toenails or nails that are thick or tend to split when cut should be cared for by a foot care specialist.

FOOT CARE GUIDELINES *continued*

CORNS AND CALLUSES

- After washing your feet, gently rub any corns and callused areas with an emery board or pumice stone to control buildup.
- Avoid using do-it-yourself corn or callus removers. These can cause burns and may harm healthy skin around the problem area.
- Never cut your corns and calluses with a razor blade. This can lead to infections.
- Use pads on corns to reduce pressure.

SOCKS

- Socks should fit well and be free of seams and darns that might reduce the blood supply.
- Wear socks that are mostly natural fibers, such as cotton or wool, to allow skin to breathe.

SHOES

- Wear shoes or hard-soled slippers to cover and protect your feet. Avoid going barefoot, and use common sense about wearing sandals. Thong sandals can cause blisters between your toes, and you can step out of them and injure your feet.
- At the beach, avoid walking barefoot on hot sand or shells, wear water shoes, and put sunscreen on the tops of your feet.
- Choose the shoes that are most comfortable for your activities each day.
- Before you put on your shoes, shake them out and then carefully feel inside for stones or rough spots that might hurt your feet.
- The top part of the shoe should be soft and pliable. The lining should not have ridges, wrinkles, or seams. The toe area should be round and high to fit your toes. You may need to see an orthotic specialist for inserts, for special shoes, or to have your shoes adapted to your feet.
- Shop for shoes in midafternoon when feet are larger. Buy shoes that feel good and have room for all the toes to wiggle and be in their natural place. Avoid shoes that are too tight or pinch. Try on both shoes, and if one of your feet is slightly larger than the other, buy for the bigger foot. Shoes that don't fit well can lead to sores, blisters, and calluses.

FOOT CARE GUIDLEINES *continued*

- If your feet are numb, you can't rely on how shoes feel to know if you have a good fit. Make an outline of each foot from stiff paper to insert in shoes when you are shopping for new ones.
- Break in new shoes slowly by wearing them for 1–2 hours a day at first. Change your shoes at least once during the day.

CIRCULATION (BLOOD FLOW)

- Exercise each day.
- If you smoke, plan to quit or cut down.
- Wear wool socks and warm, waterproof shoes or boots for outside winter activities.
- Avoid heating pads, hot water bottles, or microwavable warmers. These can burn the skin. Instead, use wool socks to keep your feet warm.

TREATMENT OF INJURIES

- Look at your feet if you stumble or bump a hard object to be sure that there is no damage.
- If your foot is hurt, don't keep walking on it—that can cause more damage.
- Treat blisters, cuts, and scratches right away. Wash with soap and water and apply a mild antiseptic. Never use strong chemicals such as boric acid, epsom salts, or any antiseptic that contains a dye. Remember, opening blisters yourself can lead to infections.
- Cover all injuries with an adhesive bandage or dry sterile dressing.
- If sores do not begin to heal within 2 days, or look worse after the first day, call your doctor.

Foot Care Plan

Name _____   Date _____

It is especially important for me to:

_____

_____

_____

_____

_____

_____

Referral

Podiatrist:

Other:

Reason for referral:

Signature _____

Phone _____   Hours _____

#14	Long-Term Complications

STATEMENT OF PURPOSE

This session is intended to provide information about the chronic complications that can occur with diabetes.

PREREQUISITES

It is recommended that each participant have basic knowledge about diabetes and self-care, from either personal experience or from attending previous sessions. Readiness to learn about complications should be carefully assessed before this content is presented.

OBJECTIVES

At the end of this session, participants will be able to:

1. state that blood glucose and blood pressure control reduces risks for complications;

2. describe the major consequences of small blood vessel disease;

3. describe the symptoms that may occur with diabetic retinopathy and with diabetic nephropathy;

4. list treatments for diabetic retinopathy and diabetic nephropathy;

5. state the value of annual ophthalmologic and renal function examinations;

6. describe what happens to large blood vessels in arteriosclerosis;

7. list the risk factors and ways to decrease the risk for developing arteriosclerosis;

8. list consequences and symptoms of diabetic neuropathy;

9. list one treatment for neuropathy;

10. state that research into treatment for complications continues.

CONTENT

Chronic Complications.

MATERIALS NEEDED

VISUALS PROVIDED	ADDITIONAL
1. Circulatory System 2. Normal Eye 3. Microaneurysms 4. Proliferative Retinopathy 5. Retinal Detachment 6. Normal Kidney 7. Large-Vessel Disease 8. Nervous System 9. Wound Healing	■ Information about local support groups and local resources for those with complications

Handouts (one per participant)
1. Resources for Diabetes Complications

METHOD OF PRESENTATION

Start by introducing yourself and telling what you do. Ask participants to introduce themselves. Explain that the purpose of this session is to provide an overview of the long-term complications of diabetes so participants can identify symptoms early and seek treatment if complications occur.

Present material in a question/discussion format. Begin by asking how they did with their short-term goal and what they learned from it. When presenting this material, it is important to be sensitive to the participants' readiness to hear about complications and to their emotional responses to this difficult topic.

CONTENT OUTLINE

CONCEPT	DETAIL	INSTRUCTOR'S NOTES
1. Occurrence of long-term complications	1.1 In this session, you will learn some of the long-term problems people with diabetes can face, and you will be given information about prevention, symptoms, and treatment options.	State that you understand this is a difficult topic to talk about, but it is needed so that they can identify symptoms early and get treatment. Ask, "What questions or concerns do you have about complications?"
	1.2 Even though it may be hard to hear this information, you need to know for three reasons: ■ to make decisions about personal blood glucose goals ■ to do all you can to prevent the complications ■ to recognize early signs or obtain screening for complications so they can be treated early	Emphasize that causes for the development of complications are unclear, but are related to: ■ duration of diabetes ■ hyperglycemia and hypertension ■ type of diabetes (to some extent)

CONTENT OUTLINE

CONCEPT	DETAIL	INSTRUCTOR'S NOTES
	1.3 People with both type 1 and type 2 diabetes are at risk for all of the long-term complications.	Ask, "Do you know what some of the complications are? Have you known people with complications?"
	1.4 Some people get none of the complications, while others get one or more than one.	
	1.5 Evidence shows that some of the problems can be delayed or prevented with improved glucose control. You are giving yourself the best chance for good health by keeping your blood glucose near the normal range.	Review results of the Diabetes Control and Complications Trial (DCCT) and the United Kingdom Prospective Diabetes Study (UKPDS) from Outline #11, *Managing Blood Glucose.*
	1.6 Some of the problems are reversible or their progress can be slowed, if they are found and treated early.	The experiences of others in the past with complications don't have to happen to you.
	1.7 There is good news: more and better treatments are now available. This is also an area of great research interest.	
2. Systems affected	2.1 Complications affect various systems of your body.	
	2.2 In the large-vessel circulatory system, the heart, legs, feet, and toes are affected.	
	2.3 In the small-vessel circulatory system, the kidneys and eyes are affected.	
	2.4 In the nervous system, both peripheral and autonomic, many functions are affected.	This does not mean that you feel nervous.
3. Circulatory system	3.1 You have large and small blood vessels in your body. Small blood vessels are called capillaries. Veins and arteries are large blood vessels.	Use Visual #1, Circulatory System. Arteries carry blood and oxygen from your heart and lungs out to your cells. Veins then bring the blood back to get more oxygen and other needed nutrients.

CONTENT OUTLINE

CONCEPT	DETAIL	INSTRUCTOR'S NOTES
	3.2 The large vessels move large amounts of blood into and out of your heart and lungs and supply blood to the arms, legs, and brain.	
	3.3 The small vessels provide blood to the eyes, kidneys, fingers, and toes.	
	3.4 In diabetes, both large and small vessels can be affected.	
4. Eyes (diabetic retinopathy)	4.1 When you look at an object, the image is sent from the lens through the vitreous (area filled with clear gel-like fluid) to the retina.	Ask, "What questions do you have about diabetic eye disease?" Use Visual #2, Normal Eye. Point out that blurred vision is often a symptom of high blood glucose and that the vision will return to normal with better glucose control.
	4.2 The retina is a thin membrane at the back of the eye that receives the image.	Use the analogy of a camera: the retina is the film receiving the image from the lens.
	4.3 It is possible to look into the eye using an ophthalmoscope. The optic nerve, many small blood vessels, and the macula (the center of vision of the retina) can be seen.	Point out the blood vessels, optic nerve, and macula on Visual #2, Normal Eye.
	4.4 In diabetes, weak spots develop in the walls of the smallest blood vessels. Balloon-like outpouchings occur (microaneurysms). This is *diabetic retinopathy*.	Use Visual #3, Microaneurysms. Blurred vision from elevated glucose levels is not the same as retinopathy.
	4.5 These areas can leak, and fluid escapes. As these areas heal, scarring occurs.	This is called nonproliferative retinopathy and may occur without any change in vision.
	4.6 This interruption of the circulation causes formation of new, smaller blood vessels (neovascularization) in an attempt to provide blood flow to these areas.	This is called proliferative retinopathy. Use Visual #4, Proliferative Retinopathy.
	4.7 These new vessels are very fragile and can easily break. When this	

CONTENT OUTLINE

CONCEPT	DETAIL	INSTRUCTOR'S NOTES

happens, blood leaks into the space between the retina and the vitreous (the clear gel that fills the eyeball) and sometimes out into the vitreous itself.

4.8 When a hemorrhage occurs into the gel, it is like looking through a pool of blood or a spider web. This blood and the vision may eventually clear or partially clear. The scarring that results also causes some loss of vision. If bleeding occurs in or near the macula, visual loss can be severe; if untreated, total blindness may result.

4.9 If scars develop, they may form fibrous attachments between the retina and vitreous. If these scars contract, the retina can be torn away from the back surface of the eye. This is *retinal detachment*—if this happens, there is a rapidly developing partial or complete loss of vision. People have described this as being like a torn curtain in the eye, or dark streaks, or a black curtain coming across the eye. If this happens to you, SEE AN OPHTHALMOLOGIST OR GO TO THE EMERGENCY ROOM!

Use Visual #5, Retinal Detachment.

Blurred vision often occurs with high or low blood glucose levels. This is not related to detached retina.

Immediate care is necessary.

4.10 Treatment for proliferative retinopathy consists of laser therapy to the retina. The laser produces a finely focused beam of light to cause microscopic-sized burns on the retina. This slows or prevents the development of abnormal new blood vessels or causes their disappearance. The laser can also be used to destroy nests of new blood vessels, which is especially important if they are bleeding.

Point out that laser therapy is not painful, but it is uncomfortable.

CONTENT OUTLINE

CONCEPT	DETAIL	INSTRUCTOR'S NOTES

4.11 Glasses do not help to restore the vision lost in retinopathy. Glasses can only help when the problem is in the lens of the eye, and in retinopathy the problem is with the retina.

Use the analogy of the camera again; if the film is fogged, changing the lens won't help.

4.12 There may be no symptoms at the time damage is occurring. The only way to find out is to have a dilated eye exam by an eye specialist who can look into the back of your eye and see very early changes.

Emphasize that this eye exam is more than just a refraction or glaucoma test. It must be done with the pupils dilated.

4.13 Treatment at an early stage can often prevent severe visual loss and blindness. Regular eye exams are one of the most important things people with diabetes can do to protect their eyesight. Keeping your blood pressure within recommended limits is another way to help avoid retinopathy.

People with type 1 diabetes should get an exam within 3–5 years after diagnosis and yearly thereafter; people with type 2 diabetes should get an exam at diagnosis and yearly thereafter. Exams may be recommended less often for those with no abnormalities.

4.14 Diabetes is the leading cause of new blindness in this country, but most of it is preventable. In the DCCT, risk for retinopathy was decreased by 76% with intensive therapy. The UKPDS demonstrated reductions in risk for visual loss with improved glucose and blood pressure levels.

Provide information about eye specialists in your area and/or encourage patients to seek a referral.

5. Eyes (cataracts)

5.1 Another problem that can occur is cataracts. These have nothing to do with circulation, but are the result of the accumulation of sugars in the lens of the eye. This causes swelling and clouding.

There are two kinds of cataracts. Senile cataracts are not preventable and have a different cause. Metabolic cataracts are often seen in younger people with diabetes.

5.2 This is often an early complication of diabetes.

CONTENT OUTLINE

CONCEPT	DETAIL	INSTRUCTOR'S NOTES
6. Kidneys (diabetic nephropathy)	6.1 Small blood vessels in the kidneys filter the blood; needed components are kept, and waste products including water are disposed of as urine.	Ask, "What questions do you have about diabetic kidney disease?" Use Visual #6, Normal Kidney.
	6.2 Sometimes in diabetes, the small vessels thicken and the kidneys do not filter as they should. Necessary blood components such as protein are lost in the urine; waste products are not adequately filtered out and eventually build up in the blood.	No symptoms are noticeable early in the development of diabetic kidney disease.
	6.3 To test kidney function, a spot, overnight, or 24-hour urine sample should be tested once a year for the presence of protein and for the amount of creatinine excreted. Blood tests for blood urea nitrogen (BUN) and creatinine can also be done.	Explain these tests and normal results if appropriate. Encourage participants to request these tests.
	6.4 The kidneys normally have a large reserve function. They can handle the needs of the body without causing any symptoms, until only 10% of the kidney function remains.	
	6.5 Two groups of medicines (called angiotensin-converting enzyme [ACE] inhibitors and angiotensin II receptor blockers [ARBs]) can delay the progression of diabetic nephropathy. In addition, keeping the blood pressure close to normal can slow the course of kidney damage.	List ACE inhibitors and ARBs used in your setting. Ask, "Are you taking any of these?" Review side effects, if appropriate. Beta-blockers are effective for participants with uncomplicated hypertension, but their protective effect on the kidneys isn't clear.
	6.6 Treatment for diagnosed nephropathy may include eating less protein. Some signs and symptoms (edema and hypertension) can be treated by improved glucose control, eating less salt, and with medicines such as ACE inhibitors and ARBs.	Byproducts of protein metabolism are part of the waste products filtered by the kidney.

CONTENT OUTLINE

CONCEPT	DETAIL	INSTRUCTOR'S NOTES

6.7 Later symptoms are nausea, poor appetite, irregular heart action, fatigue, dry and itchy skin, slow thinking, confusion and memory failure, numbness and tingling in hands and feet, poor balance, depression, and irritability.

6.8 In the DCCT, intensive therapy decreased the risk for nephropathy by 35–56%. The UKPDS also demonstrated reductions in risk for nephropathy. You can help prevent or delay kidney failure by keeping your blood glucose and blood pressure close to normal and treating high blood pressure and bladder infections promptly.

Cautions: Untreated urinary tract infections can progress to kidney infection and damage; high blood pressure makes diabetic kidney disease worse.

6.9 If kidney disease becomes worse, the kidneys may fail. The three treatment options are:
- hemodialysis (a machine is used to filter the blood two to three times per week)
- peritoneal dialysis (fluid flows into and out of the abdomen, and the peritoneum is used as a filter)
- kidney transplantation

These options are the same regardless of the cause of kidney failure.

7. Heart

7.1 Large-vessel problems in diabetes especially affect the heart, legs, and feet.

Ask, "What questions or concerns do you have about diabetes and heart disease?"

7.2 Fats (cholesterol and triglycerides) are deposited along the walls of the vessels. This is called arteriosclerosis.

Use Visual #7, Large-Vessel Disease. Heart disease is the leading cause of death among people with diabetes.

7.3 The vessels become stiff and less elastic, and the diameter of the vessel is smaller.

7.4 When this occurs in the coronary arteries, it can lead to heart attacks caused by not enough blood getting to the heart or to sections of the heart.

Arteriosclerosis is two to four times more common in men with diabetes and four to eight times more common in women with diabetes.

CONTENT OUTLINE

CONCEPT	DETAIL	INSTRUCTOR'S NOTES
	7.5 When this occurs in cerebral arteries, it can lead to strokes.	Strokes are two to four times more common in people with diabetes.
	7.6 When this occurs in the large vessels of the general circulation, especially those leading to the legs and feet, many problems can result, such as calf pain (claudication), ulcers, and delayed healing of injuries.	These complications are four to forty times more common in people with diabetes.
	7.7 Hyperglycemia raises triglyceride levels.	
8. Risk factors for heart disease	8.1 The risk factors for heart disease are:	Ask, "What are risk factors for heart disease?"
	■ diabetes	Say, "You already have one of these risk factors, and you can't do anything about that. But you can do things about other risk factors to help delay or prevent problems."
	■ high blood fats (lipids)—your cholesterol level should be measured once a year	Ask, "Do you know your cholesterol level?" Review normal results, if appropriate. Encourage participants to request this test. (See Outline #18, *Eating for a Healthy Heart.*)
	■ high blood pressure (hypertension—your blood pressure should be checked at every visit to your provider	Ask, "Do you know your blood pressure?" The goal in diabetes is <130/80 mmHg. Stress the importance of blood pressure control to protect heart and kidneys.
	■ smoking ■ heredity ■ gender	Males have higher risk for heart disease than females.
	■ stress ■ inactivity ■ obesity (more than 20% over ideal weight)	These are contributing factors, although not proven to be direct causes of large-vessel disease.

CONTENT OUTLINE

CONCEPT	DETAIL	INSTRUCTOR'S NOTES
9. Prevention, detection, and treatment of heart disease	9.1 Prevent heart disease by eliminating risk factors that are preventable. Smoking is one of the most important risk factors you can eliminate.	Ask, "Do you have any risk factors on which you would like to work?" Nicotine patches, gum, or medications may be helpful in smoking cessation.
	9.2 Lowering your cholesterol and blood glucose levels also decreases your risk. The UKPDS showed reductions of risk for heart failure and strokes with reductions in blood pressure.	Current cholesterol recommendations are: HDL (men) $\geq$40 mg/dl HDL (women) $\geq$50 mg/dl LDL <100 mg/dl Triglycerides <150 mg/dl
	9.3 Problems can be detected through electrocardiogram and Doppler studies.	
	9.4 Treatment is the same as in people without diabetes.	
10. Nervous system	10.1 Nerves conduct impulses (send messages) from one part of your body to another and back and forth to your brain.	Ask, "What questions or concerns do you have about nerve damage and diabetes?" Use Visual #8, Nervous System. Neuropathy is the most common complication of diabetes. Much research is currently being done in this area.
	10.2 The peripheral nerves connect your brain and spinal cord to all other parts of your body, including the skin, muscles, and organs.	
	10.3 The peripheral nerves are named based on what they do. There are three types of these nerves. ■ Sensory nerves send information to the brain about how things feel. For example, the sensory nerves tell the brain that the stove is hot when you touch it. ■ Motor nerves send commands from the brain to the body about movements. For example, motor nerves cause you to take your hand off the hot stove.	

CONTENT OUTLINE

CONCEPT	DETAIL	INSTRUCTOR'S NOTES
	■ Autonomic nerves control the things your body does automatically. For example, autonomic nerves control digestion, heart rate and blood pressure, the bladder, and sexual function.	
	10.4 Diabetic neuropathy is classified by the type of nerves that are affected. Damage to the sensory nerves causes pain or a loss of feeling. Damage to the motor nerves causes muscle weakness. Damage to the autonomic nerves causes changes in the way your body controls certain functions.	Point out that having damage to one type of nerve doesn't mean that you will have other types of nerve damage. However, they often occur in combination.
	10.5 Diabetes can affect all types of nerves. Why this happens is unclear, but the rate of conduction of impulses in the nerves is decreased, the nerve endings are damaged, and other disturbances occur.	
11. Feet, legs, and hands	11.1 Peripheral neuropathy (damage to the peripheral nerves) affects legs, feet, and, to a lesser extent, hands.	
	11.2 Symptoms are increased sensitivity with numbness or tingling, pain and burning, decreased sensation, and sometimes muscle weakness.	Symptoms depend on the type of nerves and the extent of the damage.
	11.3 Symptoms tend to come and go and decrease with lower blood glucose levels.	
	11.4 If sensation is decreased, you can hurt yourself without realizing it because of an inability to sense heat or pain.	Pain is a protective mechanism.
	11.5 Another problem of the feet and legs involves large-vessel circulation. Decreased blood flow to the feet and legs means that wounds will not heal as quickly as they should.	Use Visual #9, Wound Healing. Point out the narrowed vessels with arteriosclerosis.

CONTENT OUTLINE

CONCEPT	DETAIL	INSTRUCTOR'S NOTES
	11.6 The combination of circulatory and nerve problems in the legs can result in severe impairment. If you get a cut, you may not feel it. The decreased blood flow means that the wound will not heal quickly and may become infected.	Stress the importance of daily foot inspection and foot care to prevent amputations. Refer to Outline #13, *Personal Health Habits*.
	11.7 Increased sensitivity can lead to severe pain.	
	11.8 Treatment for pain includes: ■ medications	Narcotics are generally not used for long-term treatment. Drugs may include tramadol, tricyclic antidepressants (e.g., amitriptiyline [Elavil]) antiseizure medicines (e.g., gabapentin [Neurontin] and lidocaine 5% patch and opioids.
	■ an analgesic balm such as capsaicin (Zostrix-HP)	The high-potency form is recommended and is available without a prescription.
	■ walking to decrease leg pains ■ relaxation exercises, hypnosis, or biofeedback training ■ transcutaneous nerve stimulation (TENS) unit ■ acupressure and acupuncture	A TENS unit is a battery-powered device that sends an electric current to the painful areas. The current blocks the pain message from going to the brain, which decreases the pain. These units are costly but may be covered by insurance.
	Pain clinics are also available in many cities.	
	11.9 In the DCCT, risk for neuropathy was decreased by 60% with intensive therapy.	
12. Autonomic neuropathy	12.1 Damage to stomach nerves can cause delayed emptying, which causes nausea, stomach distention, and vomiting.	This is called *gastroparesis diabeticorum*. An early sign may be erratic blood glucose values.
	12.2 Damage to intestinal nerves leads to delayed emptying, causing a buildup of bacteria, constipation, and diarrhea.	Constipation and diarrhea may alternate, and nocturnal fecal incontinence may occur.

CONTENT OUTLINE

CONCEPT	DETAIL	INSTRUCTOR'S NOTES
	12.3 Dizziness and unsteadiness on standing can occur as a result of a drop in blood pressure (postural hypotension).	
	12.4 Incontinence (leaking of urine) or retention and difficulty urinating may occur.	Emphasize that frequent emptying of the bladder may help prevent urinary retention and stretching of the bladder.
	12.5 Damage to the nerves that control sexual function can also occur.	Ask, "Have you heard about this before? Do you have any questions?" Discuss according to the interest and needs of the group. Refer to Outline #23, *Sexual Health and Diabetes.*
	12.6 Men may experience impotence. Treatments are available for impotence.	Of males who have had diabetes for 10+ years, 40–50% have impaired sexual function. Stress the importance of discussing this with your provider or other professional to get treatment.
	12.7 Women may have diminished orgasms or none at all. Sexual problems in women are often related to genital infections (vaginitis) or lack of lubrication (which can be hormonal after menopause).	
	12.8 Treatment is available for all aspects of neuropathy. Talk with your health care professional about your symptoms and concerns.	
13. What can you do?	13.1 There are things you can do to prevent or delay complications or to detect them and get early treatment.	Present this section as positive actions participants can take.
	13.2 Keeping your blood glucose levels near normal will help prevent or delay eye, kidney, and nerve complications. Every improvement in blood glucose control helps in preventing complications.	Review the results of the DCCT and UKPDS.

CONTENT OUTLINE

CONCEPT	DETAIL	INSTRUCTOR'S NOTES
	13.3 Eliminate those risk factors that you can. Take care of yourself. Pay attention to little things, and treat them carefully.	Have information on smoking cessation, weight loss, and other programs in your area.
	13.4 Take care of your feet.	
	13.5 See your eye specialist annually for a dilated eye exam.	
	13.6 Most of the complications can be treated more effectively early. Regular examinations are needed, especially of the eyes, kidneys, feet, and heart. Ask your provider for these exams and tests.	Review referrals and tests to request.
	13.7 Research is being done on causes and treatment for complications that offers great hope for the future.	
	13.8 Living with the complications of diabetes—even with the *possibility* of complications—is very hard. If you find that you feel sad and depressed, find a health care provider or counselor you can talk to about your feelings. Help is available.	Have information available regarding local support groups. Distribute Handout #1, Resources for Diabetes Complications. Choose a short-term goal to try before the next session.

SKILLS CHECKLIST

None.

EVALUATION PLAN

Knowledge will be evaluated by achievement of learning objectives and by responses to questions during the session. The ability to apply knowledge will be evaluated by appropriate screening for complications and through program outcome measures.

DOCUMENTATION PLAN

Record class attendance and achieved objectives as appropriate.

SUGGESTED READINGS

Overview

Al-Delaimy WK, Willett WC, Manson JE, Speizer FE, Hu FB. Smoking and mortality among women with type 2 diabetes. *Diabetes Care.* 2001;24:2043–2048.

Braunstein JB. Exercise: the healthy alternative to smoking. *Diabetes Forecast.* 2002; 55(5):30–32.

Canga N, DeIrala J, Vara E, Duaso MJ, Ferrer A, Marinez-Gonzalez MA. Intervention study for smoking cessation in diabetic patients: a randomized controlled trial in both clinical and primary care settings. *Diabetes Care.* 2000;23:1455–1460.

Clark WL. Preventing and treating the complications of diabetes. *Diabetes Self-Management.* 2000;17(3):81–86.

De Groot M, Anderson R, Freedland KE, Clouse RE, Lustman PJ. Association of depression and diabetes complications: a meta-analysis. *Psychosom Med.* 2001;63:619–30.

Gabriel AR. Complications care. *Diabetes Forecast.* 2004;57(2):63–65.

Glasgow RE, Haire-Joshu D. Why you should kick butts. *Diabetes Forecast.* 2000; 53(8):46–50.

Haire-Joshu D, Tibbs T, Glasgow R. Smoking and diabetes. *Practical Diabetology.* 2001; 20(1):16–20.

Haire-Joshu D, Glasgow RE, Tibbs TL. Smoking and diabetes: a technical review. *Diabetes Care.* 1999;22:1887–1898.

Hillier TA, Pedula KL. Complications in young adults with early-onset type 2 diabetes. *Diabetes Care.* 2003;26:2999–3005.

Levin ME, Pfeifer MA. *The Uncomplicated Guide to Diabetes Complications.* Alexandria, VA: American Diabetes Association, 1997.

O'Connell B. Herbal therapies and diabetes complications. *Diabetes Self-Management.* 2001;18(1):87–98.

Peppa M, Uribarri J, Vlassara H. Glucose, advanced glycation end products, and diabetes complications: what is new and what works. *Clinical Diabetes.* 2003;21:186–188.

Retinopathy

AADE Visually Impaired Persons Specialty Practice Group. Guidelines for the practice of adaptive diabetes education for visually impaired persons (ADEVIP). *The Diabetes Educator.* 1994;20:111–112, 115–116, 118.

Aiello LP, Gardner TW, King GL, Blankenship G, Cavallerano JD, Ferris FL III, Klein R. Technical review: Diabetic retinopathy. *Diabetes Care.* 1998;21:143–156.

Albert, SG, Bernbaum, M. Exercise for patients with diabetic retinopathy. *Diabetes Care.* 1995;18:130–132.

American Diabetes Association. Position statement: Diabetic retinopathy. *Diabetes Care.* 2004;27(Suppl 1):S84–S87.

Cavallerano JD. Protect your vision. *Diabetes Forecast.* 1999;52(9):53–58.

Ciulla TA, Amador AG, Zinman B. Diabetic retinopathy and diabetic macular edema. *Diabetes Care.* 2003;26:2653–2664.

Fong DS, Aiello L, Gardner TW, King GL, Blankenship G, Cavallerano JD, Ferris FL, Klein R. Position Statement: diabetic retinopathy. *Diabetes Care.* 2003;26:226–229.

Hirsch IB. The eyes have it. *Diabetes Forecast.* 2002;55(10):68–70.

Kass M. The other eye disease: glaucoma. *Diabetes Forecast.* 1994;47(11):50–53.

Legorreta AP, Hasan MM, Peters AL, Pelletier KR, Leung K-M. An intervention for enhancing compliance with screening recommendations for diabetic retinopathy. *Diabetes Care.* 1997;20:520–523.

Petzinger RA. Tools for people with eye problems. *Diabetes Forecast.* 1995; 48(5):48–53.

Rogell GD. All about laser eye surgery. *Diabetes Forecast.* 2004;57(2):50–52.

Rogell GD. Save your sight. *Diabetes Forecast.* 2001;54(12):54–59.

Williams AS. A focus group study of accessibility and related psychosocial issues in diabetes education for people with visual impairment. *The Diabetes Educator.* 2002; 28:999–1008.

SUGGESTED READINGS *continued*

Retinopathy *continued*

Williams AS. Accessible diabetes education materials in a low-vision format. *The Diabetes Educator.* 1999;25:695–715.

Williams AS. Recommendations for desirable features of adaptive diabetes self-care equipment for visually impaired persons. *Diabetes Care.* 1994;17:451–452.

Nephropathy

Alzaid AA. Microalbuminuria in patients with NIDDM: an overview. *Diabetes Care.* 1996;19:79–89.

American Diabetes Association. Consensus statement: Consensus development conference on the diagnosis and management of nephropathy in patients with diabetes mellitus. *Diabetes Care.* 1996;19 (Suppl 1):103–106.

American Diabetes Association: Position statement: Diabetic nephropathy. *Diabetes Care* 2004;27(Suppl 1):S79–S83.

Bloomgarden ZT. Nephropathy. *Diabetes Care.* 1995;18:1402–1405.

Brennan DT, ed. *Diabetic Nephropathy: A Monograph for Diabetes Educators and Nephrology Nurses.* Chicago, IL: American Association of Diabetes Educators,1995.

Burr RA. All about dialysis. *Diabetes Forecast.* 2003;56(7):70–73.

Cannon JD. Recognizing chronic renal failure. *Nursing.* 2004;34(1):50–53.

D'Arrigo T. Kidney care 101. *Diabetes Forecast.* 2000;53(11):63–66.

Evans TC, Capell P. Diabetic nephropathy. *Clinical Diabetes.* 2000;18(1):7–13.

Kelly M. Chronic renal failure. *American Journal of Nursing.* 1996;96(1):36–37.

Kshirsagar AV, Joy MS, Hogan SL, Falk RJ, Colindres RE. Effect of ACE inhibitors in diabetic and nondiabetic chronic renal disease: a systematic overview of randomized placebo-controlled trials. *The American Journal of Kidney Disease.* 2000;35:695–707.

Rais-Keely P. Nutrition interventions in early diabetic renal disease. *The Diabetes Educator.* 2002;28:62–70.

Rodby RA. Fabulous filters. *Diabetes Forecast.* 1997;50(3):32–36.

Still WJP. 6 ways to beat kidney disease. *Diabetes Forecast.* 1999;52(3):56–58.

Wheeler ML, Fineberg SE, Fineberg NS, Gibson RG, Hackward LL. Animal versus plant protein meals in individuals with type 2 diabetes and microalbuminuria: effects on renal, glycemic and lipid parameters. *Diabetes Care.* 2002;25:1271–1276.

Hypertension

American Diabetes Association. Hypertension management in adults with diabetes. *Diabetes Care.* 2004;27(Suppl 1): S65–S67.

Aruz-Pacheco C, Parrott MA, Raskin P. The treatment of hypertension in adult patients with diabetes: technical review. *Diabetes Care.* 2002;25:134–147.

Bell DSH. Beta-blockers in the diabetic patient. *Practical Diabetology.* 2003;22(1):20–23.

Egede LE. Lifestyle modification to improve blood pressure control in individuals with diabetes. *Diabetes Care.* 2003;26:602–607.

Gottlieb SH. Hypertension essentials. *Diabetes Forecast.* 2002;55(7):40–43.

Hieronymus L, Griffin S. Blood pressure drugs: what are the options? *Diabetes Self-Management.* 2003;20(5):6–15.

Padawal R, Laupacis. Antihypertensive therapy and incidence of type 2 diabetes: a systematic review. *Diabetes Care.* 2004;27:247–255.

Schaars CF, Genig P, Kasje WN, Stewart RE, Colfeenbuttel BHR, Haajer-Ruskamp FM. Physician, organizational and patient factors association with suboptimal blood pressure management in type 2 diabetes patients in primary care. *Diabetes Care.* 2004;27:123–128.

Cardiovascular

Adler AI, Stevens RJ, Neil A, Stratton IM, Bouton AJM, Holman RR, and the UK Prospective Diabetes Study Group. UKPDS 59: hyperglycemia and other potentially modifiable risk factors for peripheral vascular disease in type 2 diabetes. *Diabetes Care.* 2002;25:894–899.

SUGGESTED READINGS *continued*

Alexander CM, Antonello S, Heggan C, Calder RA. NCDEP ATPIII guidelines. *Practical Diabetology.* 2002;21(1):21–28.

American Diabetes Association. Consensus statement: role of cardiovascular risk factors in prevention and treatment of macrovascular disease in diabetes. *Diabetes Care.* 1989; 12:573–579.

American Diabetes Association. Consensus statement: peripheral arterial disease in people with diabetes. *Diabetes Care.* 2003;26:3333–3341.

American Diabetes Association. Consensus Statement: management of dyslipidemia in children and adolescents with diabetes. *Diabetes Care.* 2003;26:2194–2197.

American Diabetes Association, National Health, Lung, and Blood Institute, the Juvenile Diabetes Foundation International; The National Institutes of Diabetes and Digestive and Kidney Diseases; and the American Heart Association. Joint Editorial Statement: Diabetes mellitus: a major risk facet for cardiovascular disease in diabetes. *Circulation.* 1999;100:1132–1133.

American Diabetes Association. Position statement: Management of dyslipidemia in adults with diabetes. *Diabetes Care.* 2000;23 (Suppl 1):S57–S60.

Braunstein JB. PAD: the vascular in cardiovascular disease. *Diabetes Forecast.* 2002; 55(9):46–48.

Braunstein JB. Working to mend a broken heart. *Diabetes Forecast.* 2000;53(8):29–33.

Buse JB. Lipid changes associated with diabetes therapy. *Practical Diabetology.* 2003; 22(1):24–30.

Buse JB. Statin treatment in diabetes mellitus. *Clinical Diabetes.* 2003;21:168–172.

Cho E, Manson JE, Stampfer MJ, Solomon CG, Colditz GA, Speizer FE, Willett WC, Hu FB. A prospective study of obesity and risk of coronary heart disease among diabetic women. *Diabetes Care.* 2002;25:1142–1148.

Colwell JA. Aspirin therapy in diabetes: a technical review. *Diabetes Care.* 1997;20:1767–1771.

D'Arrigo T. Cholesterol: the good, the bad, and the ugly. *Diabetes Forecast.* 1999;52(8), 54–59.

D'Arrigo T. Counting down cholesterol. *Diabetes Forecast.* 2001;54(9):73–76.

D'Arrigo T. Women, type 2, and cardiovascular risk. *Diabetes Forecast.* 1999;52(1):31–33.

Davis ED, Rodgers PT. Supporting post-MI recovery in patients with diabetes. *Nursing.* 2004;34(1):29.

Dinsmoor R. Cardiac testing: what to expect. *Diabetes Self-Management.* 2002;19(2):23–29.

Fox CS, Sullivan L, D'Argostino RB, Wilson PWF. The significant effects of diabetes duration on coronary heart disease mortality. *Diabetes Care.* 2004;27:704–708.

Gaillard TR, Schyuster DP, Bossetti BM, Green PA, Osei K. The impact of socioeconomic status on cardiovascular risk factors in African-Americans at high risk for type II diabetes. *Diabetes Care.* 1997;20:745–752.

George EL, Tasota FJ. Predicting heart disease with C-reactive protein. *Nursing.* 2003; 33(5):70–71.

Goldberg RB. Cardiovascular disease in diabetic patients. *Medical Clinics of North America.* 2000;84:81–93.

Gottleib SH. Dr. Quick's aspirin fix. *Diabetes Forecast.* 2001;54(10):38–40.

Hagberg L. Cardiac rehabilitation. *Diabetes Self-Management.* 2003;20(1):59–62.

Haines ST, Zeolla MM. Stroke. *Diabetes Forecast.* 2000;53(9):58–62.

Hinson J, Riordan K, Hemphill D, Randolph C, Foneseca V. Hypertension education: a neglected part of the diabetes education curriculum. *The Diabetes Educator.* 1997; 23:166–170.

Hu FB, Stampfer MJ, Haffner SM, Solomon CG, Willet WC, Manson JE. Elevated risk of cardiovsacular disease prior to clinical diagnosis of type 2 diabetes. *Diabetes Care.* 2002; 25:1129–1134.

Jenkins A, Lyons T. Preventing vascular disease in diabetes. *Practical Diabetology.* 2000; 19(1):19–29.

King DE, Mainous AG, Buchanan TA, Pearson WS. C-reactive protein and glycemic control in adults with diabetes. *Diabetes Care.* 2003; 26:1535–1529.

SUGGESTED READINGS *continued*

Cardiovascular *continued*

Kordella T. C-reactive protein. *Diabetes Forecast.* 2004;56(6):51–54.

Krein SL, Vijan S, Pogach LM, Hogan MM, Kerr EA. Aspirin use and counseling about aspirin among patients with diabetes. *Diabetes Care.* 2002;25:965–970.

Kuncl N, Nelson KM. Getting the skinny on lipid-lowering drugs. *Nursing.* 2000;30(7):52–54.

Lacey KO, Chyum DA, Grey M. An integrative literature review of cardiac risk factor management in diabetes education interventions. *The Diabetes Educator.* 2000;26:812–820.

Lopez JAG, Marker CL, Holloway RM. Caring for your cardiovascular system. *Diabetes Forecast.* 2001;54(11):73–75.

Lopez JAG. Tests for your heart. *Diabetes Forecast.* 1999;52(6):56–59.

McAllister FA, Man J, Bistritz L, Amad H, Tandon P. Diabetes and coronary artery bypass surgery. *Diabetes Care.* 2003; 26:1518–1524.

Merrill J. Don't sweat a stress test. *Diabetes Forecast.* 1996;49(10):32–36.

Nesto RW. Screening for asymptomatic coronary artery disease in diabetes. *Diabetes Care.* 1999;22:1393–1396.

Platnik AM. How cardiac drugs do what they do. *Nursing.* 2001;31(5):54–58.

Roberts SS. Aspirin therapy. *Diabetes Forecast.* 2003;56(10):31–32.

Streja D. Drug therapy for dyslipidemia in diabetes. *Practical Diabetology.* 2000;19(1):14–18.

Vinik AI, Erbas T, Park TS, Nolan R, Pittenger GL. Platelet dysfunction in type 2 diabetes. *Diabetes Care.* 2001;24:1476–1485.

Wakabayashi I, Kobaba-Wakabayashi R, Masuda H. Relation of drinking alcohol to atherosclerotic risk in type 2 diabetes. *Diabetes Care.* 2002;25:1223–1228.

Williams KV, Erbey, JF, Becker, D, Orchard, TJ. Improved glycemic control reduces the impact of weight gain on cardiovascular risk factors in type 1 diabetes. *Diabetes Care.* 1999;22:1084–1091.

Neuropathy

American Diabetes Association. Consensus statement: diabetic neuropathy. *Diabetes Care.* 1996;19(Supplement 1):S67–S71.

American Diabetes Association. Consensus statement: standardized measures in diabetic neuropathy. *Diabetes Care.* 1996;19 (Supplement 1):S72–S92.

Bernstein G. The diabetic stomach: management strategies for clinicians and patients. *Diabetes Spectrum.* 2000;13:11–15.

Breite ID. Diabetic gastroparesis. Practical Diabetology. 2004;22(4):6–9.

De Csepel J, Goldfarb B, Jordan C. Gastric electrical stimulation. *Practical Diabetology.* 2004;22(4):14–18.

Dworkin RH, Backonja M, Towbotham MC, Allen RR, Argoff CR, Bennett GJ, Bushell MC. Advances in neuropathic pain. *Archives of Neurology.* 2003;60:1524–1534.

Dyck J, Davies JL, Wilson DM, Service FJ, Melton LJ III, O'Brien PC. Risk factors for the severity of diabetic polyneuropathy. *Diabetes Care.* 1999;22:1479–1486.

Gilden JL. Treating orthostatic hypotension. *Practical Diabetology.* 1996;15(3):28–31, 34.

Gordis A, Scuffham P, Shearer A, Oglesby A, Tobian JA. The health care costs of diabetic periphral neuropathy in the US. *Diabetes Care.* 2003;26:1790–1795.

Kong MF, Horowitz M, Jones KL, Wishart JM, Harding PE. Natural history of diabetic gastroparesis. *Diabetes Care.* 1999;22:503–507.

Kordella T. Frozen shoulder and diabetes. *Diabetes Forecast.* 2002;55(8):60–62.

LaCava EC. Diabetes and your nerves. *Diabetes Forecast.* 2003;55(2):66–69.

Meijer JWG, van Sonderen E, Blaauwwiekel EE, Smit AJ, Goothoff JW, Eisma WH, Links TP. Diabetic neuropathy examination. *Diabetes Care.* 2000;23:750–753.

Mendell JR, Sahenk Z. Painful sensory neuropathy. *NEJM.* 2003;348:1243–1255.

Merio R, Festa A, Bergmann H, Eder T, Eibl N, et al. Slow gastric emptying in type I diabetes:

SUGGESTED READINGS *continued*

relation to autonomic and peripheral neuropathy, blood glucose, and glycemic control. *Diabetes Care.* 1997;20:419–422.

O'Leary C, Quigley EMM. Evaluation of upper-gastrointestinal symptoms in the diabetic patient. *Practical Diabetology.* 2000; 19(2):7–14.

Partanen J, Niskanen L, Lehtinen S, Mervaala E, Siitonen O, Uusitupa M. Natural history of peripheral neuropathy in patients with non-insulin-dependent diabetes mellitus. *The New England Journal of Medicine.* 1995;333:89–94.

Pendergast JJ. Diabetes autonomic neuropathy: early detection. *Practical Diabetology.* 2001; 20(1):7–14.

Pendergast JJ. Diabetes autonomic neuropathy: treatment. *Practical Diabetology.* 2001; 20(2):30–36.

Sacerdote AS, Wasserman I, Enenajor G. Treatment of diabetic gastroparesis. *Practical Diabetology.* 2004;22(4):10–13.

Siegel LB, Huang SR. Get a grip: diabetes and your hands. *Diabetes Forecast.* 2003; 56(4):62–64.

Simmons Z, Feldman EL. The pharmacological treatment of painful diabetic neuropathy. *Clinical Diabetes.* 2000;18(3):116–118.

The SYDNEY Trial Authors for the SYDNEY Study Trial group. The sensory symptoms of diabetic polyneuropathy are improved with alpha-lipoic acid. *Diabetes Care.* 2003; 26:770–776.

Tanenberg RJ, Pfeifer MA. Neuropathy: the forgotten complication. *Diabetes Forecast.* 2000;53(12):58–69.

Thomas-Dobersen D, Ryan-Turek T. Gastroparesis: a case of unexplained lows. *Diabetes Forecast.* 2003;56(9):69–72.

Vileikyte L, Peyrot M, Bundy C, Rubin RR, Leventhal W, Mora P, Shaw JE, Baker P, Boulton AJM. The development and validation of a neuropathy- and foot ulcer-specific quality of life instrument. *Diabetes Care.* 2003;26:2549–2555.

Vinik AI, Maser RE, Mitchell BD, Freeman R. Diabetic autonomic neuropathy: a technical review. *Diabetes Care.* 2003;26:1553–1579.

Welch AC. Constipation and diabetes. *Diabetes Forecast.* 2003;56(8):65–68.

Ziegler D. Cardiovascular autonomic neuropathy: clinical manifestations and measurements. *Diabetes Reviews.* 1999;7:300–315.

Risk-Factor Reduction

American Diabetes Association. Position statement: Aspirin therapy in diabetes. *Diabetes Care.* 2004;27(Suppl 1):S72–S73.

American Diabetes Association. Position statement: Management of dyslipidemia in adults with diabetes. *Diabetes Care.* 2004;27 (Suppl 1):S68–S71.

University of New Mexico Diabetes Team. *101 Tips for Staying Healthy with Diabetes,* 2nd Edition. Alexandria, VA: American Diabetes Association, 1999.

➲ Circulatory System

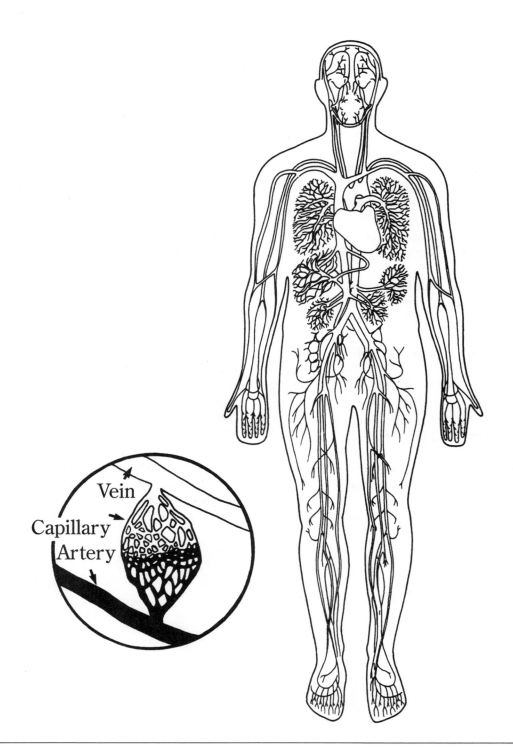

Vein

Capillary

Artery

➡ Normal Eye

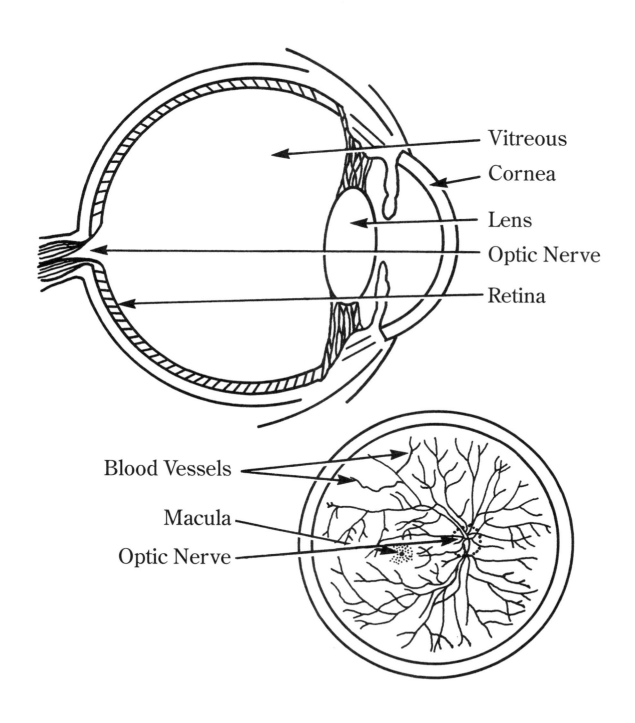

Vitreous

Cornea

Lens

Optic Nerve

Retina

Blood Vessels

Macula

Optic Nerve

➡ Microaneurysms

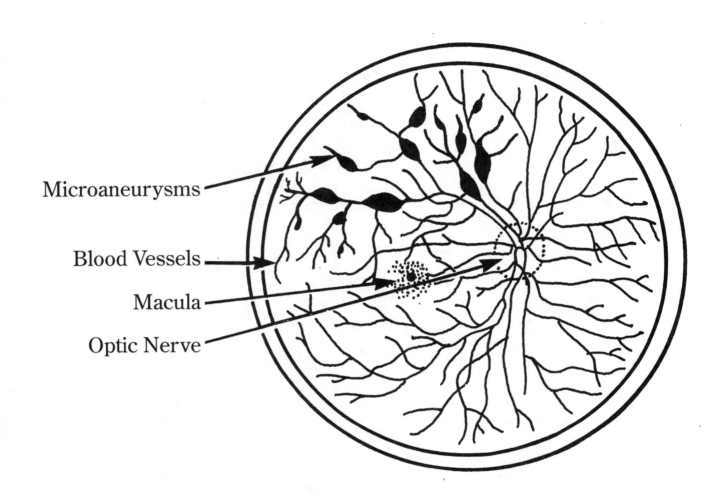

Microaneurysms

Blood Vessels

Macula

Optic Nerve

➲ Proliferative Retinopathy

Microaneurysms

New Blood Vessels

Blood Vessels

Macula

Optic Nerve

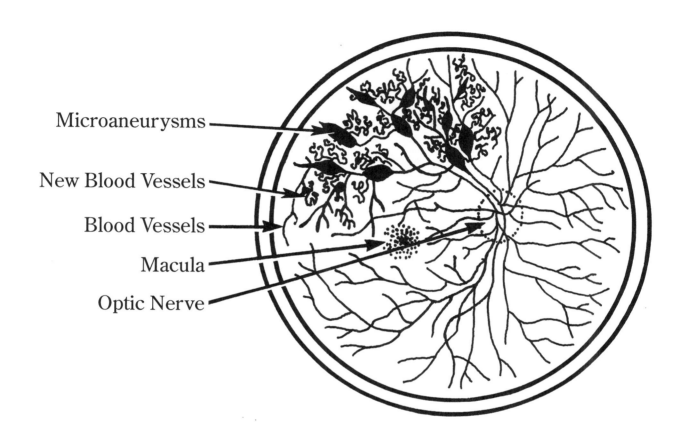

➡ Retinal Detachment

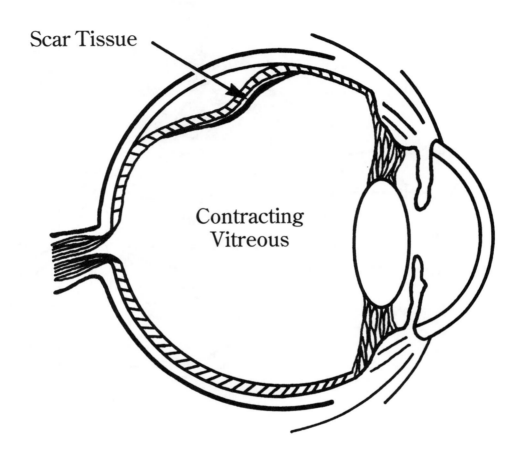

Scar Tissue

Contracting
Vitreous

➡ **Normal Kidney**

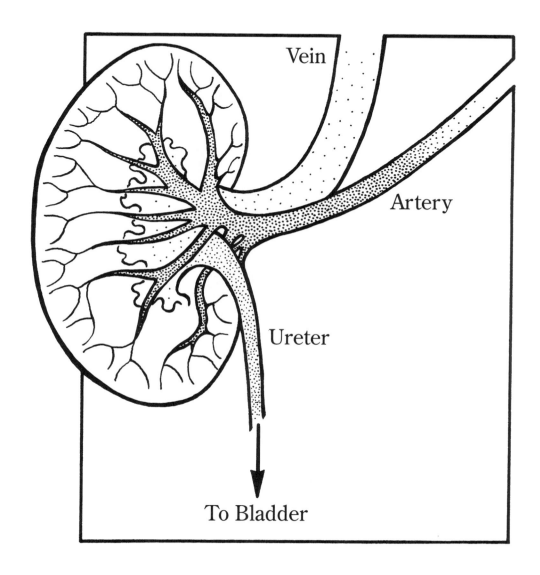

Vein

Artery

Ureter

To Bladder

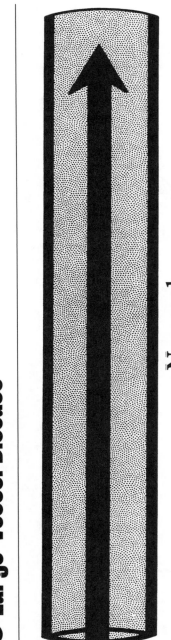

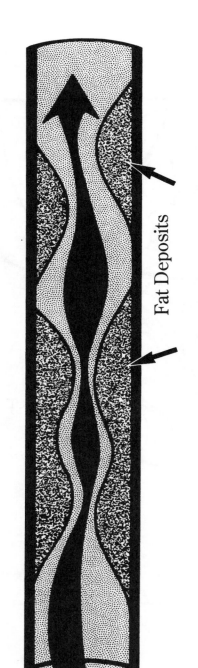

Large-Vessel Disease

Normal

Fat Deposits

Arteriosclerosis

➲ Nervous System

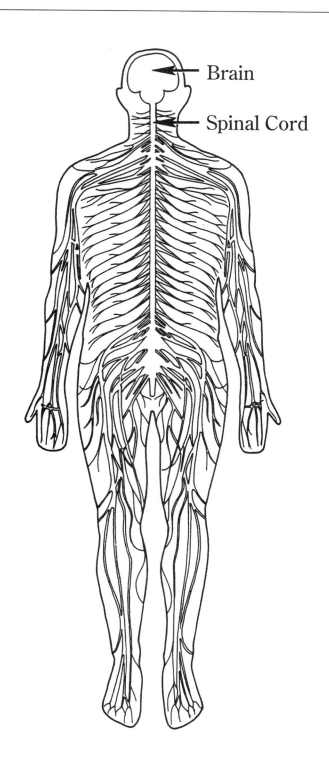

Brain

Spinal Cord

➡ Wound Healing

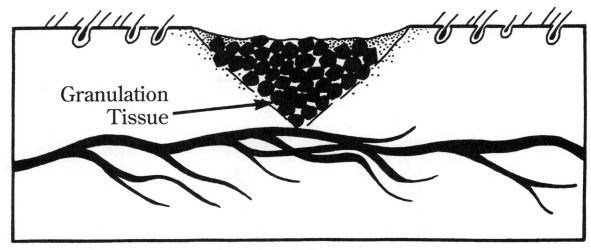

Granulation Tissue

Normal Circulation

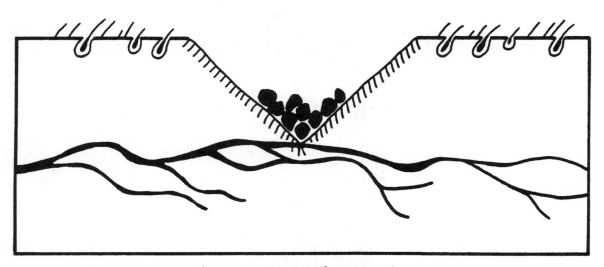

Arteriosclerosis

➔ Resources for Diabetes Complications

When people begin to experience the complications that can occur with diabetes, they often find that they need support and resources. There is help available. The following is a list of national organizations. Ask your health care team for more information about resources in your area.

VISION PROBLEMS

Services for the Blind is an agency that offers vocational or job training to legally blind persons. They can be contacted through the county Social Services Office (listed under "county government" in the white pages). They offer medical and surgical services and vocational training, including college, on-the-job, tutorial, and adjustment teaching.

Other service agencies

American Council of the Blind
1155 15th Street, NW
Washington, DC 20005
800-424-8666
www.acb.org

Lions Club International
300 West 22nd Street
Oakbrook, IL 60523-8842
630-571-5466
www.lionsclub.org

National Eye Institute
Information Specialist
Building 31, Room 6A32
Bethesda, MD 20892
301-496-5248
www.nei.nih.org

National Federation of the Blind
1800 Johnson Street
Baltimore, MD 21230
410-659-9314
www.nfb.org

Prevent Blindness America
500 East Remington Road
Schaumburg, IL 60173-5611
800-331-2020
www.preventblindness.org

Sources for tapes or reading material

National Library Service for the Blind and Physically Handicapped
Library of Congress
1291 Taylor Street, NW
Washington, DC 20542
202-707-5100
www.loc.gov/nls/

Braille Exchange Lists
Braille Institute
741 N. Vermont Avenue
Los Angeles, CA 90029
323-663-1111
www.braillelibrary.org

American Printing House for the Blind
1839 Frankfort Avenue
Louisville, KY 40206
502-895-2405
www.aph.org

Correspondence course

Hadley School for the Blind
700 Elm Street
Winnetka, IL 60093
847-446-8111
www.hadley-school.org

RESOURCES FOR DIABETES COMPLICATIONS *continued*

Kidney disease

National Kidney Foundation
30 East 33rd Street
New York, NY 10016
212-889-2210
www.kidney.org

American Association of Kidney Patients
3505 E. Frontage Road
Suite 315
Tampa, FL 33607
800-749-2257
www.aakp.org

Kidney Directions
http://www.kidneydirections.com
Baxter health-care corporation online resource for education materials.

Heart disease

American Heart Association
7272 Greenville Avenue
Dallas, TX 75231
800-242-8721
www.americanheart.org

Amputations

National Amputation Foundation
40 Church Street
Malverne, NY 11565
516-887-3600
www.nationalamputation.org

Impotence

Erection Devices
ErecAid: 800-344-9688
VED: 800-531-3333
Pos-T-Vac: 800-627-7434

Neuropathy

The Neuropathy Association
60 East 42nd Street
Suite 942
New York, NY 10165
800-247-6968
www.neuropathy.org

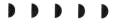

| #15 | Changing Behavior |

STATEMENT OF PURPOSE

This session is intended to present a problem-solving approach to diabetes self-care and general health habits. Behavior change strategies and goal setting are included. This content is most useful if presented during the first or second session and participants are encouraged to choose a short-term behavioral goal as an experiment at each session. The goal-setting form can be used during the last class as a way of helping participants establish new goals or sustain the changes they made.

PREREQUISITES

None.

OBJECTIVES

At the end of this session, participants will be able to:

1. state a specific strategy for making behavior changes;

2. identify a personal long-term goal related to diabetes;

3. make a behavior change plan;

4. set a behavior change goal;

5. make a commitment to carry out behavior change goals.

CONTENT

Goal Setting; Problem Solving.

MATERIALS NEEDED

VISUALS PROVIDED	ADDITIONAL
None.	■ Pencils for participants
	■ Chalkboard and chalk
Handout (one per participant)	
1. Behavior Change Plan	

METHOD OF PRESENTATION

Start by introducing yourself and telling what you do. Ask participants to introduce themselves and tell what they are currently doing to care for their diabetes. Explain that the purpose of this session is for participants to develop a clear plan for working on a problem they want to solve or a behavior they want to change.

Present material in a question/discussion format. Elicit and incorporate as many patient experiences and suggestions as possible into the discussion. The Behavior Change Plan handout can be used either as an in-class activity or at home by each participant. In either case, it is very important to review it with the participants so that they can choose a behavior change they believe will be helpful to them. Help participants break down large goals into smaller, more achievable steps. Help them to feel that they can do it and not feel overwhelmed. End with the visualization, if desired.

Encourage family members and friends of participants to take part in the session, either by making a personal behavior change plan or by identifying how they will provide support.

CONTENT OUTLINE

CONCEPT	DETAIL	INSTRUCTOR'S NOTES
1. Health habits	1.1 The ways that you eat, exercise, and take care of your health are habits, or behaviors. You have had these habits for many years, and they are rarely easy to change.	Ask, "How did you do with your short-term goal? What did you learn from it?"
	1.2 Taking care of diabetes may mean changes in your health habits.	Ask, "What changes have you made as a result of diabetes? What changes have been hard? Easy?"
	1.3 You will not be able to make a lot of changes overnight—no matter how much "willpower" you have.	Ask, "What questions or concerns do you have about making changes in your health habits?"
	1.4 But you can make changes in your life. First you need to be ready, then learn how to make changes, then choose what you want to change, and then make a plan for change.	Emphasize that not being ready to change, not planning for change, not setting clear goals, setting a goal that's too hard, and lack of commitment are more likely reasons for not achieving goals than lack of "willpower."
2. Strategies for making changes	2.1 There are strategies that you can use in making behavior changes.	Ask, "What changes have you made in your habits in the past? What helped or hindered you in making these changes or reaching your goals?"

CONTENT OUTLINE

CONCEPT	DETAIL	INSTRUCTOR'S NOTES
	2.2 Start with something you feel you can do and will be meaningful for you. Success will help you feel that you can make changes.	Ask, "What is hardest or the worst part for you about caring for your diabetes?"
	2.3 Start with something you feel ready to change.	Frustration can also serve as a source of motivation.
	2.4 Because diabetes involves multiple changes in various aspects of your lifestyle, you may feel differently about different health habits. For example, you can be ready to exercise, but not ready to change your meal plan.	
	2.5 Start by adding one new habit. It is easier to add a new habit than to give up one that you already have. For example, if you want to exercise, start with that behavior.	Ask, "How ready do you feel to make this change? How sure do you feel you can make this change?"
	2.6 Write down your new habits. Records, such as food diaries and weight charts, can help you see how you are doing.	Point out that some people find weight charts frustrating, because things other than behavior can influence results.
	2.7 Make it easy to remember your new habits. For example, if it's hard for you to remember to take your pills before breakfast, put the bottle on the kitchen table or by the alarm clock.	Ask, "What other things have you done that serve as reminders to yourself to do things?"
	2.8 Get rid of reminders of habits you want to break. If you want to stop smoking, get rid of your ashtrays.	Ask, "Can you think of anything that reminds you of habits that you are trying to break?"
	2.9 Changing your daily routine may also help eliminate cues for certain behaviors or help you add a behavior.	Ask, "Are there ways to change your routine that will help?"
	2.10 Ask for help from your family and friends. Tell them how they can be most helpful to you.	
	2.11 Write a contract or agreement with your family or care team about the behavior changes you want to make.	

CONTENT OUTLINE

CONCEPT	DETAIL	INSTRUCTOR'S NOTES
	2.12 Reward yourself when you make progress. Treat yourself to something when you reach each step toward your long-term goal. This isn't childish, but is a proven way to change habits.	A reward could be taking time to do something you enjoy, such as reading a book or doing a hobby.
3. Choices for behavior change	3.1 During the next part of the class, you can use some of these strategies to make a behavior change plan. The first step is deciding what you want to do. Think about your overall goals of caring for your diabetes. These are considered your long-term goals or outcomes. Personal blood glucose and weight loss goals are in this category.	Distribute Handout #1, Behavior Change Plan. Have each participant work through the steps as you review them, or work through the handout as a group on the chalkboard, then have participants develop a personal plan. Point out that they may not have responses in all categories. If done in the group, ask the class to choose an area or situation that is relevant for most, such as blood glucose control or weight loss.

Encourage participants to choose goals that are both meaningful and attainable. For example, maintaining normal blood glucose levels at all times is not realistic for most people with diabetes. |
	3.2 Make a list of all your long-term goals related to diabetes.	Point out that a participant's goals may be different than those of the health care provider. It is critical that the goal be selected by the participant.
	3.3 What parts of living with diabetes are hardest for you?	This helps participants focus on their concerns about living with and caring for diabetes.
	How does that make you feel?	"Negative" feelings about a situation are often powerful motivators for change. Help participants identify and use the energy these emotions create.

CONTENT OUTLINE

CONCEPT	DETAIL	INSTRUCTOR'S NOTES
	3.4 How does this need to change for you to reach your goals or feel better about it?	Ask, "What will happen if you don't do anything? How will you feel?"
	3.5 Where would you like to be in achieving this goal in a year? Six months from now? Three months?	Help participants evaluate appropriate time frames based on long-term goals.
	3.6 What would you like to accomplish in the next month? Week? This is your short-term goal.	Help participants set achievable short-term goals. For example, if the concern is lack of exercise, and the long-term goal is to walk a mile every day, the short-term goal may be to walk $\frac{1}{4}$ mile three times a week by the end of the month, and two blocks by the end of the week.
	3.7 There are costs and benefits to any action or change that you want to make.	If participants aren't ready to make any changes, responding to question #5 in Handout #1 and listing costs and benefits of making changes may help to clarify their feelings.
	3.8 What would be the costs to you of taking action or achieving this goal? For example, for weight loss, the costs may be giving up foods you enjoy, less flexibility, discomfort in social situations involving food, or changing the way you cook.	Do this with participants in an accepting, nonjudgmental way with participants. Avoid pointing out benefits or strategies yourself.
	3.9 What would be the benefits to you of taking action or achieving this goal? For example, if the goal is losing weight, the benefits may be that you will look better, feel better, or have better blood glucose control.	Point out that the benefits listed need to be personally meaningful. This provides the needed motivation.
	3.10 Think about the costs and benefits. Is it worth it to you to make this change? If the costs outweigh the benefits, you need to decide if you are still ready and willing to take action to improve this situation or achieve this goal.	Ask, "On a scale of 1–10, how important is this goal to you?" Recognize that choosing to do nothing is an option. Only you can decide if the benefit is worth the cost.

CONTENT OUTLINE

CONCEPT	DETAIL	INSTRUCTOR'S NOTES
	3.11 Make a commitment to yourself or another person.	
4. Making a plan	4.1 What are some steps you could take to improve this situation or move closer to your goal? Think of all the possible options you have and what you can do. In the weight loss example, options related to social situations may include saving meat and fat exchanges, not going, meeting with the dietitian specifically to discuss this topic, ignoring the meal plan on that occasion and monitoring more closely, taking extra insulin, or increasing activity that day.	Options need to be generated by the participants to be meaningful. Encourage participants to choose behavior change strategies over which they have control (e.g., skipping dessert three times a week rather than losing a specific number of pounds, or testing blood three times a day rather than achieving a certain blood glucose number).
	4.2 What are ways you can change your environment at home or work?	Ask, "Are there barriers to overcome?" Examples: Remove tempting foods from the house, place them out of sight, bring a lunch to work.
	4.3 What are ways you believe your family or friends can be most helpful to you? Think of how you will ask for help, and practice in your mind.	Ask, "Are there people who can help you?" Examples: Eat similar food, exercise with you, not eat tempting foods in front of you.
5. Setting behavior-change goals	5.1 Now, look at all the steps and options that you have identified and choose one to three steps that you will take toward achieving your short-term goal when you leave here. These are your behavior-change goals.	These steps need to be readily achievable and specific. For example, if a morning exercise program is a goal, getting up half an hour earlier or buying comfortable shoes is an appropriate step.
	5.2 Think of these as experiments. The benefit of an experiment is that whether it works or does not work, you can still learn something.	
	5.3 Make a commitment that you will carry out this behavior change or step.	This can be verbal or written, with the educator, a partner, or significant other.

CONTENT OUTLINE

CONCEPT	DETAIL	INSTRUCTOR'S NOTES
	5.4 What is your time frame? Choose a deadline for starting or identify the number of times per week you will do the behavior.	Again, this needs to be realistic given the other demands and priorities that participants have. It may not be realistic to do something every day.
	5.5 How will you keep track of your new behavior?	Record keeping can be a very reinforcing part of behavior change. The system should be simple and easy to do, so that it is not a deterrent to change.
	5.6 Decide how you will reward yourself for achieving your long-term goal and short-term goal and for trying each behavior-change goal or step along the way.	This is a very important part of the behavior-change process that is often neglected. Having better health or preventing long-term complications is too elusive and futuristic to be rewarding for most people. Encourage patients to choose a reward that is meaningful enough so that it offers an incentive at times when the goal seems too hard to achieve, such as a reward for staying with behavior changes for 1 week.
6. Problem-solving	6.1 Are there any problems or issues that you can anticipate and plan for? For example, do you have a place to exercise in good and bad weather?	Ask, "Are there barriers that you can anticipate? What can you do to make a plan to overcome them?"
	6.2 If the plan doesn't work, think about what you learned from your experiments. The first step in solving problems is to identify the problem. Go back over the steps to see what you could do differently.	Encourage participants to think of these as problems to be solved, not failures.
	6.3 It could be that your goal is too big, you might be trying to do too much at one time, a different option will work better, the costs outweigh the benefits, or this goal isn't relevant for you at this time.	

CONTENT OUTLINE

CONCEPT	DETAIL	INSTRUCTOR'S NOTES
	6.4 You may decide on a different long-term or short-term goal or choose a different option or behavior-change goal as your next experiment.	
	6.5 If you have a day when you don't meet your goals, try not to let it get you down. Think about what problems you encountered, what you learned, and what you might do differently the next time.	
7. Visualization	7.1 One technique that sometimes helps is visualization: imagining yourself as successful in meeting your goals. If you find this exercise helpful, you can do it yourself each day or when you feel discouraged.	After reviewing the plans, one way to end this session is by having the participants visualize themselves as successful at meeting their goals.
		Speak slowly and in a relaxing manner as you go through the exercise, pausing between requests.

Visualization Exercise

Ask participants to close their eyes and picture themselves in 3 months or a year when they have met their goal. Suggest that they picture:

- how they look
- how they feel physically
- how their family and friends feel about them
- how they feel about themselves

Ask that they keep their eyes closed for as long as they like and enjoy these feelings. Then, slowly open their eyes and come back into the present.

SKILLS CHECKLIST

Each participant will be able to identify a long-term diabetes-related goal and develop a behavior-change plan.

EVALUATION PLAN

Knowledge will be evaluated by achievement of learning and skill objectives and by responses to questions during the session. The ability to apply knowledge will be evaluated by development of personal long-term and behavior-change goals, by the development and implementation of a plan to achieve those goals, and through program outcome measures.

DOCUMENTATION PLAN

Record class attendance and achieved objectives as appropriate.

SUGGESTED READINGS

Behavior Change

American Diabetes Association. *Facilitating Lifestyle Change: A Resource Manual.* Alexandria, VA: American Diabetes Association, 1997.

Anderson RM, Funnell MM, Butler PM, Arnold MS, Feste CC. Patient empowerment: results of a randomized controlled trial. *Diabetes Care.* 1995;18:943–949.

Delahanty LM. Evidence-based trends for achieving weight loss and increased physical activity: applications for diabetes prevention and treatment. *Diabetes Spectrum.* 2002;15:183–196.

The Diabetes Prevention Program (DPP) Research Group. The diabetes prevention program: description of lifestyle intervention. *Diabetes Care.* 2002;25:2165–2171.

Earles J. Time to get motivated. *Diabetes Forecast.* 2003;56(12):50–53.

Faulk JS. Several habits of highly successful self-advocates. *Diabetes Self-Management.* 2001;18(1):38–44.

Fisher EB, Walker EA, Bostrom A, Fischhoff B, Haire-Joshu D, Johnson SB. Behavioral science research in the prevention of diabetes. *Diabetes Care.* 2002;25:599–606.

Funnell MM, Anderson RM. Patient empowerment: a look back, a look ahead. *The Diabetes Educator.* 2003;29:454–464.

Funnell MM. Lessons learned as a diabetes educator. *Diabetes Spectrum.* 2000;13:69–70.

Glasgow RE, Anderson RM. In diabetes care, moving from compliance to adherence is not enough. *Diabetes Care.* 1999;2090–2091.

Glasgow RE. Behavioral and psychosocial measures for diabetes care: what's important to assess? *Diabetes Spectrum.* 1997;10:12–17.

Glasgow RE, Hiss RG, Anderson RM, Friedman NM, Hayward RA, Marrero DG, Taylor CB, Vinicor F. Report of the health care delivery work group: behavioral research related to the establishment of a chronic disease model for diabetes care. *Diabetes Care.* 2001; 24:124–130.

Haddad LG, Hoeman SP. Development of the Arabic language readiness to stop smoking questionnaire A-RSSQ. *Image.* 2001; 33:355–359.

Heisler M, Smith DM, Hayward RA, Krein SL, Kerr EA. How well do patients' assessments of their diabetes self-management correlate with actual glycemic control and receipt of recommended diabetes services. *Diabetes Care.* 2003;26:738–743.

Kennedy JAE, Erb C. Prescription noncompliance due to cost among adults with disabilities in the US. *AJPH.* 2002;92:1120–1124.

Krichbaum K, Aarestad V, Buethe M. Exploring the connection between self-efficacy and

SUGGESTED READINGS *continued*

Behavior Change *continued*

effective diabetes self-management. *The Diabetes Educator.* 2003; 29:653–662.

Lorenz RA, Bubb J, Davis D, Jacobson A, Jannasch K, Kramer J, Lipps J, Schlundt D. Changing behavior: practical lessons from the Diabetes Control and Complications Trial. *Diabetes Care.* 1996;19:648–652.

Nelson KM, Reiber G, Boyko EJ. Diet and exercise among adults with type 2 diabetes. *Diabetes Care.* 2002;25:1722–1728.

Nies MA, Hepworth JT, Wallston KA, Kershaw TC. Evaluation of an instrument for assessing behavioral change in sedentary women. *Image.* 2001;33:349–354.

Peyrot M. Behavior change in diabetes education. *The Diabetes Educator.* 1999; 25(Suppl):62–74.

Peyrot MF. Theory of behavioral diabetes research. *Diabetes Care.* 2001;24:1703–1705.

Satterfield DW, Volansky M, Caspersen CJ, Engelgau MM, Bwman BA, Gregg EW, Geiss LS, Gosey GM, May J, Vinicor F. Community-based lifestyle interventions to prevent type 2 diabetes. *Diabetes Care.* 2003;26:2643–2652.

Thorne SE, Paterson BL. Health care professional support for self-care management in chronic illness: insights from diabetes research. *Patient Education and Counseling.* 2001;42:81–90.

Tupling H, Webb K, Harris G, Sulway M. *You've Got to Get Through the Outside Layer.* Sydney: Bloxam and Chambers, 1981. (Available from the American Association of Diabetes Educators.)

Walker EA. Health behavior: from paradox to paradigm. *Diabetes Spectrum.* 2001;14:6–9.

Welch G, Guthrie DW. Lifestyle and behavior: supporting lifestyle change with a computerized psychosocial assessment tool. *Diabetes Spectrum.* 2002;15:203–208.

Whitlock EP, Orleans T, Pender N, Allan J. Evaluating primary care behavioral counseling interventions: an evidence-based approach. *American Journal of Preventive Medicine.* 2002;22:267–284.

Whittemore R. Strategies to facilitate lifestyle change associated with diabetes mellitus. *Image.* 2000;32:225–232.

Williams GC, Zeldman A. Patient-centered diabetes self-management education. *Current Medicine.* 2002;2:145–152.

Wittemore R, Sullian A, Bak PS. Working within boundaries: a patient-centered approach to lifestyle change. *The Diabetes Educator.* 2003;29:69–74.

Wolpert HA, Anderson BJ Management of diabetes: are doctors framing the benefits from the wrong perspective? *BMJ.* 2000; 320:994–996.

Wing RR, Goldstein MG, Acton KJ, Birch LL, et al: Behavioral science research in diabetes. *Diabetes Care.* 2001; 24:117–123.

Problem-Solving and Goal-Setting

Anderson BJ. Cowboys and horse whisperers: changing paradigms of diabetes education and care. *Diabetes Spectrum.* 2003; 16:245–252.

Anderson BJ. Diabetes self-care: lessons from research on the family and broader contexts. *Current Diabetes Reports.* 2003;3:134–140.

Bartol T. Putting the patient with diabetes in the driver's seat. *Nursing.* 2002;32(2)53–55.

Brock DW, Wartman SA. When competent patients make irrational choices. *The New England Journal of Medicine.* 1990;322: 1595–1598.

Davis ED, Vander Meer JM, Yarborough PC, Roth SM. Using solution-focused therapy strategies in empowerment-based education. *The Diabetes Educator.* 1999;25:249–257.

Faulk JS. Going from compliance to collaboration. *Diabetes Self-Management.* 2000;17(2):47–53.

Funnell MM. Helping patients take charge of their chronic illnesses. *Family Practice Management.* 2000;7(3):47–51.

Mitchell GJ, Lawton C. Living with the consequences of personal choices for persons with diabetes: implications for educators and practitioners. *Canadian Journal of Diabetes Care.* 2000;24(2)23–30.

SUGGESTED READINGS *continued*

Montori VM, Bryant SC, O'Connor AM, Jorgensen NW, Walsh EE, Smith SA. Decisional attributes of patients with diabetes: the aspirin choice. *Diabetes Care*. 2003;26:2804–2809.

Morrow IS. What I learned from Rosa: a story of poverty and empowerment. *The Diabetes Educator*. 2002;28:750–754.

Roberts SS. Why you shouldn't be a good patient. *Diabetes Forecast*. 2002;55(5):23–24.

Rubin RR. Facilitating self-care in people with diabetes. *Diabetes Spectrum*. 2001;14:55–57.

Rubin RR, Anderson RM, Funnell MM. Collaborative diabetes care. *Practical Diabetology*. 2002;21(1):29–32.

Skinner TC, Cradock S, Arundel F, Graham W. Lifestyle and behavior: Four theories and a philosophy: self-management education for individuals newly diagnosed with type 2 diabetes. *Diabetes Spectrum*. 2003;16:75–80.

➡ Behavior Change Plan

---

1. What are all of your goals related to diabetes and its care?

2. What part of living with diabetes is hardest for you? How does that make you feel?

3. How does this situation need to change for you to reach your goals or feel better about it?

4. Where would you like to be regarding this situation or your goals a year from now?

   Six months from now?

   Three months from now?

   One month from now?

   Next week?

BEHAVIOR CHANGE PLAN *continued*

5. What are the costs and benefits of taking action to improve this situation or reach your goals?

Benefits	Costs

6. What are some steps you could take to improve this situation or bring you closer to your goal?

7. In what ways can you change your environment (setting) at home or work (that is, eliminate negative triggers or change your routine)?

8. What are ways your family and friends can help you?

9. Write down one to three steps or behaviors that you will do when you leave here to change the situation or reach your goal.

BEHAVIOR CHANGE PLAN *continued*

10. How often will you do this behavior? When is your deadline?

11. Write down how you will keep track of your new behavior.

12. Write down how you will reward yourself for achieving this behavior.

13. Commitment:

I, _____ , will _____

_____

_____

_____

_____   _____
Signature   Date

| #16 | **Putting the Pieces Together** |

STATEMENT OF PURPOSE

This session is intended to help participants find and use information to deal with common situations, to provide information about resources available for people with diabetes, and to obtain desired family and social support.

PREREQUISITES

It is recommended that each participant have basic knowledge about diabetes and self-care, from either personal experience or attending previous sessions.

OBJECTIVES

At the end of this session, participants will be able to:

1. identify strategies to cope with a variety of diabetes-related issues and situations;

2. find resources appropriate to particular situations;

3. state how to obtain a driver's license;

4. list strategies for dealing with possible problems associated with social activities and with traveling;

5. list strategies for obtaining desired family and social support.

CONTENT

Problem-Solving.

MATERIALS NEEDED

WORKSHEETS PROVIDED	ADDITIONAL
1–11. Problem Situations	• Membership brochures from the American Diabetes Association • Magazines and other information for people with diabetes • Information about local community resources • Information about obtaining a driver's license • Information about local syringe-disposal policies

METHOD OF PRESENTATION

Start by introducing yourself and telling what you do. Ask participants to introduce themselves. Explain that the purposes of the class are to discuss a variety of issues that are common for people with diabetes and to provide information about social, vocational, medical, and financial resources that are available.

Eleven situations can be discussed. Choose only the situations and issues that are appropriate for the participants. These situations can also be used for discussion as part of other sessions. An alternative is to ask participants to describe situations or dilemmas they have encountered. Begin by asking how they did with their short-term goal and what they learned from it.

Read each situation to the class, or ask each person in turn to read a situation aloud. Ask the participants to suggest ideas for dealing with the issue and resources that are available. Encourage participants to brainstorm ideas and discuss experiences. Point out that there are usually a variety of ways to deal with issues and problems and that no one way will work for everyone. Supply additional information from the instructor's resources sheets. Distribute pamphlets, membership blanks, and so on, as indicated. Then move on to the next situation. End by asking participants to choose a short-term goal to try before the next session.

SKILLS CHECKLIST

Each participant will be able to suggest a strategy or resource for an issue or problem situation.

EVALUATION PLAN

Knowledge will be evaluated by achievement of learning objectives and by strategies and resources suggested during the session. The ability to apply knowledge will be evaluated by the ability to identify strategies for personal diabetes-related issues or problems, by the use of appropriate resources, and through program outcome measures.

DOCUMENTATION PLAN

Record class attendance and achieved objectives as appropriate.

SUGGESTED READINGS

Resources

Albright A. Diabetes advocacy. *Diabetes Spectrum*. 1999;12:212–245.

American Association of Diabetes Educators. The educators guide to diabetes resources. *The Diabetes Educator*. 2003;29:933–948.

American Diabetes Association. Economic costs of diabetes in the US in 2002. *Diabetes Care*. 2003;26:917–931.

American Diabetes Association. Position statement: Unproven therapies. *Diabetes Care*. 2004;27(Suppl 1):S135.

SUGGESTED READINGS *continued*

American Diabetes Association. Position statement: Third-party reimbursement for outpatient diabetes education and counseling. *Diabetes Care.* 2004;27(Suppl 1):S136–S137.

American Diabetes Association. Resource Guide 2004. Supplement to *Diabetes Forecast.* 2004.

Beddoe SS. Reachable moment. *Image: Journal of Nursing Scholarship.* 1999;31:248–249.

Caro JJ, Ward AJ, O'Brien JA. Lifetime costs of complications resulting from type 2 diabetes in the United States. *Diabetes Care.* 2002; 25:476–481.

Corbett CF, Cook D, Setter SM. Oasis and beyond: improving outcomes for home health patients. *The Diabetes Educator.* 2003; 29:83–89.

Evans JMM, MacDonald TM, Leese, GP, Ruta DA, Morris AD. Impact of type 1 and type 2 diabetes on patterns and costs of prescribing. *Diabetes Care.* 2000;23:770–774.

Klawuhn G. Learning to empower patients: a journey in, a journey out. *The Diabetes Educator.* 1997;23:457–462.

Peele PB, Lave JR, Songer TJ. Diabetes in employer-sponsored health insurance. *Diabetes Care.* 2002;25:1964–1968.

Roberts SL. Medicare, Medicaid and diabetes. *Diabetes Forecast.* 2000;53(9):53–54.

Roberts SL. Pharmacy assistance programs help the needy. *Diabetes Forecast.* 2001; 54(11):67–70.

Roberts SL. Saving money: a dozen prescription price tips. *Diabetes Forecast.* 2003;56(8):73–75.

Roberts SS. When your insurance company denies a claim. *Diabetes Forecast.* 2002; 55(7):60–62.

Ryerson B, Tierney EF, Thompson TJ, Engelgau MM, Wang J, Gregg EW, Geiss LS. Excess physical limitations among adults with diabetes in the US population, 1997–1999. *Diabetes Care.* 2003;26:206–210.

Travel

Bailey LE. Flying smart. *Diabetes Forecast.* 1995;48(1):40–45.

Casale M, Keystone JS. Traveling far and wide with diabetes. *Diabetes Forecast.* 2000; 54(5):46–52.

Gustaitus J. Taking to the air with diabetes. *Diabetes Self-Management.* 2002;19(2):36–37.

Hernandez CL. Traveling with diabetes. *Diabetes Self-Management.* 2004;20(6):118–122.

Hieronymus L, Cherolis J. On the road: driving safely with diabetes. *Diabetes Self-Management.* 2001;18(6):1925.

Rosenbaum M. Welcome aboard (cruises). *Diabetes Forecast.* 1994;48(3):47–50.

Sebastian O, Friesen FG, Frank GJ, et al. Travel-related morbidity in travelers with insulin dependent diabetes mellitus. *J Travel Med.* 1999;6:12–15.

Work Issues

AADE Position Statement. Diabetes education for people with disabilities. *The Diabetes Educator.* 2002;28:916–921.

American Diabetes Association. Position statement: Hypoglycemia and employment/ licensure. *Diabetes Care.* 2004;27 (Suppl 1):S134.

Arent S. The role of diabetes healthcare professionals in diabetes discrimination issues in work and school. *The Diabetes Educator.* 2002;28:1021–1027; *Diabetes Spectrum.* 2002;15:217–221.

Bell DSH. The graveyard shift. *Diabetes Forecast.* 1994;48(2):47–49.

Dominguez CM. Diabetes, the Americans with Disabilities Act, and the EEOC. *Diabetes Forecast.* 2003;56(7):66–68.

Kordella T. Diabetes at work. *Diabetes Forecast.* 2003;56(8):45–48.

Padgett DL, Nord WR, Heins JM, Arfken C. Managing diabetes in the workplace: clinical factors. *Diabetes Spectrum.* 1996;9:13–19.

Ramsey S, Summers KH, Leong SA, Birnbaum HG, Kemner JE, Greenberg P. Productivity and medical costs of diabetes in a large employer population. *Diabetes Care.* 2002; 25:23–29.

SUGGESTED READINGS *continued*

Relationships with Health Care Professionals

Freeman J, Loewe R. Barriers to communication about diabetes mellitus. *The Journal of Family Practice*. 2000;49:507–512.

Frohna JG, Frohna Al Gahagan, Anderson RM. Tips for communicating with patients in managed care. *Seminars in Medical Practice*. 2001;4(2):29–36.

Funnell MM, Anderson RM. Changing office practice and health care systems to facilitate diabetes self-management. *Current Diabetes Reports*. 2003;3:127–133.

Heisler M, Bouknight RR, Hasyward RA, Smith DM, Kerr EA. The relative importance of physician communication, participatory decision making, and patient understanding in diabetes self-mangement. *JGIM*. 2003; 2:17:243–253.

Levinson W, Gorawara-Bhat R, Lamb J. A study of patient clues and physician responses in primary care and surgical settings. *JAMA*. 2000;284:1021–1027.

Marvel MK, Epstein RM, Flowers K, Beckman HB. Soliciting the patient's agenda: have we improved? *JAMA*. 1999;281:283–287.

Sidorov J, Harris R. The integrated approach to diabetes mellitus: the impact of clinical information systems, consumerism, and managed care. *Diabetes Spectrum*. 1996;9:158–163.

Research

American Diabetes Association. Pancreas transplantation in type 1 diabetes. *Diabetes Care*. 2004;27(Suppl 1):S105.

American Diabetes Association. Position statement: Prevention of type 1 diabetes mellitus. *Diabetes Care*. 2004;27(Suppl 1): S133.

Anderson RM, Fitzgerald JT. Should you do it? *Diabetes Forecast*. 1993;46(2):32–33.

Davidson JA, Wilkinson A. On behalf of the Panel on New-Onset Diabetes after Transplantation. *Diabetes Care*. 2004; 27:805–812.

Kordella T. The Edmonton Protocol. *Diabetes Forecast*. 2003;56(3):59–62.

Nakamoto M. Clinical Trials: should you sign up? *Diabetes Self-Management*. 2002; 19(5):72–78.

Shapiro AMJ, Lake JRT, Ryan EA, Korbutt GS, Toth E, Warnock GL, Kneteman, NM, Rajotte RV. Islet transplantation in seven patient with type 1 diabetes mellitus using a gluco-corticoid-free immunosuppressive regimen. *NEJM*. 2000;343:230–239.

SITUATION ONE

MEDICAL/COMMUNITY

You and your family have just moved to another state and you are unfamiliar with the town. You take two pills and NPH insulin at bedtime for your diabetes. You realize that your medications are getting low. You don't have a local doctor.

1. Brainstorm ideas such as calling your former health care team for written or telephone prescriptions, contacting local urgent or emergency care centers, or calling the local health department. If you use a chain pharmacy and have refills left, you can call a local branch for refills.

2. To find a new health care team:

    a. Have your current team refer you to one in your new community. If they can't do this, ask for a copy of your chart or a letter to introduce you to your new provider when you do locate one.

    b. Call or write to the local chapter of the American Diabetes Association (ADA), and request a list of health care professionals in your new location who are members of the ADA.

    c. Contact the American Association of Diabetes Educators for an educator in your area who can refer you to a provider and help you find other needed resources.

    d. Look in the phone book to see if there is a diabetes clinic or other diabetes-related services nearby.

    e. Call the local hospital in the new community for names of providers.

    f. Write to the appropriate medical association or society in your new location for recommendations.

    g. When you get to your new town, ask friends or coworkers whose judgment you trust to recommend a care provider.

3. In some states, a prescription is not needed to buy syringes, needles, or monitoring equipment. Some health insurance plans have prescription coverage, however, and your diabetes supplies may be covered if they are ordered by prescription. Review local syringe disposal policies.

4. Laws that can affect people with diabetes include those regarding a driver's license, medical insurance, life insurance, and employment compensation. Review the specifics for your state. People with diabetes are protected under the Americans with Disabilities Act. For information about a driver's license, call the Bureau of Motor Vehicles or the Secretary of State in your new location. Some states put a notation on your driver's license to indicate that you have diabetes. Some reserve the right to deny or revoke licensure if an accident happens that is due to hypoglycemia.

SITUATION TWO

SOCIAL (FAMILY)

You are a 50-year-old woman with newly diagnosed type 2 diabetes. You have decided you want to lose one pound a week. You take insulin, but your provider says if you lose weight, there's a chance you may not need to stay on it.

Because you've always cooked all the meals for the family, your husband and sons expect you to keep doing so. Your teenage sons have already told you they do not want to eat "rabbit food." Your husband has kept on eating his snack foods in front of you. He makes a point of telling you that you shouldn't have "even a taste."

1. This person may not get much support at home. Lack of support may take the following forms:
   a. Trying to get the person with diabetes to indulge in food so other family members won't feel guilty
   b. Asking the person with diabetes to "try just a taste" of food because they feel sorry for the person
   c. Monitoring eating—being a "parent" to the adult person with diabetes
   d. Teasing about food or weight
   e. Refusing to make any changes in their eating habits
2. Some possible ways to handle this lack of support are:
   a. Start with one area at a time and gradually ask for support in each area.
   b. Have family members attend classes or talk with the health care team to gain a greater understanding of diabetes.
   c. Cook the same meals for all family members, and limit portion size for the person with diabetes.
   d. Ask nonsupportive family members to cook their own food.
   e. Work on assertiveness skills. Use "I" statements to ask for support ("I really need help staying with my diet," or, "It's really hard for me to avoid snack foods when they are around me," or, "I feel so much better when you are helping me").
   f. Join a diabetes support group in your area.
   g. Remember, in most cases, family members are trying to help the person with diabetes. Try to provide your family with positive ways they can help you, such as:
      - ignore eating
      - notice weight loss
      - ask family members to help plan menus
      - ask family members to eat their snack foods away from you
   h. Consider joining a weight loss program or support group.

Weight Watchers International
The Jericho Atrium
175 Crossways Park West
Woodbury, NY 11797-2055
800-651-6000
www.weightwatchers.com

TOPS
4575 South Fifth Street
Milwaukee, WI 53207
414-482-4620
Chapter location:
800-932-8677
www.tops.org

Overeaters Anonymous
PO Box 44020
Rio Rancho, NM 87174
505-891-2664
www.oa.org

i. Purchase a diabetes cookbook that offers recipes the whole family can enjoy. Check your local bookstore, or contact the American Diabetes Association at 800-232-6733.

SITUATION THREE
_____

SOCIAL
_____

You are attending a family birthday dinner at your sister's house. Your sister, who takes pride in her cooking, has prepared a special meal with several courses. Most of the foods are combination dishes with sauces and gravies. After dinner, your sister personally hands you the dessert tray, insisting that you take some. She says, "I know several people with diabetes, and they eat anything."
_____

1. Some ways to handle this situation are:

   a. Eat smaller portions of the food that is served; don't take seconds.

   b. Avoid obviously sweet foods, high-fat foods, sauces, gravies, and alcohol.

   c. Take dessert, but eat none, eat only a small amount, or take it home and throw it away.

   d. Take a walk after eating.

2. Some ways to plan ahead are:

   a. Make a conscious decision before you go about how you will handle the situation. Weigh the costs, benefits, and barriers. If you decide to have dessert, think of it as a choice you have made, not as cheating. Realize that all choices have positive and negative consequences.

   b. Remind your sister before you go that you have diabetes, and talk about the kinds of food you prefer to eat and those you'd rather avoid.

   c. Tell your sister how she can be of the most help to you. Do this at a time other than during the event.

   d. Offer to bring a dessert or other dish that fits your way of eating.

   e. Plan ahead for the special meal (for example, eat less fat that day). Don't take tempting leftovers home.

   f. Find out what the menu will be, then plan ahead what you will and will not eat. Reward yourself with something other than food for doing what you planned.

3. Other strategies for dealing with this type of situation are:

   a. Discuss assertiveness and how to develop it. Practice statements such as, "I appreciate the offer, but I can't possibly eat more," or, "I will feel better if I don't eat that."

   b. Talk about how to be appreciative without compromising health or diet, i.e., "Thank you for making this for me, I really appreciate your thoughtfulness, but. . . ."

   c. Discuss how personal attitude can influence a situation.

   d. Discuss the issue of "wasting" food versus "waisting" food.

   e. Be careful that these special days don't become a reason to overeat. On the other hand, don't let having diabetes keep you from being with your family.

   f. If one dinner doesn't go as you wanted, start over again tomorrow and think about ways to handle it differently the next time.

SITUATION FOUR

SICK DAYS

You wake up with the flu. Your body aches and you have a fever. You usually eat a hearty breakfast, but aren't sure you could keep any food down this morning.

1. Some ways to manage food intake when not feeling well are:
   a. Try to eat the same amount of carbohydrate as usual.
   b. Drink fluids in frequent sips. Try to drink at least once every 30 minutes or with every commercial break on TV.
   c. Clear liquids and soft foods may be appropriate. Consider what sounds good to you. Have the class brainstorm options.

2. Discuss changes needed in medicine or monitoring:
   a. Take your usual insulin dose even if you are unable to eat or are eating less.
   b. Check blood glucose every 2–4 hours.
   c. Check ketones every 4 hours or every time you go to the bathroom.
   d. Check fever and record every 4 hours take aspirin or Tylenol as needed.
   e. You may need extra rapid- or short-acting insulin.

3. Talk about when to call the health care team:
   a. Call if ketones persist for more than 12 hours or are rising.
   b. Call if your blood glucose is higher than 250 mg/dl or you are vomiting persistently.
   c. Call if your fever is 101.5°F or higher, if your fever is rising, or if you have a fever for longer than 24 hours.

TRAVEL

You are flying to Mexico for a vacation soon. At home, you take insulin injections twice a day, count carbohydrates, and walk 30 minutes every other day.

1. Some ways to plan ahead are:

   a. Notify your health care team of your approaching trip. If possible, carry enough insulin and monitoring supplies with you. Get a prescription for insulin and syringes before you leave. Get a letter from your provider about your diabetes, especially if you will be taking syringes through customs. Find out about the availability of insulin and monitoring supplies in the country where you will be traveling by writing to the manufacturer or asking your pharmacist.

   b. An address for locating English-speaking physicians in foreign countries can be found in most travel books specific to the country you plan to visit. Bookstores or the local library may have books that provide this information.

   c. Airlines can provide special meals. You need to notify the airline 24 hours in advance if you would like a special meal.

   d. Wear diabetes identification. Carry a telephone number and instructions to call that number if health care information about you is needed. Travel with someone, if possible.

   e. Take medication with you to control vomiting (especially if you get motion sickness) or diarrhea, and bring antacids to counteract new foods that might irritate your stomach.

   f. Write down the phrases for "Please get me a doctor," "Please get me some sugar or juice," "I have diabetes," "Where is a pharmacy?," "I need some insulin," and "I need to buy a syringe" in English and in the language of the country where you will be traveling. These can be found in a travel guidebook or dictionary of phrases.

   g. Carry your insulin and syringes with you. Do not pack them in your suitcase. Luggage compartments of airplanes are not insulated and the insulin may freeze. Take along more insulin than you will need, in case a bottle is lost or broken. You'll need to keep it cool (below 86°F) in your hotel room. Be sure to take along your monitoring supplies.

   h. Find out what foods are available at your destination. Think through how your usual meal plan may have to be modified for these foods.

   i. Your diet and activity will be different, and your blood glucose can quickly get out of control. You will need to plan for testing your blood glucose more often than at home. Take extra supplies so you can monitor as often as you need.

   j. Realize that with all of your efforts, things will probably not always go as planned. Do the best you can and enjoy the trip.

   k. Talk with your health care team to determine if immunizations or other special precautions are needed for the country or climate where you are going.

SITUATION FIVE *continued*

2. To make adjustments for time zone changes, ask your health care team about using multiple injections of rapid- or short-acting insulin before each meal while actually en route and converting back to the usual schedule when settled. Other options are to stay on your home schedule for short trips, or to gradually change to the new time zone before you go by changing your meal/insulin times 30 minutes per day.

3. To handle delayed meals, carry some food in case of unexpected delays such as packaged peanut butter or cheese and crackers, juice boxes, and peanuts. If a meal is delayed and you have no emergency food, ½ cup of fruit juice or non-diet soft drink every 30 minutes until food is served should keep your blood glucose from going too low.

SPECIAL EVENTS

You feel good about the way you have been caring for your diabetes. You want to keep doing well, but the holidays are coming. You know that both your schedule and usual meals will be different.

1. Strategies to manage diabetes during unusual or special times are:
   a. Set realistic blood glucose and exercise goals for the holidays and plan accordingly. Make conscious decisions about your self-care behaviors, weighing costs, benefits, and barriers.
   b. Write down what you plan to eat at the beginning of each day. You may want to share that plan with another person. Save fats and meats to "spend" at a special meal.
   c. If you don't have time for your regular exercise program, try to increase your daily activity level.
   d. Limit alcohol.
   e. Test blood glucose more often.
   f. Take extra insulin to cover additional food, or increase your activity level.
   g. Make a plan for meals at different times.
   h. If going to a gathering where a meal will be served, offer to contribute food that fits with your meal plan, such as vegetables, homemade bread, or diet soft drinks. Suggest a walk after the meal.
   i. If things don't go well, plan how you will do better tomorrow.

You usually take your evening NPH and regular insulin at about 5:30, eat dinner at 6:00, and have a snack before bedtime at about 10:00 p.m. Today you have been invited to a dinner at a friend's home at 8:00 p.m.

1. Strategies to handle a schedule change are:
   a. If your friend knows that you have diabetes, discuss the evening plans together.
   b. Test your blood glucose at 5:30 p.m.
      - If greater than 200 mg/dl, delay both insulin and food. Test again at 7:30. If still greater than 200 mg/dl, take insulin.
      - If between 100 and 200 mg/dl, take insulin and a snack.
      - If less than 100 mg/dl, eat a snack and bring your insulin to your friend's house to take before you eat dinner.

FINANCIAL

Diabetes is expensive. You have figured out what you want to do to take care of your diabetes but are concerned about how you will be able to afford to pay for some of your medicines or monitoring supplies.

1. Ways to economize are:
   a. On diabetes supplies:
      - Shop wisely and compare prices. They can vary a great deal from store to store.
      - Check prices of mail-order pharmacies—they are sometimes less expensive.
      - Reuse lancets and syringes.
   b. On food:
      - Shop wisely and plan ahead; use lists, coupons, and specials; buy fewer prepared or fast foods; or buy generic brands when possible.
      - Explore food cooperatives, community meal programs, low-cost meals through Meals-on-Wheels, and so on.
      - Grow a garden—some communities offer gardening plots if you don't have space.
2. Options for financial help are:
   a. Talk to someone in your hospital social services department about your financial problems (have the telephone number available).
   b. Contact the Department of Social Services, which is a state agency (have the telephone number available).
      - Apply for Medicaid. Financial eligibility requirements change, so you will need to check. The public library has copies of the eligibility manuals. Coverage varies greatly. If you are financially eligible and over 21 years old, you'll need to be medically approved by the Department of Social Services. If you are under 21, you just need to qualify financially.
      - Apply for food stamps. Eligibility is based on income and size of family. Generally, those who qualify for Medicaid also qualify for food stamps.
   c. Some pharmaceutical companies or service organizations may be able to offer help.
   d. Apply for disability assistance.
      - Social Security disability benefits provide monthly checks to workers who are disabled. The amount paid is based on average earnings under Social Security over a period of years. Services offered are counseling, job retraining, and job placement. Call the Social Security office or your hospital social worker.
      - Supplemental Security Income (SSI) is provided to people in need who are over 65 years old or to blind and disabled people of any age. This is a supplement, an addition to your income, and is not meant to meet all of your living expenses. If you qualify for SSI payments, you can also usually qualify for Medicaid.

FINANCIAL (HEALTH INSURANCE/EMPLOYMENT POLICIES)

Your spouse has retired and you are moving. Your spouse is now eligible for Medicare, but you are not. Your group coverage at work has paid for your medical bills, diabetes medicines, and supplies, which have been quite expensive at times. You need to have health insurance coverage until you can find a new job. You are also concerned that you are less likely to be hired because of your diabetes.

1. **Health insurance.** The Health Insurance Portability and Accountability Act of 1996 helps people with chronic health conditions obtain and keep health insurance.

   a. Federal government.

      ■ *Medicare:* beneficiaries are retired or are disabled according to the Social Security Act.

      ■ *Veterans Administration (VA):* payment for care within the VA Medical System only.

      ■ *Public Health Service and Indian Health Service:* federally funded care for specific small groups.

      ■ *Champus:* a program for reimbursing health care providers in the private sector for care of members of the armed forces and their dependents.

   b. State government.

      ■ *Medicaid:* test criteria and coverage vary greatly.

   c. Fee-for-service insurance.

      ■ *Blue Cross/Blue Shield (BC/BS):* various plans with coverage for groups or individuals.

      ■ *Commercial Insurance Companies:* each makes its own decisions about coverage and to whom they will offer insurance.

      ■ *Self-Insuring Groups (e.g., companies and unions):* insure their members while employing BC/BS or commercial carriers as administrators.

   d. Prepaid health plans.

      ■ *Health Maintenance Organization (HMO):* a health care plan with its own coverage policy. There are a variety of HMOs with different provider models.

   e. Group coverage.

      ■ A group insurer may only refuse or limit coverage of a new enrollee with a health condition treated or diagnosed in the 6-month period before enrollment for a maximum of 12 months. Having once met the 12-month waiting period, a person cannot be denied coverage when changing jobs as long as he or she has had continuous coverage.

      ■ Make the most of group coverage wherever you get it. See that all eligible family members are included in your plan so they can take advantage of the conversion privilege if you leave the plan. For them to exercise the privilege, you will probably have to convert as well.

SITUATION EIGHT *continued*

- If you are covered on someone else's group plan, such as your spouse's, familiarize yourself with all conversion possibilities. This is critical if the person who has primary coverage is planning to leave the job.

f. Single policies.

- You may be able to purchase individual health insurance from the company that provided your group coverage at a reduced rate for a period of time (COBRA).

- You can convert from a group policy to an individual one, free from preexisting condition exclusions, if you have had continuous coverage for the previous 10 months, are not eligible for group coverage, and have exhausted your COBRA coverage.

- If you buy a policy on your own, look for one with guaranteed (not optional) renewability and unlimited or very high major medical benefits.

- Many states require companies to offer "pooled risk" policies for people with diabetes. This decreases the cost of premiums. Contact your State Insurance Commissioner.

g. If you cannot get regular health insurance.

- Look for policies that have liberal preexisting condition rules. Those are the clauses that exclude claims resulting from health problems that you were treated for before you took out the policy. Two years is a typical exclusion time, but some plans offer 1 year or less.

- Compare coverage, costs, and preexisting rules for several mail-order plans. These do not require a medical exam, but you may be asked specific questions about your health—whether you've been hospitalized recently and why—to exclude certain conditions.

- When you're between jobs, shop for interim health insurance for coverage. Typical interims are 30, 60, or 90 or more days. These are generally open enrollment plans (no medical exam) and have liberal preexisting condition clauses.

- Contact the American Diabetes Association for information about obtaining health insurance or other assistance.

2. Find out about the coverage for diabetes.

a. Treatment: How often can I see my doctor? Can I see a dietitian and nurse educator?

b. Education: Are diabetes education programs covered?

c. Supplies: Are insulin, syringes, and diabetes pills covered? Monitoring supplies? Insulin pump? Supplies for the insulin pump?

d. Complications: Are screening and treatments for complications covered?

e. Specialty referral practices: Can I see an endocrinologist? An ophthalmologist? A podiatrist? A mental health specialist? An obstetrician who manages high-risk pregnancies? Other specialists as needed?

3. **Employment policies.** Americans with diabetes have been protected under the Americans with Disabilities Act since 1992. A fact sheet is available from the Equal Employment Opportunity Commission (EEOC) (www.eeoc.gov) and from the American Diabetes Association.

a. The law guarantees equal opportunity for individuals with disabilities in employment, public accommodations, transportation, state and local government services, and telecommunications.

SITUATION EIGHT *continued*

   b. The law covers employment practices, including job application procedures, hiring, firing, advancement, compensation, training, and other terms, conditions, and privileges of employment (e.g., tenure, layoff, leave, fringe benefits, and so on).

   c. During an interview, you cannot be asked if you are disabled. An employer can only ask if you can perform the particular job functions. This is also true if the employer already knows that you have diabetes.

   d. Once you have been offered the job, you must disclose the fact of your diabetes to be protected under the Act. You need to explain that you need to do certain diabetes-related things during work hours. Then you need to negotiate with your new employer about how the job requirements and your diabetes management needs can both be "reasonably accommodated."

   e. If you feel you are discriminated against because of your diabetes, you may be able to receive free counseling through a federally mandated program called the National Association of Protection and Advocacy Systems (NAPAS). Each state has a representative. For more information, call 202-408-9514.

FINANCIAL (LIFE INSURANCE)

You never worried about life insurance before, but now you're getting married and feel you should offer this security to your spouse. You call your friendly agent to find out what "a piece of the rock" is going to cost you and learn that it will cost almost 50% more than it costs a friend of yours who does not have diabetes.

1. To obtain life insurance at reasonable cost:
   a. Before you assume you're not insurable at reasonable cost, ask your agent to investigate.
   b. Group life insurance coverage is less expensive and often does not require a medical exam. Coverage is automatic after you join the group and meet certain time limits or employment standards.
      - If you're covered at work, you may be able to take on more insurance under the same plan, for a fee. It's about the cheapest way available to get more insurance.
      - Seek out other groups, whether or not you have on-the-job coverage. Often unions, credit unions, fraternal societies, and the like offer group life insurance to members.
      - Convert your group coverage when you leave your job. Many employers offer up to 30 days to get a new, individual policy from the same company, with no medical exam required and no medical questions asked. You may have a choice of converting to a whole-life policy or to a less costly 1-year term policy that you could convert later into whole life. Either will cost you more than group coverage. The 30-day conversion is your best recourse if you fear a health problem will cause an insurer to turn you down or "rate" you for more expensive premiums than normal for your age. Compare the facts about other plans as soon as you know you'll be leaving your job.
   c. Buy insurance with a "waiver of premium" clause (cost: about 38–40¢ a year per $1000 face value for a 30-year-old man) so that your premiums will be paid and your insurance kept in force even if you become disabled and can no longer work.
   d. Some companies offer life insurance to people with diabetes at group rates providing they meet certain requirements. For example:

      John W. Hall & Assoc., Inc.   This policy is underwritten by the Sentry Life
      P.O. Box 14868   Insurance Company.
      Shawnee Mission, KS 66285-4868
      913-268-7878

   e. Look into policies that allow you to use the dividends to purchase additional insurance.
   f. Consider buying a "convertible term" that can be converted to permanent insurance without a physical exam. Rates are pegged to your age when you convert.

g. Investigate whole-life policies that will permit additional purchases up to set amounts in future years—again, without a medical exam.

2. "Graded death benefit" life insurance (sometimes called "modified" or "guaranteed issue life") is written by a few companies in most states. The key to this insurance is its terms: open enrollment with no medical exam required. Depending on the coverage and the company, premiums can run about 10–50% higher than regular policies—but the insurance may be your only protection. Terms and costs vary. Your best approach is to write several of these companies for more information.

FOR SPOUSES

*Your spouse has diabetes and you want to show your support. You are also
worried about your ability to handle the situation and about your own health.*

1. It's not always easy to live with someone who has diabetes. Discuss some of the situations that
   class members describe. Ways that spouses and family members can be helpful are to:
   - Learn about diabetes.
   - Ask the person who has diabetes for ways you can be helpful.
   - Recognize and reinforce positive changes.
   - Eat the same foods as your spouse.
   - Exercise with your spouse.
   - Avoid nagging, "policing," and taking over the responsibility.
   - Listen when your spouse needs to talk about his or her diabetes.
   - Attend diabetes classes and/or a support group with your spouse.
2. Ways that spouses can get the support they need are:
   - Talk with friends or family.
   - Do what you need to take care of yourself and your health.
   - Consider joining a support group.

STAYING ON TRACK

Congratulations! You are a graduate of a diabetes education program, and you are ready to start doing the best you can to take care of yourself. However, you are concerned about staying up-to-date and motivated.

1. Reassure participants that it is not always easy to make a lot of changes at one time. Therefore, they should try not to get discouraged and should recognize each step of progress along the way. Their health care team is also available to offer support.

   a. Have the participants review all of the aspects of self-care (medication, monitoring, exercise, foot care, diet) and how they plan to fit it into their daily schedules. Suggest that they couple these new self-care behaviors with something they already do routinely (such as doing foot care along with their daily shower). Also, keeping records and diaries (such as a graph of blood glucose levels or a food diary) can reinforce progress.

   b. Other suggestions may include:

   - Make a plan for change. Select a goal, then break it down into smaller steps.
   - Start by adding one new habit. It is easier to add a new habit than to break one that you already have.
   - Write down your new habits. Make them easy to remember by using reminders.
   - To change an old habit, choose the habit that is easiest for you to change. Success will help you feel that you *can* make changes.
   - Get rid of reminders of habits that you want to break and of tempting foods, too.
   - Join a diabetes support group. (Have information about local groups available.)
   - Ask for help from your family and friends. Tell them how they can be most helpful.
   - Write a contract or an agreement with a family member, friend, or health care giver about the changes you want to make.
   - Reward yourself when you make progress. Treat yourself to something you enjoy when you reach each step toward your larger goal.

   c. Motivation comes from commitment to goals. Reevaluate your goals and your treatment plan now and then, and reaffirm your commitment.

2. People can continue learning about diabetes in many ways. Some ideas are:

   a. Join the American Diabetes Association (ADA). Have membership forms and information about your local chapter and other local groups available. To find a local group of the ADA, write to the chapter in your state. Some local groups offer educational programs for people with diabetes. Newsletters for adults and for young people may be available. Many groups offer summer camping experiences for young people.

   b. Read periodicals. The ADA provides a subscription to *Diabetes Forecast* when you become a member. Other periodicals are available.

SITUATION ELEVEN *continued*

c. Use the Internet to get information from reputable websites.

d. Read books. Many books are available for people with diabetes at bookstores or your local library. For a current listing, contact:

American Diabetes Association
1701 N. Beauregard Street
Alexandria, VA 22311
800-ADA-ORDER (800-232-6733)

National Diabetes Information Clearinghouse
One Information Way
Bethesda, MD 20892-3560
800-860-8747

e. Continue your diabetes education. Provide information about follow-up plans for your program or other local options.

➡ Situation One

MEDICAL/COMMUNITY

You and your family have just moved to another state, and you are unfamiliar with the town.

You take two pills and NPH insulin at bedtime for your diabetes. You realize that your medications are getting low. You don't have a local doctor.

1. How can you get a prescription?

2. How do you find a new health care team?

3. You realize that state laws can vary. What are your state's laws about purchasing syringes and insulin? About disposing of used syringes?

4. What other laws can affect you as a person with diabetes? What are your state's laws about people with diabetes having a driver's license?

➡ Situation Two

SOCIAL (FAMILY)

You are a 50-year-old woman with newly diagnosed type 2 diabetes. You have decided you want to lose one pound a week. You take insulin, but your provider says if you lose weight, there's a chance you may not need to stay on it.

Because you've always cooked all the meals for the family, your husband and sons expect you to keep doing so. Your sons have already told you they do not want to eat "rabbit food." Your husband has kept on eating his snack foods in front of you. He makes a point of telling you that you shouldn't have "even a taste."

1. What problems might happen when you get home?

2. What are some ways to handle this situation?

➲ Situation Three

SOCIAL

You are attending a family birthday dinner at your sister's house. Your sister, who takes pride in her cooking, has prepared a special meal with several courses. Most of the foods are combination dishes with sauces and gravies. After dinner, your sister personally hands you the dessert tray, insisting that you take some. She says, "I know several people with diabetes, and they eat anything."

1. What are some ways to handle this situation?

2. What are some ways you can plan ahead for these special events?

3. What are other ideas for dealing with this type of situation?

➲ Situation Four

SICK DAYS

You wake up with the flu. Your body aches and you have a fever. You usually eat a hearty breakfast, but aren't sure you could keep any food down this morning.

1. What can you do to take care of yourself and your diabetes when you feel so awful?

2. When should you call your health care team?

➔ Situation Five

TRAVEL

You are flying to Mexico for a vacation soon. At home, you take insulin twice a day, count carbohydrates, and walk 30 minutes every other day.

1. What plans do you need to make for your diabetes care as you travel and once you arrive?

2. What adjustments will be necessary for time zone changes?

3. You have stopped over in Houston to refuel. It is your suppertime, but the plane is delayed by severe thunderstorms. The flight crew will not serve a meal until the plane is in flight. What can you do?

➡ Situation Six

SPECIAL EVENTS

You feel good about the way you have been caring for your diabetes. You want to keep doing well, but the holidays are coming. You know that both your schedule and usual meals will be different.

1. What are strategies you can use so that you stay on track?

You usually take your evening NPH and regular insulin at about 5:30, eat dinner at 6:00, and have a snack before bedtime at about 10:00 p.m. Today you have been invited to a dinner at a friend's home at 8:00 p.m.

1. How might you handle this change in your schedule?

➡ Situation Seven

FINANCIAL

Diabetes is expensive. You have figured out what you want to do to take care of your diabetes and are concerned about how you will be able to afford to pay for some of your medicines or monitoring supplies.

1. What can you do to economize?

2. Where can you go for help?

➲ Situation Eight

FINANCIAL (HEALTH INSURANCE/ EMPLOYMENT POLICIES)

Your spouse has retired and you are moving. Your spouse is now eligible for Medicare, but you are not. Your group coverage at work has paid for your medical bills, diabetes medicines, and supplies, which have been quite expensive at times. You need to have health insurance coverage until you can find a new job. You are also concerned that you are less likely to be hired because of your diabetes.

1. What options do you have to obtain health insurance?

2. What questions should you ask to get the best coverage?

3. During an interview for a new job, what are the employer's legal responsibilities related to your diabetes? What are your responsibilities?

➲ Situation Nine

FINANCIAL (LIFE INSURANCE)

You never worried about life insurance before, but now you're getting married and feel you should offer this security to your spouse. You call your friendly agent to find out what "a piece of the rock" is going to cost you and learn that it will cost almost 50% more than it costs a friend of yours who does not have diabetes.

1. How can you get life insurance without paying so much?

2. What can you do if your agent tells you that you can't get life insurance?

➡ Situation Ten

FOR SPOUSES

Your spouse has diabetes and you want to show your support. You are also worried about your ability to handle the situation and about your own health.

1. What are some ways you can be helpful?

2. What are ways you can get the support that YOU need?

➡ Situation Eleven

STAYING ON TRACK

Congratulations! You are a graduate of a diabetes education program, and you are ready to start doing the best you can to take care of yourself. However, you are concerned about staying up-to-date and motivated.

1. What are some ways you can include diabetes care in your daily routine?

2. You also want to keep learning about diabetes, new treatments, and new research. List some ways you can continue learning about diabetes.

›››››Supplementary Outlines

#17	Food and Weight

STATEMENT OF PURPOSE

This session is intended to provide an understanding of how different foods affect body weight. Information about nutrients and food groups introduced in Outline #4, *Food and Blood Glucose*, will be reviewed and expanded to predict the caloric density of foods. Weight reduction is one means to lower blood glucose levels and reduce cardiovascular risks (high LDL cholesterol and triglyceride levels and elevated blood pressure). The information may be appropriate for anyone interested in losing weight, in avoiding the weight gain that occurs with better blood glucose control and that is common with intensive insulin regimens, or in decreasing their cardiovascular disease risk factors. Understanding caloric density can also be applied to weight gain efforts or to maintaining calorie intake during periods of poor appetite. The focus in this session is on helping participants identify and develop strategies to change food behaviors to reach personal weight goals.

PREREQUISITES

It is recommended that participants have attended session #4, *Food and Blood Glucose*, or have achieved those objectives.

OBJECTIVES

At the end of this session, participants will be able to:

1. name the six basic food groups and the nutrients in each group;

2. name the nutrient that supplies the most calories;

3. give examples of foods high in calories and low in calories;

4. identify one behavior change they could make to work toward achieving their weight goals.

CONTENT

Nutritional Management.

MATERIALS NEEDED

VISUALS PROVIDED	ADDITIONAL
None. **Handouts** (one per participant) 1. Nutrients and Calories in Food Groups	■ Chalkboard and chalk ■ Food models or pictures of foods ■ Commercial food product containers or labels that show foods of various caloric densities ■ *Exchange Lists for Meal Planning* (booklet available from the American Diabetes Association, 800-232-6733) ■ *Exchange Lists for Weight Loss* (booklet available from the American Diabetes Association, 800-232-6733) ■ *Living in a Healthy Body* (booklet available from Krames Communication, 800-333-3032, www.krames.com)

METHOD OF PRESENTATION

Start by introducing yourself and telling what you do. Ask participants to introduce themselves. Explain that the purpose of the session is to expand the information about different groups of foods and the nutrients in each group from session #4, *Food and Blood Glucose*, to learn how different foods affect body weight. This information can be used by participants to make food choices that help them reach their personal weight goals.

Present material in a question/discussion format. Begin by asking how they did with their short-term goal and what they learned from it.

CONTENT OUTLINE

CONCEPT	DETAIL	INSTRUCTOR'S NOTES
1. Diabetes and weight management	1.1 Weight loss is one way to lower blood glucose and to reduce risks for heart and blood vessel disease.	Ask, "What questions or concerns do you have about diabetes and weight?"
	1.2 For most people, weight loss is difficult. Losing 10–20% of your body weight can have a big impact on your blood glucose levels.	Ask, "Have you ever tried to lose weight? What worked or did not work for you? What did you learn?" Acknowledge any struggle implied in their comments. Most people feel self-conscious and guilty about their excess weight.
	1.3 Keeping weight off once you lose it can also be difficult. If you lose weight too quickly, it often returns.	Ask, "Have you ever lost weight and then regained it? Why do you think that happened?"

CONTENT OUTLINE

CONCEPT	DETAIL	INSTRUCTOR'S NOTES
	1.4 Your weight is determined by: ■ food eaten ■ activity level ■ heredity and body build ■ body chemistry ■ medicines Some things you can change and some things you cannot change.	Point out the benefits of healthy eating regardless of body size. The booklets *Living in a Healthy Body* and *Exchange Lists for Meal Planning* may be useful supplements to keep the focus on health rather than weight.
2. Calories	2.1 Eating fewer calories is one way to lose weight.	A calorie is a measure of stored energy.
	2.2 The minimum recommended calories to obtain needed vitamins and minerals is 1200 for adult females and 1500 for adult males. Fad diets and quick weight loss plans can harm health and interfere with diabetes management. Weight loss of no more than 1 lb per week is recommended.	Very-low-calorie diets are sometimes prescribed to improve pancreatic function in type 2 diabetes. They should be attempted only under medical supervision.
	2.3 Awareness of the calorie content of food can help you choose foods to lose weight or to avoid weight gain. Because glucose calories are lost in the urine when blood glucose levels are high, it is easy to gain weight when you lower your blood glucose.	
	2.4 Awareness of the calorie content of food can also help you choose foods to gain weight or avoid weight loss.	
3. Role of carbohydrate, protein, and fat in weight management	3.1 Carbohydrate, protein, and fat all contribute calories when digested.	Review information about nutrients and food groups in Outline #4, *Food and Blood Glucose,* as needed. Use Handout #1, Nutrients and Calories in Food Groups.
	3.2 Fat provides more calories per gram than carbohydrate or protein and is most easily changed into body fat. However, too much of any nutrient is stored as fat.	Counting fat grams has been a successful way for some to limit total calories.

CONTENT OUTLINE

CONCEPT	DETAIL	INSTRUCTOR'S NOTES
	3.3 Excess fat intake leads to excess fat on our bodies. Fat can be stored almost directly on the body.	A total of 97% of excess dietary fat is converted to body fat.
	3.4 Foods high in water and/or fiber have fewer calories per bite. Fresh fruits, vegetables, and whole grains have the fewest calories per bite. These foods tend to require more chewing, take longer to eat, and help you feel full and satisfied without a lot of calories.	Ask, "What foods are low in calories?" Use food models or pictures of food to illustrate. See Outline #18, *Eating for a Healthy Heart,* for more detailed information about fiber.
	3.5 Calories from high-fat foods, such as regular salad dressing and peanut butter, can add up quickly. Both approach 100 calories per tablespoon.	From a pitcher with ½ cup (8 Tbsp) salad dressing, pour dressing onto lettuce or crinkled-up paper. From a shallow container with ¼ cup peanut butter, spread some on a piece of bread. Ask participants to estimate the amounts used. Measure the amount left in each container and calculate the calories in the portions used.
	3.6 Meat, cheese, and milk contain valuable nutrients but can be high in fat (e.g., sausage, cheddar cheese, and whole milk). You can obtain the nutrients and limit fat and calories by choosing lean meat, fish, poultry without skin, low-fat cheese, and skim milk.	Compare the calorie level of equal amounts of high- and low-fat milk and meats. Refer to *Exchange Lists for Meal Planning* or *Exchange Lists for Weight Loss* for lists of very lean, lean, medium-fat, and high-fat meats.
	3.7 Fried chicken, french fries, cream sauce, some frozen dinners, and snack chips are examples of foods that are high in fat.	Ask participants to name other high-fat foods. Show food models or labels.
	3.8 Foods with added sugar (e.g., cookies and candy) or compact foods (e.g., Grape Nuts or dried fruit) are high in calories as well as carbohydrate per bite.	The makers of some low-fat dessert and snack items have replaced fat with extra sugar. The products tend to be high in carbohydrate and may have as many calories as the higher-fat versions.

CONTENT OUTLINE

CONCEPT	DETAIL	INSTRUCTOR'S NOTES

3.9 Most dessert items are high in both sugar and fat. Examples are cake, cookies, pies, ice cream, chocolate, and candy.

Instructor's Notes: Ask, "What foods are high in sugar and fat?" Research shows that people are born enjoying foods that combine sugar and fat.

3.10 In summary, to decrease calories without eating less total food:
- Emphasize fresh fruits, vegetables, and whole grains.
- Choose measured amounts of lean meat, fish, poultry, and skim milk.
- Limit added-fat and high-fat foods.
- Limit calories from liquids.

Instructor's Notes: Note that this is the recommended way of eating for everyone.

3.11 You don't have to give up your favorite foods. To decrease calories without eliminating types of food:
- Limit portion sizes.
- Choose a low-fat version of the food.
- Limit number of portions per day or week.
- Limit between-meal snacking.
- Eat high-calorie foods less often.

Instructor's Notes: For selection of lower-calorie prepared foods, see Outline #6, *Stocking the Cupboard.* Illustrate with commercial food products or labels. For example, if a participant likes a cheese and bologna sandwich for lunch each day, he or she could:
- have half a sandwich and a salad
- use low-fat bologna, cheese, and/or mayonnaise
- have it 1 or 2 days a week
- give up another high-fat food item he or she wants less

3.12 A calculated meal plan can include all of these ways to limit calories.

Instructor's Notes: See Outlines #20, *Diabetes Exchange Lists* and #21, *Using Exchanges to Plan Meals.*

4. Tips for changing behaviors to eat fewer calories

4.1 Changing a series of behaviors is usually required before new food choices are habits. You can use several strategies to help.

Instructor's Notes: Ask, "What helps you change? What strategies have you used to help you lose weight?" Brainstorm a list of ideas for changing behavior. Ask, "Would any of these work for you?" Offer information from sections 4 and 5 not included on the brainstorm list.

CONTENT OUTLINE

CONCEPT	DETAIL	INSTRUCTOR'S NOTES
	4.2 Recording everything you eat or drink for a week can help you see patterns you want to change. Writing down the time, place, and your feelings can make you more aware of situations that affect your food choices.	Ask, "Do you know what you want to change?" Offer copies of Handout #2, Food Diary, from Outline #3, *The Basics of Eating*.
	4.3 Planning meals and snacks ahead may help avoid overeating (a bag lunch avoids temptation in the cafeteria, a snack after work may avoid nibbling through dinner preparations, and regular grocery shopping helps prevent fast food meals).	Different approaches to overall meal plans are covered in Outlines #5, *Planning Meals*, #19, *Carbohydrate Counting*, and #20–22 about the exchange system.
	4.4 Water, coffee, tea, diet soda, sugar-free KoolAid, club soda, and bottled water may help you feel full and satisfied, but provide few (or no) calories. Because beverages can be quickly consumed, it is easy to "overeat" when drinking fruit juice, punch, and regular soft drinks.	
	4.5 Planning for small amounts of your favorite foods (even if they are high in carbohydrate, fat, and calories) helps some people stick with their overall meal plan. Others overeat sweets once they start and do better avoiding them. If you crave certain foods, you may be cutting back too much on a particular nutrient.	Ask, "Is there a food you crave when on a diet? What approach would work best for you?" A dietitian can help find ways to include favorite foods and reduce cravings.
	4.6 Buy high-fat foods in single-portion sizes—"economy packs" can encourage overeating or eating when not hungry. There are many ways to eat less fat: ■ Choose high-fat foods less often. ■ Eat smaller amounts of the same foods you eat now. ■ Omit some high-fat foods. ■ Substitute a similar food with less fat per bite; many lower-fat and	Ask, "Do you think eating less fat would help you reach your goal(s)? What ways could you eat less fat?" Help participants identify specific changes they could make. Examples: Eat peanuts once a week instead of every night; eat one slice of cheese instead of two; stop buying bacon. Examples: Substitute ground sirloin for hamburger; eat regular

350

CONTENT OUTLINE

CONCEPT	DETAIL	INSTRUCTOR'S NOTES
	lower-calorie alternatives are now available at restaurants and in the grocery store.	instead of premium ice cream; use lite instead of regular salad dressings; buy low-fat crackers; choose a grilled instead of a deep-fried chicken sandwich.
5. Other ways to help manage weight	5.1 Look for other things to do if you eat when you are not hungry. Examples: Go for a walk, call a friend, drink water or diet soft drinks, chew sugarless gum, or knit. Urges to eat do pass.	Ask, "Do you ever eat when you are not really hungry?" Ask participants to identify other reasons for eating and suggest alternate activities.
	5.2 Individual counseling from a dietitian or joining a support group may help you reach your goals.	Refer individuals with suspected eating disorders, anxiety, or depression to a mental health professional.
	5.3 Test before treating symptoms of a reaction. Frequent eating to avoid or treat reactions is a common source of excess calories for persons treated with insulin and means your dose needs to be adjusted.	Refer to Outline #11, *Managing Blood Glucose*, for information about appropriate treatment for hypoglycemia.
	5.4 As you lose weight, you may notice that your blood glucose levels are lower. Talk with your provider if you think you need less insulin or oral medication.	Low blood glucose reactions are one sign less medication is needed.
	5.5 Exercise helps with weight management by burning calories, relieving stress, and maintaining muscle mass.	See Outline #7, *Physical Activity and Exercise.*
	5.6 Exercise helps people with type 2 diabetes improve blood glucose levels by helping insulin to work better and decreasing glucose output from the liver.	
	5.7 Medicines to help with weight loss are available. These may help people lose and maintain a modest weight loss when combined with a reduced-calorie diet. Consult your provider about the benefits and risks of these drugs.	One medication, Xenical (Orlistat), blocks absorption of fat. It prevents about 30% of dietary fat from being absorbed. Patients can expect a loss of 10% of their body weight. The main side effect is cramping and

CONTENT OUTLINE

CONCEPT	DETAIL	INSTRUCTOR'S NOTES
		diarrhea. Sibutramine (Meridia) is an appetite suppressant. The average weight loss is 10–14 lb. Common side effects are dry mouth, constipation, and insomnia. Serotonin-uptake inhibitors can be used to promote weight loss. These are not stimulants, but help decrease appetite and improve insulin sensitivity. These may be recommended for people who are at least 20–30% over their desirable body weight. Usually mild and short-term side effects include dry mouth, drowsiness, and diarrhea. An acute side effect is primary pulmonary hypertension. Neurotoxicity is another concern. Other medications are also available and under development (Rimonabant).
	5.8 Surgical options are becoming more widely available, but have risks as well as benefits.	A thorough physical assessment and extensive education is needed as part of the decision-making process.
6. Planning for change	6.1 There are many approaches to managing weight through your food choices: ■ Set a long-range goal that is important to you and is realistic. ■ Assess the way you are eating now. ■ Develop a plan on which you are willing and able to work. ■ Choose one behavior change you can do before the next class. ■ Commit to that behavior change for the next week.	Examples: In the next 4 months, lower glycated hemoglobin by 1–2%; reduce reactions from eight to four per week; lose 10 lb; or lower your cholesterol by 30 points. See Outline #15, *Changing Behavior.* Choose a short-term goal to try before the next session. Examples: Try diet soft drinks; carry your snack; measure amount of cereal eaten; and drink 2% instead of whole milk.

SKILLS CHECKLIST

None.

EVALUATION PLAN

Knowledge will be evaluated by achievement of learning objectives and by responses to questions during the session. The ability to apply knowledge will be evaluated by development of personal weight goals, by the development and implementation of a plan to achieve those goals, and through program outcome measures.

DOCUMENTATION PLAN

Record class attendance and achieved objectives as appropriate.

SUGGESTED READINGS

Agnew B. Rethinking Atkins. *Diabetes Forecast.* 2004;57(4):64–70.

American Diabetes Association, The American Dietetic Association. *Exchange Lists for Weight Management.* Chicago, IL: The American Dietetic Association, and Alexandria, VA: American Diabetes Association, 1999.

Beebe CA. Body weight issues in preventing and treating type 2 diabetes. *Diabetes Spectrum.* 2003;16:261–265.

Fentress: A guide to healthy weight loss. *Diabetes Forecast.* 2002;55(5):49–86.

Fentress D: Weight loss: get real. *Diabetes Forecast.* 2004;57(4):51–63.

Fitzgerald JT, Anderson RA, Funnell MM, Arnold MS, Davis WK, Aman LC, Jacober SJ, Grunberger G. Differences in the impact of dietary restrictions on African Americans and Caucasians with NIDDM. *The Diabetes Educator.* 23:41–47, 1997.

Gallagher S. Taking the weight off with bariatric surgery. *Nursing.* 2004;34(3): 59–63.

Glasgow RE, Toobert DJ, Hampson SE. Effects of a brief office-based intervention to facilitate diabetes dietary self-management. *Diabetes Care.* 1996;19:834–842.

Gregg EW, Gersoff RB, Thompson TJ, Williamson DF. Trying to lose weight, losing weight, and 9-year mortality in overweight US adults with diabetes. *Diabetes Care.* 2004; 27:657–662.

Hansen BC, Roberts SS. *The Commonsense Guide to Weight Loss.* Alexandria, VA: American Diabetes Association, 1998.

Henry B, Kalynovskyi S. Reversing diabetes and obesity naturally: a NEWSTART lifestyle program. *The Diabetes Educator.* 2004; 30:48–59.

Holzmeister LA. *The Diabetes Carbohydrate and Fat Gram Guide.* Alexandria, VA: American Diabetes Association, 1998.

Polivy J. Psychological consequences of food restriction. *Journal of the American Dietetic Association.* 1996;96:589–592.

Vanwormer JJ, Boucher JL. Counseling diabetic patients about weight management. *Practical Diabetology.* 2003;22(2):30–35.

Wing RR, Anglin K. Effectiveness of a behavioral weight control program for blacks and whites with NIDDM. *Diabetes Care.* 1996;19:409–413.

Wing RR, Hill JO. Successful weight loss maintenance. *Annual Review in Nutrition.* 2001;21:323–341.

Wylie-Rossett J, Swencionis C, Caba A, Friedler AJ, Schaffer N. *The Complete Weight Loss Workbook.* Alexandria, VA: American Diabetes Association, 1997.

➡ Nutrients and Calories in Food Groups

Food Group	Nutrient(s)	Effect on Blood Glucose*	Calories per Bite
Starch	**Carbohydrate** Protein	Large	Low
Fruit	**Carbohydrate**	Large	Low
Milk	**Carbohydrate** Protein Fat	Large	Low (higher if 2% or whole milk)
Vegetable	**Carbohydrate** Protein	Small	Low
Meat	**Protein** Fat	—	High (lower if very low fat)
Fat	**Fat**	—	High

* Within 2 hours of eating.

| #18 | **Eating for a Healthy Heart** |

▶ ▶ ▶ ▶ ▶

STATEMENT OF PURPOSE

This session is intended to provide information about fats, fiber, and sodium and their impact on the risks for cardiovascular complications. Sources and effects of the different types of dietary fat and fiber are included.

PREREQUISITES

It is recommended that each participant have attended session #5, *Planning Meals*, or have achieved those objectives. This session also builds on information about the food label in session #6, *Stocking the Cupboard*.

OBJECTIVES

At the end of this session, participants will be able to:

1. define lipids;

2. identify factors that influence blood lipids;

3. state the benefits of controlling blood lipids for people with diabetes;

4. explain the effect of dietary cholesterol on blood cholesterol;

5. identify foods high in cholesterol;

6. distinguish between the effects of saturated and unsaturated dietary fat on blood lipids;

7. identify two sources of each of the three types of dietary fat;

8. explain the two types of dietary fiber and give two examples of foods high in each;

9. state two benefits and two reasons for caution in the use of dietary fiber;

10. state the rationale for limiting sodium in the diet;

11. identify foods high in sodium;

12. identify personal food habits or behaviors that may contribute to increasing risk for cardiovascular complications;

13. identify one behavior change they could make to work toward risk reduction for cardiovascular complications.

CONTENT

Nutritional Management.

MATERIALS NEEDED

VISUALS PROVIDED	ADDITIONAL
1. Reasons for Meal Planning 2. Types of Fat in Blood 3. Types of Fat in Food	■ Commercial food product containers or labels

Handouts (one per participant)
1. Sources of Cholesterol and Fat
2. Sources of Fiber
3. High-Sodium Foods
4. Alternative Seasonings

METHOD OF PRESENTATION

Start by introducing yourself and telling what you do. Ask participants to introduce themselves. Explain that the purpose of this session is to provide information about blood fats and the reasons why it is important for people with diabetes to work toward normal levels.

Present material in a question/discussion format. Begin by asking how they did with their short-term goal and what they learned from it.

Guidelines for maintaining normal blood fat levels are consistent with guidelines for healthy eating. Although designed for people with diabetes, this content can be used by anyone to improve blood lipid levels.

CONTENT OUTLINE

CONCEPT	DETAIL	INSTRUCTOR'S NOTES
1. Review goals for meal planning	1.1 Control of blood fats or lipids is a major reason for meal planning.	Review goals for meal planning. Use Visual #1, Reasons for Meal Planning. Ask, "What reason is most important for you?"
	1.2 *Lipid* is a medical term used for fat and/or cholesterol.	
	1.3 Your weight and your blood glucose levels affect the fat in your blood. Staying at a desirable weight and in your target blood glucose range helps keep your blood lipids at the right level. Heredity and exercise also affect blood lipid levels.	Refer to Outline #4, *Food and Blood Glucose.*

CONTENT OUTLINE

CONCEPT	DETAIL	INSTRUCTOR'S NOTES
	1.4 People with diabetes are two to four times more likely to have heart and circulation (blood flow) problems. Normal blood lipids and blood pressure can help lower that risk.	Lipid management is aimed at lowering LDL cholesterol and triglycerides and raising HDL cholesterol.
	1.5 Reducing saturated fat and cholesterol intake, weight loss, and physical activity have been shown to improve lipids among people with diabetes.	
2. Tests for blood lipids	2.1 Three kinds of lipids are present in your blood: ■ low-density lipoprotein (LDL) cholesterol ■ high-density lipoprotein (HDL) cholesterol ■ triglycerides Each of these lipids in your blood can be measured, and your total cholesterol level can be determined.	Ask, "How do you know if your blood lipids are normal? Do you know your cholesterol level?" Use Visual #2, Types of Fat in Blood.
	2.2 The total cholesterol level is used as a screening tool.	A fasting lipid profile is recommended for all people with diabetes. Atherosclerotic disease is not seen in people with cholesterol levels lower than 150 mg/dl.
	2.3 LDL cholesterol is the lipid that builds up inside your blood vessels and slows or blocks blood flow. It is called the "bad" or "lousy" cholesterol. Recommended LDL level for people with diabetes is less than 100 mg/dl.	$LDL = \text{total cholesterol} - HDL - \dfrac{triglycerides}{5}$ Currently, LDL cholesterol is considered the measure most predictive of atherosclerosis. As research continues, other tests may be recommended to better evaluate lipid abnormalities in diabetes.
	2.4 Decreasing saturated and trans fat intake may help to lower LDL cholesterol.	

CONTENT OUTLINE

CONCEPT	DETAIL	INSTRUCTOR'S NOTES
	2.5 HDL cholesterol is the lipid that helps remove cholesterol from the blood. It is called the "good" or "helpful" cholesterol. The higher your HDL level, the lower your risk of heart disease. The recommended HDL level is more than 40 mg/dl.	Maximal medical nutrition therapy typically reduces HDL by 15–25 mg/dl. HDL level is not directly affected by diet, but may be increased by exercise and weight reduction. It may be desirable for women to have an HDL level of 50mg/dl. HDL levels above 60 mg/dl are considered protective.
	2.6 Triglycerides in the blood tend to be high when blood glucose is high. High triglycerides also tend to lower HDL cholesterol. The recommended triglyceride level is less than 150 mg/dl.	Triglycerides are used to calculate LDL cholesterol. Point out that some people are particularly sensitive to the effects of carbohydrates, sugar, alcohol, dietary fat, or large meals. These factors can also elevate triglyceride levels even without high blood glucose levels.
3. Cholesterol	3.1 The amount of cholesterol and, primarily, the amount and type of fat in your diet affect the level of cholesterol in your blood.	To some extent, lipid abnormalities associated with diabetes are thought to be part of the disease. Genetics may also influence a person's response to diet.
	3.2 Fat and cholesterol are two types of lipids (fatty substances) found in food.	Use Visual #3, Types of Fat in Food.
	3.3 Cholesterol in your food may increase the cholesterol in your blood.	
	3.4 Cholesterol is a soft, waxy substance made by all animals, including humans. It is essential for life, but the body makes all it needs.	Ask, "What is cholesterol?" Cholesterol is made in the liver. It is used to make bile acid, hormones, and vitamin D.
	3.5 Cholesterol is found in all foods that come from animals. Examples are meat, cheese, egg yolk, whole or 2% milk, and ice cream. The American Diabetes Association and The American Dietetic Association	Ask, "What foods contain cholesterol?" Use Handout #1, Sources of Cholesterol and Fat. Ask, "Which foods high in cholesterol do you eat often?" Note that cholesterol is part of

CONTENT OUTLINE

CONCEPT	DETAIL	INSTRUCTOR'S NOTES
	recommend limiting cholesterol to 300 mg/day.	meat and cannot be trimmed off as fat can and that cholesterol is not present in egg whites. Some people (e.g., those with an LDL cholesterol >100 mg/dl) may benefit from lowering cholesterol intake to <200 mg/day.
4. Fat	4.1 All fats are high in calories and can contribute to excess weight.	1 gram of fat = 9 calories.
	4.2 Different people need different amounts of fat depending on their weight, blood glucose goals, and lipid goals. A dietitian can help you learn the best amount for you.	A total of 30% of total calories or 50–70 gm of fat per day is a reasonable initial target for most people. Optimal levels for most individuals range from 20 to 40%.
	4.3 Fat contributes flavor and texture to foods and gives you a sense of fullness.	Fat transports the fat-soluble vitamins A, D, E, and K and provides linoleic acid, an essential fatty acid.
	4.4 Only some fats in food can directly increase the cholesterol in blood.	
	4.5 Saturated, trans, and unsaturated are the three types of fat in food.	Refer again to Visual #3, Types of Fat in Food.
5. Saturated fat and hydrogenated and trans fatty acids	5.1 Saturated fat and trans fatty acids increase blood cholesterol levels because your body makes cholesterol from these fats. This fat is solid at room temperature.	Limiting saturated fat to less than 10% of total calories is recommended. For patients with elevated LDL, less than 7% is recommended. Eliminating trans fatty acids is recommended.
	5.2 All animal products contain saturated fat. Examples are whole milk, meat, bacon, butter, sour cream, and cheese.	Ask, "What foods contain saturated fat?" Less expensive *cuts* of meat contain less marbling and are lower in fat, but more expensive *ground* meat is lower in fat.
	5.3 Some vegetable products are high in saturated fat. Palm and coconut oil are vegetable fats naturally high in saturated fat.	Coconut oil is not an oil, but is solid at room temperature.

CONTENT OUTLINE

CONCEPT	DETAIL	INSTRUCTOR'S NOTES
	5.4 Vegetable oils that have been processed to become solid are trans fats. Trans fats are not listed on food labels. They are listed in the ingredients as hydrogenated or partially hydrogenated fat (trans fatty acids). To determine the amount of trans fats, add the grams of saturated, mono-unsaturated, and polyunsaturated fat. If this is less than the total grams of fat, the remainder are trans fats.	Shortening is an example of hydrogenated vegetable oil. Foods listing this first on the label contain higher amounts. Most margarine, commercial baked goods, and snack foods contain trans fats. Show examples (or labels) of these products. Trans fatty acids are believed to have a more negative impact than saturated fat. Labels will list trans fats in 2004.
	5.5 A product may contain saturated fat even though the label truthfully says that it contains no cholesterol. Since 1990, an item labeled "cholesterol-free" can contain no more than 2 mg saturated fat per serving.	Illustrate with commercial food products (or labels) that contain saturated fat but no cholesterol.
	5.6 To reduce saturated and trans fats in your diet, you can eat fewer or smaller portions of these foods or substitute other products.	Ask, "How could you lower saturated and trans fats in your diet?" Show examples of products or labels such as reduced-fat cheeses, imitation or low-fat sour cream, and baked goods made with liquid oils.
	5.7 Many low- and no-fat products can be found in the grocery store. However, they may be higher in carbohydrate and may be no lower in calories than foods they are meant to replace.	Show examples of products low in fat but high in carbohydrate. Ask, "How might this product fit into your meal plan?"
6. Monounsaturated and Polyunsaturated fats	6.1 Unsaturated fat lowers blood cholesterol. These fats are liquid at room temperature. Unsaturated fats are either polyunsaturated or monounsaturated.	The more liquid the fat, the more unsaturated it is—tub margarine is more unsaturated than stick margarine; liquid is more unsaturated than tub.
	6.2 Polyunsaturated fats lower both LDL and HDL cholesterol. Some polyunsaturated fat is essential to life.	Linoleic acid, the essential fatty acid, is a polyunsaturated fat.

CONTENT OUTLINE

CONCEPT	DETAIL	INSTRUCTOR'S NOTES
	6.3 Polyunsaturated fats are found in safflower, sunflower, corn, and soybean oil; margarines made from these liquid oils; mayonnaise; and nuts such as brazil nuts and walnuts.	Ask, "What foods contain polyunsaturated fats?" It is recommended that polyunsaturated fat intake be <8% of total fat intake. Monounsaturated fat intake should be >12% of total fat intake.
	6.4 Monounsaturated fats are liquid at room temperature but become too thick to pour when cold.	
	6.5 Monounsaturated fats are found in olive, peanut, and canola oil; olives and avocados; and almonds, cashews, peanuts, and pistachios.	Ask, "What foods contain monounsaturated fat?"
	6.6 Monounsaturated fat lowers LDL cholesterol without lowering HDL cholesterol.	Replacing some carbohydrate with added monounsaturated fat may help to lower blood glucose and triglycerides in some people without worsening lipid levels.
	6.7 Omega-3 fats are found in fish oil, flaxseed, and soybean oil. These lower triglycerides and protect the heart.	Ask, "What foods contain omega-3 fats? Tuna, salmon, lake trout, and sardines are high in omega-3 fats. Eating two to three servings per week is recommended. Taking omega-3 oil pills has not been found to be protective.
	6.8 New food products are available that may help to lower cholesterol levels, if eaten in therapeutic amounts.	Show examples of products (i.e., margarine). Plant products are added to decrease absorption of the cholesterol and saturated fat.
7. Guidelines for choosing foods lower in fat	7.1 Guidelines for limiting fat: ■ Choose lean meats, fish, and poultry. ■ Use skim or low-fat milk. ■ Limit egg yolks and organ meats.	Ask, "What are some ideas for limiting fat in your meal plan?" Write down responses on the board and add to the list as needed.

CONTENT OUTLINE

CONCEPT	DETAIL	INSTRUCTOR'S NOTES
	■ Limit high-fat animal products such as bacon, hot dogs, cheese, and butter. ■ Limit commercially prepared baked and snack foods. ■ Use monounsaturated fat for cooking and to replace other oils when making salad dressing or baking.	To eat less than 300 mg cholesterol and less than 30% total fat: ■ Eat 4–6 oz lean meat per day. ■ Drink skim milk only. ■ Eat no more than three to four egg yolks per week. ■ Use small amounts of monounsaturated oil for cooking and as a substitute oil in food preparation. Note that this way of eating is recommended for all people. Fruits and vegetables contain antioxidant vitamins A, D, and E, which may reduce risks for heart disease and other complications.
8. Fiber	8.1 Fiber is the undigestible part of plant food. It provides bulk but no calories.	Ask, "What is fiber?"
	8.2 There are two types of fiber. The coarse or stringy kind called insoluble fiber helps prevent constipation.	Insoluble fiber speeds up the passage of food through the digestive system.
	8.3 Insoluble fiber is found in whole grain bread and cereal, wheat bran, fresh fruit, and vegetables.	Ask, "What foods help prevent constipation?" Use Handout #2, Sources of Fiber.
	8.4 The other kind of fiber absorbs water like gelatin and is called soluble fiber.	Soluble fiber slows down the passage of food through the digestive system.
	8.5 Water-soluble fiber is found in okra, oat bran, rice bran, dried beans, dried peas, lentils, and most fresh fruits and vegetables.	Recent studies show mixed effects of fiber on glycemia and and lipids.
	8.6 To eat the recommended amount of fiber, you can include ■ fresh fruits ■ fresh vegetables ■ whole grains ■ bran cereal ■ legumes	The recommended goal for dietary fiber is 20–35 gm/day, the same as for the general population. Legumes are various dried beans, dried peas, and lentils.

CONTENT OUTLINE

CONCEPT	DETAIL	INSTRUCTOR'S NOTES
	8.7 Some high-fiber foods may cause gas and cramping. Gradually adding fiber into your diet helps control this problem.	Ask, "Are there any problems with eating fiber?" Drinking adequate fluid is necessary to prevent constipation.
	8.8 If the stomach empties slowly (as with autonomic neuropathy), high-fiber diets can make the problem worse.	If participants report feeling full quickly, suggest that they consult their provider before adding high-fiber foods.
	8.9 Some people find that a high-fiber diet helps them feel full and more able to limit calories.	
9. Sodium	9.1 About half of the people with diabetes also have high blood pressure. High blood pressure increases your risk for heart and blood vessel disease.	
	9.2 Reducing dietary sodium may help to reduce your blood pressure.	Sodium restrictions do not help everyone (they do help 10–20% of the general population and 60% of those with hypertension).
	9.3 Sodium recommendations for people with diabetes are the same as for the general public. If your blood pressure is: ■ normal—3000 mg of sodium per day ■ high—2400 mg of sodium per day	The goal for people requiring blood pressure medication is 2400 mg of sodium per day or sodium chloride to 6000 mg per day.
	9.4 The body needs no more than 500 mg of sodium per day (the amount in ¼ tsp of salt). The naturally occurring sodium in food and water easily supplies that amount.	
	9.5 Table salt is high in sodium, but soup, pickles, olives, canned vegetables, lunch meats, and convenience foods also tend to be very high in sodium. Restaurant food, especially fast food, is often high in sodium. Many of these items provide more than 1000 mg per serving.	Ask "What foods contain sodium?" Show Handout #3, High-Sodium Foods.

CONTENT OUTLINE

CONCEPT	DETAIL	INSTRUCTOR'S NOTES
	9.6 To reduce sodium in your diet, you can eat fewer or smaller portions of these foods or substitute other foods.	Ask, "How would you lower the sodium in your diet?" Mean effects of moderate sodium restriction is about 5 mmHg for systolic and 2 mmHg for diastolic blood pressure among hypertensive patients and about 3 and 1 mmHg among normotensive patients.
	9.7 A guideline is to choose foods that are: ■ less than 400 mg per serving ■ less than 800 mg per entree or frozen meal	Ask, "Where is information about sodium on the food label?" Show product labels; include low-salt foods. If possible, have the class taste some reduced-salt products.
	9.8 Products are now available to help lower sodium intake, such as reduced-sodium soups. Many food products are lower in sodium than they used to be; these can help you meet recommendations.	Salt substitutes contain potassium and must be used cautiously. People with renal disease and those treated with potassium-sparing diuretics should avoid them.
	9.9 Many seasonings and spices can add flavor without sodium. Several sodium-free seasoning blends are available. Try small amounts of unfamiliar herbs and spices from bulk food stores. Your ability to taste other flavors and enjoy foods without sodium improves with time.	Use Handout #4, Alternative Seasonings. If possible, offer samples of Mrs. Dash and other salt-free seasonings.
	9.10 Modest weight loss has beneficial effects on blood pressure as does moderate (e.g., 30–45 minutes of brisk walking) physical activity. Smoking cessation and limiting alcohol intake are also recommended?	There is no evidence of beneficial effects from calcium and magnesium supplementation.
10. Planning for change	10.1 If your lipid profile or blood pressure is abnormal, or if you want to change your diet to help prevent heart disease, there are many food choices you could make.	Ask, "Are there ways you could change your eating to help lower your heart disease risk?" Note that exercise is also a key factor in blood lipid control. See Outline #7, *Physical Activity and Exercise.*

CONTENT OUTLINE

CONCEPT	DETAIL	INSTRUCTOR'S NOTES
	10.2 It's important to begin making changes one step at a time. You could start by: ■ deciding what your long-term blood lipid goal is ■ planning how to work toward that goal ■ choosing one step to take right now	Ask participants to: ■ set a reasonable blood lipid goal ■ develop a plan on which they are willing and able to work ■ choose a short-term goal to try before the next session
	10.3 Counseling with a registered dietitian can help you choose and reach your goals.	

SKILLS CHECKLIST

None.

EVALUATION PLAN

Knowledge will be evaluated by achievement of learning objectives and by responses to questions during the session. The ability to apply knowledge will be evaluated by the development of personal blood lipid goals, by the development and implementation of a plan to achieve those goals, and through program outcome measures.

DOCUMENTATION PLAN

Record class attendance and achieved objectives as appropriate.

SUGGESTED READINGS

American Diabetes Association. Position statement: Management of dyslipidemia in adults with diabetes. *Diabetes Care.* 2004; 27(Suppl 1):S68–S74.

Campbell AP. Health benefits of dietary fiber for people with diabetes. *The Diabetes Educator.* 2001;27:511–514.

Gottlieb SH. About alcohol: the heart-blood glucose connection. *Diabetes Forecast.* 2004; 57(4):30–32.

Haffner SM. Technical review: Management of dyslipidemia in adults with diabetes. *Diabetes Care.* 1998;21:160–178.

Keeler A. Low-fat cooking. *Diabetes Forecast.* 1997;50(3):50–57.

Marlett JA, Cheung TF. Dietary fiber guidelines in the exchange lists for meal planning. *Diabetes Care.* 1994;17(12):1534–1541.

➡ Reasons for Meal Planning

- ■ Maintain blood glucose as close to your target range as possible.

- ■ Maintain cholesterol (blood fats) as close to your target range as possible.

- ■ Maintain blood pressure as close to your target level as possible.

- ■ Prevent, delay, or treat diabetes-related complications.

- ■ Improve health through food choices.

- ■ Meet individual nutritional needs.

➲ Types of Fat in Blood

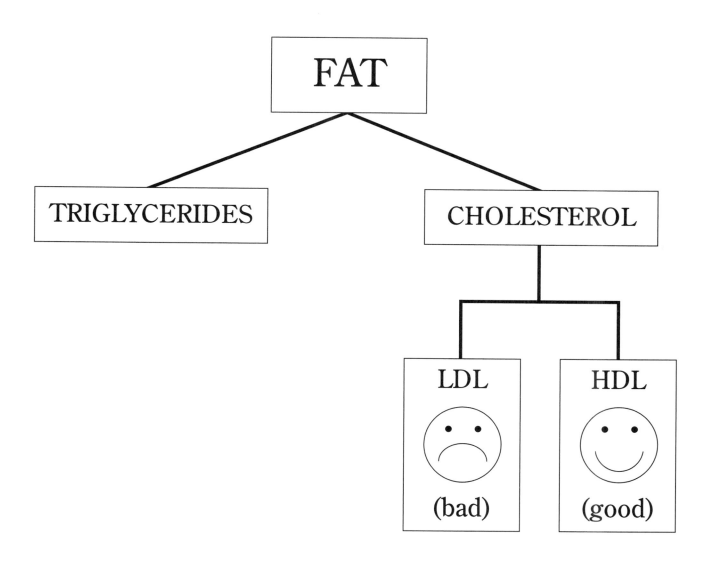

➲ Types of Fat in Food

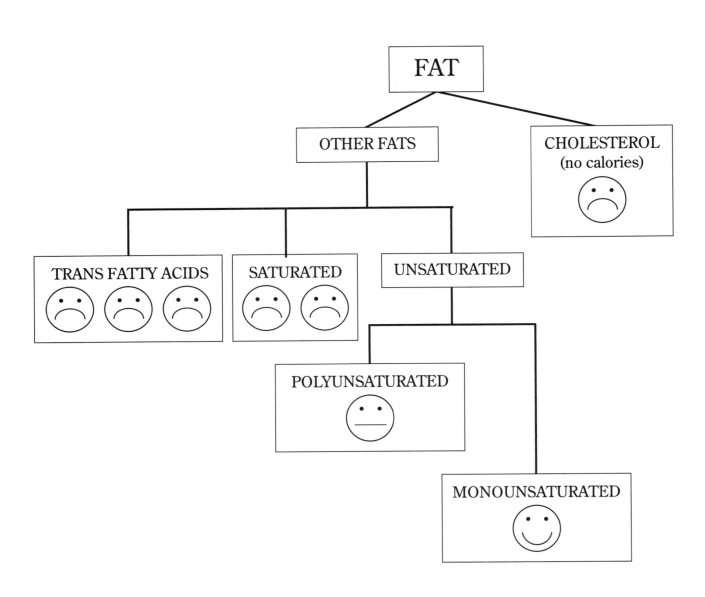

➡ Sources of Cholesterol and Fat

Cholesterol (limit these)	Saturated Trans Fat (limit these)	Unsaturated Fat	
Meat	Meat	Safflower oil	
Cheese	Cheese	Sunflower oil	
Egg yolks	Egg yolks	Corn oil	
Whole milk	Whole milk	Soybean oil	
Reduced fat (2%) milk	Reduced fat (2%) milk	Sesame oil	Polyunsaturated
Ice cream	Ice cream	Salad dressing	
Butter	Butter	Mayonnaise	
Organ meats	Cream cheese	Walnuts	
	Sour cream	Sesame seeds	
	Palm oil	Margerine (in soft tubs)	
	Coconut oil		
	Cocoa butter	Olive oil	
	Hydrogenated vegetable oil	Canola oil	
	Poultry with skin	Peanut oil	
	Fatback	Olives	
	Chitterlings	Avocados	
		Almonds	Monounsaturated (choose more often)
		Peanuts	
		Cashews	
		Pecans	
		Almonds	
		Sesame seeds	
		Peanut butter	

➡ Sources of Fiber

Soluble Fiber	Insoluble Fiber (to help prevent constipation)

Raw vegetables
Fresh fruits
Barley
Dried peas
Brown rice
Okra
Kidney beans
Lentils
Pinto beans
Black-eyed peas
Black beans
Whole-grain products:
   ■ Oat, oat bran, and rice bran cereals
   ■ Soy pasta
   ■ Oat bran, rye, and pumpernickel breads
   ■ Oat and rye crackers
	Some raw vegetables
	Wheat bran products:
	   ■ Cereal (100% bran)
	   ■ Whole grain products
	   ■ Pasta
	   ■ Bread
	   ■ Crackers

➡ High-Sodium Foods

Baking powder

Baking soda

Bouillon

Brine

Canned and dried soups

Canned meats and vegetables

Dill pickles

Disodium phosphate

Fast foods

Frozen mixed dishes

Macaroni, noodle, rice, and stuffing mixes

Monosodium glutamate (MSG)

Olives

Processed meat (corned beef, ham, frankfurters, lunch meat, and sausage)

Salty snack foods (crackers, chips, and nuts)

Sauerkraut

Seasoned salts (e.g., onion, garlic, and celery)

Sodium _____ (Any word that starts with "sodium" or has the word "sodium" in it)

Soy sauce

Steak, teriyaki, and tartar sauce

Table salt

➡ Alternative Seasonings

Herbs/Spices	Ways to Use Them
Basil	Egg, fish, tomato sauce, and vegetables
Bay leaves	Soups, stews, and boiled beef or pork
Caraway seeds	Roast pork, vegetables of the cabbage family, carrots, onions, and celery
Celery powder	Soups, salads, and deviled eggs
Curry powder	Chicken, lamb, eggs, and rice
Dill	Salads, deviled eggs, chicken, and fish
Fennel	Pork, poultry, and seafood dishes
Garlic	Meats, stews, soups, and salads
Nutmeg	Apple dishes and vegetables
Onion powder	Meat, soups, stews, and casseroles
Oregano	Italian dishes, stews, and soups
Paprika	For color; also aids browning of roasted chicken and turkey
Parsley	Eggs, soups, stews, and vegetables
Pepper, black	Salads, fish, meat, eggs, and vegetables
Pepper, red	Meats, sauces, gravies, eggs, fish, vegetable dishes, and stews (this is a strong spice)
Rosemary	Potatoes, peas, squash, lamb, veal, duck, pork stews, and salmon
Sage	Stuffing, poultry, pork, lamb, and veal
Thyme	Italian dishes, meat, and vegetables

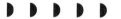

| #19 | Carbohydrate Counting |

STATEMENT OF PURPOSE

This session is intended to provide information on three methods of carbohydrate counting as a meal-planning approach. Using carbohydrate counting may improve blood glucose levels regardless of whether diabetes medications are also used. It is important for participants to work with a dietitian to develop a meal plan with the amount and distribution of carbohydrate that helps them reach their goals.

PREREQUISITES

This session builds on the basic carbohydrate-counting information in session #5, *Planning Meals.* It is recommended that each participant have attended sessions #3, *The Basics of Eating*, #4, *Food and Blood Glucose*, and #5, *Planning Meals*, or have achieved those objectives. This session is intended for individuals who have some experience living with diabetes and who want a more calculated meal plan to meet their goals. It is suggested that participants who have meal-planning booklets and meal plans bring them to class.

OBJECTIVES

At the end of this session, participants will be able to:

1. describe carbohydrate counting;

2. state the rationale for using carbohydrate counting for meal planning;

3. name three food groups high in carbohydrate;

4. describe two methods of carbohydrate counting;

5. identify three sources of information on the carbohydrate content of food;

6. list 12 food items they often eat or drink and the carbohydrate content of each;

7. calculate the amount of carbohydrate in their serving size from a food label;

8. define pattern management and carbohydrate/insulin ratios.

CONTENT

Nutritional Management.

MATERIALS NEEDED

VISUALS PROVIDED

1. Carbohydrate Servings

Handouts Provided (one per participant)
1. Carbohydrate Foods
2. Counting Carbohydrate Servings
3. Exchange and Food Composition References
4. Practice Worksheet
5. How to Calculate Carbohydrate Grams in Your Serving
6. Tips for Counting Carbohydrate Servings
7. Carbohydrate in My Food

ADDITIONAL

- Chalkboard and chalk
- Food models or pictures of foods
- Commercial food product containers or labels
- *Basic Carbohydrate Counting* and *Advanced Carbohydrate Counting* (available from the American Diabetes Association, 800-232-6733)
- *Exchange Lists for Meal Planning, Exchanges for All Occasions*, other references for exchange information (available from the American Diabetes Association, 800-232-6733)
- Food composition references (see Handout #3)

METHOD OF PRESENTATION

Start by introducing yourself and telling what you do. Ask participants to introduce themselves. Explain that the purpose of this session is to provide information about the carbohydrate-counting method for meal planning.

Present material in a discussion/question format. Begin by asking how they did with their short-term goal and what they learned from it.

CONTENT OUTLINE

CONCEPT	DETAIL	INSTRUCTOR'S NOTES
1. What is carbohydrate counting?	1.1 Counting just the carbohydrate in the food you eat is one method for meal planning that works well for many people. With this method, you count only the amount of carbohydrate at each meal and snack.	Additional information or modifications may be needed to address weight, cardiovascular health, renal disease, or the overall nutritional value of the diet.
	1.2 Carbohydrate counting focuses the attention on food choices that most affect blood glucose levels.	This method only addresses blood glucose management—the reason for meal planning unique to diabetes. Other nutrition issues, such as the levels of fat, protein, vitamins, and minerals, can be addressed after blood glucose levels are stable. This is one way to encourage the practice of an underlying educational principle: changes need

CONTENT OUTLINE

CONCEPT	DETAIL	INSTRUCTOR'S NOTES
		to be made in steps. Optimal nutrition may need to wait until blood glucose levels are in the goal range.
	1.3 Carbohydrate counting does not mean reducing the total amount of carbohydrate, but keeping track of the amount in any one meal or snack.	
	1.4 The amount of carbohydrate at each meal or snack may be consistent from day to day or flexible, depending on the type of carbohydrate-counting meal plan used.	
	1.5 This approach can be used as part of blood glucose self-management. You can learn to eat more or fewer carbohydrate foods based on your blood glucose responses.	Stress the value of blood glucose monitoring with this approach to meal planning.
	1.6 Some people calculate their premeal bolus insulin dose based on the amount of carbohydrate they plan to eat at that meal and their premeal blood glucose.	The amount of bolus (rapid-acting or short-acting) insulin needed before a meal is closely related to the amount of carbohydrate eaten at that meal.
	1.7 Each carbohydrate-counting meal plan differs based on calorie needs, blood glucose goals, food preferences, daily schedule, diabetes medicines, exercise plans, monitoring, and desire for flexibility. Ask a dietitian to help you find a plan that works for you.	Offer referral as needed.
2. Why use carbohydrate counting?	2.1 Carbohydrate affects blood glucose more than any other nutrient.	Review the material from Outline #4, *Food and Blood Glucose*, as needed.
	2.2 Carbohydrate counting may offer better blood glucose control with more ease and flexibility in food choices than other meal-planning methods.	Many think it is easier to use than the exchange system. The carbohydrate content of various foods is more often published than the exchange value.

CONTENT OUTLINE

CONCEPT	DETAIL	INSTRUCTOR'S NOTES
	2.3 Using carbohydrate counting to distribute carbohydrate throughout the day can improve blood glucose levels regardless of whether you also take diabetes pills or insulin.	If participants do not understand why their blood glucose is high after some meals, carbohydrate counting may help them learn why.
3. Planning to use carbohydrate counting	3.1 To use carbohydrate counting, you need to be familiar with foods that contain carbohydrate and with your carbohydrate needs.	
	3.2 Food groups high in carbohydrate: ■ starch ■ fruit ■ milk ■ any foods that contain sugar, honey, molasses, or syrup	Ask, "What foods are high in carbohydrate?" Use Handout #1, Carbohydrate Foods. Review information from Outline #4, *Food and Blood Glucose*, as needed.
	3.3 The vegetable group is low in carbohydrate. Vegetables usually can be ignored unless you have 1½ cups or more at a meal or snack (cooked). Remember starchy vegetables are in the starch/bread group.	Hold up containers or models of several different foods and ask participants to identify whether they are high in carbohydrate. Ask whether each item fits into the starch, fruit, milk, vegetable, or other carbohydrate category.
	3.4 The carbohydrate content of foods in the other carbohydrates group varies.	
	3.5 Carbohydrate needs usually range from 40 to 60% of total calorie needs.	To estimate carbohydrate needs, assume that 50% of the day's calories come from carbohydrate. Divide carbohydrate (CHO) calories by 4 calories per gram. Example: $1800 \text{ cal} \times 50\% = 900$ $\dfrac{900 \text{ CHO cal}}{4 \text{ cal/gm}} = 225 \text{ gm CHO}$
	3.6 There are two methods of carbohydrate-based meal planning: ■ basic: counting carbohydrate servings	

CONTENT OUTLINE

CONCEPT	DETAIL	INSTRUCTOR'S NOTES

- advanced: counting carbohydrate grams and using carbohydrate/insulin ratios (adjusting rapid- or short-acting insulin dose to the amount of carbohydrate you plan to eat)

4. Basic carbohydrate counting

4.1 The basic carbohydrate-counting method uses the food groups of the food guide pyramid or the exchange system. Each starch, fruit, and milk counts as one carbohydrate serving.

The basic carbohydrate-counting method was introduced in Outline #5, *Planning Meals*. Review this material and/or use the *Basic Carbohydrate Counting* booklet as needed. Learning to count both carbohydrate servings and carbohydrate grams may be confusing to participants. Review each and decide which best fits the needs of your audience.

4.2 For example, one carbohydrate serving is:
- ½ cup orange juice = 1 fruit
- 1 slice bread = 1 starch
- ½ cup corn = 1 bread
- 1 cup milk = 1 milk

Review and demonstrate with food models. Understanding food groupings and serving sizes is a helpful background for learning to use basic carbohydrate counting. It is helpful to relate carbohydrates to exchanges if participants already know or use that method.

4.3 Each carbohydrate serving is about 15 gm of carbohydrate. You can either servings or grams of carbohydrate

4.4 Servings of starch, fruit, and milk are used interchangeably to create meals with a similar carbohydrate content. For example, a lunch plan based on the food guide pyramid or an exchange plan might have 2 starches, 1 fruit, and 1 milk—this would be 4 carbohydrate servings.

2 starches = 2 carbohydrate servings
1 fruit = 1 carbohydrate serving
1 milk = 1 carbohydrate serving

4.5 A meal plan for the day might be 3 carbohydrate servings at breakfast, 4 at lunch, and 5 at dinner.

Use Handout #2, Counting Carbohydrate Servings.

CONTENT OUTLINE

CONCEPT	DETAIL	INSTRUCTOR'S NOTES
5. Changing foods to carbohydrate servings	5.1 When the food group of an item is unknown: ■ look up its exchange value and convert it to a carbohydrate serving, or ■ look up the grams of carbohydrate per serving and divide by 15, or ■ count the grams of carbohydrate	
	5.2 If you have used exchanges in the past, you may already know the number of starch, fruit, and milk exchanges in many foods. For example: ■ 1 cup noodle soup = 1 starch (1 carbohydrate serving) ■ 1 cup ice cream = 2 starches and 4 fats (2 carbohydrate servings)	Meat/protein and fat exchanges do not affect the number of carbohydrate choices.
	5.3 Several reference books are available to look up the exchange value of foods you don't know.	Demonstrate using *Exchange Lists for Meal Planning, Exchanges for All Occasions,* and other exchange references. Use Handout #3, Exchange and Food Composition References.
	5.4 When the grams of carbohydrate are available, dividing by 15 gives the number of carbohydrate servings. The carbohydrate content is listed on almost all food labels.	Demonstrate using product labels and food composition books to find the grams of carbohydrate in other food items. Show Visual #1, Carbohydrate Servings.
	5.5 Round off the number of choices to the nearest half choice. Examples: ■ Big Mac = 45 gm Carbohydrate = 3 servings ■ 16 Cheese Tidbits = 8 gm Carbohydrate = ½ serving	Use Handout #5, How to Calculate Carbohydrate Grams in Your Serving, and Handout #7, Carbohydrate in My Food. $\dfrac{45}{15} = 3$ $\dfrac{8}{15} = 0.53$
	5.6 Counting carbohydrate servings is not as precise as counting actual grams of carbohydrate, because the carbohydrate content of one serving	It is more difficult to calculate insulin doses based on carbohydrate intake with this degree of variability.

CONTENT OUTLINE

CONCEPT	DETAIL	INSTRUCTOR'S NOTES
	can range from 10 to 20 gm. This means the carbohydrate content of 3 choices could range from 30 to 60 gm.	
	5.7 For many people, this method is accurate enough to meet their goals. The smaller numbers may be easier to remember (e.g., 3–4 servings rather than 45–60 gm).	This method is most appropriate for: ■ people with type 2 diabetes ■ children ■ adults with type 1 diabetes who are new to carbohydrate counting ■ adults with type 1 diabetes for whom increased precision is not needed or wanted
	5.8 This approach will be easier for those familiar with the exchange system or who eat few foods in the other carbohydrates category.	Use *Basic Carbohydrate Counting* to reinforce information about carbohydrate servings. The booklet also discusses meat and meat substitutes, fat, measuring, and label reading and provides lists of foods equal to 1 carbohydrate serving.
6. Counting carbohydrate grams	6.1 Counting grams of carbohydrate is another carbohydrate-based method for meal planning.	Use *Basic Carbohydrate Counting* or *Advanced Carbohydrate Counting* booklets to reinforce information.
	6.2 You can plan a specific number of carbohydrate grams for each meal and snack or vary the carbohydrate content and adjust other aspects of your plan (e.g., your insulin bolus dose).	It is easier initially to eat a consistent amount of carbohydrate to establish target carbohydrate levels and insulin ratios.
	6.3 Grams of carbohydrate, the only information needed to use this method, is on every food label.	A reasonable target range when counting carbohydrate grams is ±3 gm.
	6.4 A wide variety of meals can be planned to match a given carbohydrate amount.	Any food with a known carbohydrate content can be used and still fit the plan.

CONTENT OUTLINE

CONCEPT	DETAIL	INSTRUCTOR'S NOTES
	6.5 For example, a meal equal to 60–65 carbohydrate grams could be:	Nutrient value can vary. Carbohydrate counting helps people reach blood glucose goals. Other information may be needed to address other nutrition goals.

6.5 For example, a meal equal to 60–65 carbohydrate grams could be:

- 1 cup 2% milk — 12
  ham sandwich — 32
  ½ cup applesauce — <u>17</u>
  — 61

- muffin — 24
  apple cinnamon oatmeal — <u>41</u>
  — 65

- large baked potato — 30
  1 cup broccoli — 10
  6 oz steak — 0
  2 cups tossed salad — 3
  2 Tbsp ranch dressing — 2
  ½ cup ice cream — <u>15</u>
  — 60

6.6 Foods high in sugar may easily be included using this method. However, the portion size of sugary foods will be small.

Instructor's notes: Use *Advanced Carbohydrate Counting* to reinforce and build on the information in this section. The booklet offers support for using carbohydrate counting for pattern management.

7. Using carbohydrate/ insulin ratios

7.1 Patterns are trends in your blood glucose over time. Pattern management refers to changes you make in food, medication, or physical activity based on comparing your blood glucose trends with your targets.

Instructor's notes: Ask, "What are your target blood glucose levels?"

American Diabetes Association guides for target blood plasma glucose levels are:
90–130 mg/dl preprandial
<180 mg/dl postprandial

7.2 It is easier to see trends when your records have more information than just your blood glucose levels. Other helpful information is:
- insulin time and dose
- missed meals/snacks
- extra unusual meals
- new food
- more or less physical activity than usual

Instructor's notes: Stress the importance of recording or downloading meter results.

CONTENT OUTLINE

CONCEPT	DETAIL	INSTRUCTOR'S NOTES

■ hypoglycemia and treatment
■ stress or illness
■ alcohol intake

7.3 To implement pattern management, you will need to monitor multiple times during the day.

Discuss information obtained from pre- and post-prandial readings.

7.4 When looking at your blood glucose records, ask yourself:
■ What patterns do I see?
■ What other information would help?
■ What could be causing or influencing these values?
■ What strategies could I use to address this trend?

Ask participants or provide examples. Stress the importance of reviewing trends, not just individual numbers.

8. Calculating carbohydrate/ insulin ratios

8.1 The next step is to figure out your carbohydrate/insulin ratio. In this approach, the premeal bolus insulin dose is based on the amount of carbohydrate you plan to eat at that meal. People who use this method take rapid-acting or short-acting insulin before each meal. Monitoring after the meal helps determine if the dose was adequate for the carbohydrate eaten.

8.2 Carbohyrate/insulin ratios vary with individual sensitivity. However, most people need 1–3 units of insulin per 15 gm of carbohydrate. For people taking 1 unit for every 15 gm of carbohydrate, the ratio is 1:15.

Before using carbohydrate/ insulin ratios, blood glucose needs to be in the target range using a set basal and bolus insulin program and a consistent carbohydrate intake for 3–7 days. Rapid-acting insulin may be particularly useful for carbohydrate/insulin ratios.

	Insulin units/15 gm
Weight (lb)	Carbohydrate
<150	1
150–200	2
>200	3

If the participant has a history of sensitivity to insulin, then start with 1 unit per 30 gm of carbohydrate.

CONTENT OUTLINE

CONCEPT	DETAIL	INSTRUCTOR'S NOTES
	8.3 It will be easier if you begin with a baseline meal plan and insulin dose. You can calculate your insulin/carbohydrate ratio or begin by taking 1 unit of rapid-acting or short-acting insulin for each 15 gm of carbohydrate you eat. If your blood glucose level is higher than you want it to be after the meal, increase the dose to 2 units per 15 gm carbohydrate, and higher as needed. Use your blood glucose record to look for patterns and make adjustments.	Most participants benefit from a baseline meal plan and insulin dose to establish the ratio. Participants need to develop their plans in collaboration with their health care teams and will be in frequent contact with their team initially. Review Visual #1 if participants will be calculating their own ratio. Distribute Handout #3.
	8.4 Once you know your carbohydrate/insulin ratio, you can use it to calculate your bolus dose and/or to estimate insulin needs for varying carbohydrate intake.	Stress the importance of post-prandial glucose checks.
	8.5 You may need to fine-tune your ratio over time. Remember that a ratio of 1:20 is **less** insulin per gram of carbohydrate than a ratio of 1:15.	
	8.6 Some foods require more or less insulin per 15 gm carbohydrate.	Foods usually requiring more insulin are Chinese and Italian dishes (e.g., pizza). Foods usually requiring less insulin are dishes containing large amounts of whole grains, legumes, and beans, as well as vegetarian dishes. Use *Advanced Carbohydrate Counting* to reinforce and build on this section.
9. Sources of information on carbohydrate content of food	9.1 Sources of information on the carbohydrate content of foods are: ■ food labels ■ exchange list references ■ food-composition references	
	9.2 Food labels tell the amount of carbohydrate per serving. Note that it is the total carbohydrate, not just sugar, that matters in carbohydrate counting.	Ask participants to find the carbohydrate content on several food labels.

CONTENT OUTLINE

CONCEPT	DETAIL	INSTRUCTOR'S NOTES
	9.3 If you use a food label to calculate your ratio and your blood glucose isn't where you'd predict, remember: ■ food labels can be slightly inaccurate ■ subtract fiber from total carbohydrate	Fiber is unabsorbed carbohydrate and needs to be subtracted from the carbohydrate total on the label.
	9.4 Exchange list references give the exchange value of many foods. Some use exchanges to estimate the number of carbohydrate grams: ■ starch = 15 gm ■ fruit = 15 gm ■ milk = 12 gm Some exchange references provide the carbohydrate content in grams.	Show examples of exchange list references. Use Handout #3, Exchange and Food Composition References.
	9.5 Food composition references also tell you the grams of carbohydrate in a food.	Show samples of food composition references. Provide time for participants to look up favorite foods. Continue to use Handout #3.
	9.6 If the serving size on the label is not the same as your serving size, you can calculate the amount of your carbohydrate from the information on the label.	Use Handout #5, How to Calculate Carbohydrate Grams in Your Serving, to demonstrate and practice how to calculate the carbohydrate content of different serving amounts.
10. Other factors influencing blood glucose	10.1 Even when carbohydrate, medication, stress, and exercise levels stay the same, blood glucose levels may vary. Some other factors influencing blood glucose are: ■ fiber ■ fat ■ weight change ■ glycemic index ■ gastroparesis	Review only the portions of this section that are relevant to your audience.
Fiber	10.2 Fiber cannot be broken down and absorbed by the digestive system. It does not increase blood glucose.	

CONTENT OUTLINE

CONCEPT	DETAIL	INSTRUCTOR'S NOTES
	10.3 If a food contains more than 5 gm of fiber per serving, subtract grams of fiber from the total carbohydrate to find the amount of carbohydrate that affects your blood glucose. 　　Example: All Bran 　　Total carbohydrate　22 gm 　　Fiber 13 gm 　　Sugar 5 gm 22 – 13 = 9 gm of carbohydrate that affect blood glucose.	This is most important for people using intensive insulin and adjusting their insulin dose based on the carbohydrate content of their meal.
Fat	10.4 Fat leaves your stomach more slowly and may delay the blood glucose rise after a meal up to 10 hours when eaten in large amounts.	Eating a high-fat bedtime snack may not cause a rise in blood glucose until the following morning. Participants could have a hypoglycemic reaction in the middle of the night if they take bedtime insulin.
Weight	10.5 Your carbohydrate/insulin ratio may change if you gain or lose weight.	
	10.6 The improved glucose levels and flexibility of carbohydrate counting cause some people to gain weight with this method. If that is a concern, talk with your dietitian about weight management strategies.	Ask, "Do you think weight gain will be an issue for you? Why or why not? What strategies could you use to avoid weight gain?"
Glycemic index	10.7 Glycemic index (GI) is a measure of how different foods containing the same amount of carbohydrate affect your blood glucose levels. Fat and fiber may lower the GI of a food.	At one time, the GI held promise as a meal-planning method, but responses to any one food were too variable.
	10.8 Glycemic index varies with the speed of digestion. Carbohydrates that are liquids, thoroughly cooked, or blended are absorbed faster than carbohydrates that are solid, raw, or require thorough chewing.	The type of carbohydrate also makes a difference. For example, the starch in Cornflakes is more quickly digested and has a higher GI than sucrose (glucose + fructose).
	10.9 Your blood glucose response to a given amount of a certain food will be different than the next person's response. Blood glucose monitoring is the only way to discover your response.	Thin people with type 1 diabetes tend to be more sensitive to changes in carbohydrate levels than those with type 2 diabetes who are overweight and newly diagnosed (insulin resistant).

CONTENT OUTLINE

CONCEPT	DETAIL	INSTRUCTOR'S NOTES
Gastroparesis	10.10 People with nerve damage to the digestive tract from diabetes do not absorb food the same way each time they eat. This means blood glucose levels can vary, even when exactly the same meal is eaten.	Gastroparesis is reviewed in Outline #14, *Long-Term Complications.*
11. Using carbohydrate counting	11.1 Finding and counting the carbohydrate content of the foods you eat each day takes time and effort; however, your blood glucose control may improve, and carbohydrate counting provides increased flexibility.	Ask, "What are the benefits to you for using carbohydrate counting? The barriers?"
	11.2 To use the carbohydrate-counting system: ■ Meet with a dietitian to develop a plan and obtain information about the carbohydrate content of foods. ■ Start with a baseline insulin dose. ■ Weigh or measure the amount of food you plan to eat. ■ Calculate the carbohydrate content for that amount.	
	11.3 Become familiar with the carbohydrate content of the foods you eat: ■ Make a list of 12 foods you eat regularly. ■ Record the number of carbohydrate choices and/or grams of carbohydrate in these foods. ■ Monitor pre- and postmeal blood glucose levels.	Use Handout #7, Carbohydrate in My Food, to do this activity. Review participants' plans and answer questions. This is designed to help participants begin carbohydrate counting more easily and accurately. Provide copies of *Exchange Lists for Meal Planning, Exchanges for All Occasions,* and other references for exchange information. Use product labels and food-composition books to find the grams of carbohydrate in other food items.
	11.4 Identify a step you can take to use carbohydrate counting.	Close with summary questions and comments.

SKILLS CHECKLIST

Participants will be able to calculate the carbohydrate content of foods they often eat.

EVALUATION PLAN

Knowledge will be evaluated by achievement of learning objectives and by responses to questions during the session. The ability to apply knowledge will be evaluated by the development of personal meal-planning goals, by the development and implementation of a carbohydrate-counting approach to achieve those goals, and through program outcome measures.

DOCUMENTATION PLAN

Record class attendance and achieved objectives as appropriate.

SUGGESTED READINGS

American Diabetes Association/American Dietetic Association. *Basic Carbohydrate Counting; Advanced Carbohydrate Counting.* Alexandria, VA, American Diabetes Association/Chicago, American Dietetic Association, 2003.

Holzmeister LA. *The Diabetes Carbohydrate and Fat Gram Guide.* 2nd Edition. Alexandria, VA: American Diabetes Association, 2000.

Laredo R. Carbohydrate counting: a return to basics. *Diabetes Spectrum.* 2000;13:149–164.

➡ Carbohydrate Servings

Amount	Food Item	Starch	Fruit	Milk	Other	Carbohydrate Servings
2 oz	½ Bagel	2				2
½ cup	Orange juice		1			1
1 cup	Milk			1		1
1 cup	Mashed potatoes	2				2
8 oz	Artificially sweetened yogurt			1		1
1 small	Banana		1	1		2

Combination Foods—Exchange Value Available

Amount	Food Item	Starch	Fruit	Milk	Other	Carbohydrate Servings
1 cup	Potato salad	2				2
1	Ice cream bar	1				1
2 cups	Spaghetti and meatballs	6				6
8 oz	Fat-free vanilla yogurt		1	1½		2½

Combination Foods—Exchange Value Not Available

Amount	Food Item	Starch	Fruit	Milk	Other	Carbohydrate Servings
16	Cheese Tidbits = 8 gm carbohydrate					½
1	Oreo Big Stuff cookie = 33 gm carbohydrate					2
8 oz	Stouffers Vegetable Lasagna = 28 gm carbohydrate					2
1	Big Mac = 43 gm carbohydrate					3

© 2004 American Diabetes Association

➔ Carbohydrate Foods

Food Group	Food
Starch	Bread, rolls, bagels, English muffins, tortillas, pita bread, naan, saltine crackers, and matzoh Pasta: noodles, spaghetti, and macaroni Rice Cereal: dry or cooked Legumes: lentils, dried beans (garbanzo, kidney, black, and butter beans), and dried peas (split peas and black-eyed peas) Starchy vegetables: potatoes, corn, peas, squash, yams, and taro root
Fruit	Apples, oranges, bananas, and all other fruits—fresh, frozen, canned, or juiced
Milk	All milk Yogurt (plain or artificially sweetened)
Vegetable	Carrots, green beans, broccoli, beets, greens, okra, and all other crunchy vegetables (only if 1½ cups or more)
Other	Foods that include any of the above items, such as: ■ casseroles ■ soups ■ stews ■ pizza ■ snack foods—chips, pretzels, and french fries ■ desserts—ice cream, frozen yogurt, cake, cookies, and pie ■ alcoholic beverages—beer and sweet wine

➲ Counting Carbohydrate Servings

Meal Time _____:_____

_____ carbohydrate servings OR

_____ grams carbohydrate

_____ meat or meat substitutes

_____ fats

Snack Time _____:_____

_____

_____

Meal Time _____:_____

_____ carbohydrate servings OR

_____ grams carbohydrate

_____ meat or meat substitutes

_____ fats

Snack Time _____:_____

_____

_____

Meal Time _____:_____

_____ carbohydrate servings OR

_____ grams carbohydrate

_____ meat or meat substitutes

_____ fats

Snack Time _____:_____

_____

_____

➔ Exchange and Food Composition References

SOURCES OF EXCHANGE VALUE INFORMATION

1. Diabetes Care and Education Practice Group, The American Dietetic Association. *Ethnic and Regional Food Practices Series: Food Practices, Customs and Holidays for Jewish, Mexican American, Chinese American, Hmong, Navajo, Alaska Native, Filipino American, Soul and Traditional Southern, Cajun and Creole*. Alexandria, VA: American Diabetes Association, and Chicago, IL: The American Dietetic Association, 1989.

2. Franz M. *Exchanges for All Occasions*. 4th ed. Minneapolis, MN: IDC Publishing, 2000.

3. Nutrition information brochures with exchange information are available from most chain restaurants such as McDonald's, Burger King, and Wendy's.

FOOD COMPOSITION REFERENCES

1. Kraus B. *Calories and Carbohydrates*. New York, NY: Signet, 1999.

2. Holzmeister LA. *The Diabetes Carbohydrate and Fat Gram Guide*, 2nd edition. Alexandria, VA: American Diabetes Association, 2000.

3. Netzers CT. *The Complete Book of Food Counts*. New York, NY: Dell Publishing, 2003.

4. Pennington JAT. *Bowes & Church: Food Values of Portions Commonly Used*. Philadelphia, PA: JB Lippincott, 1998.

5. Many published recipes, including those in the cookbooks on Handout #6 in the *Planning Meals* session.

6. Nutrition information brochures with the carbohydrate content of items are available from most chain restaurants such as McDonald's, Burger King, and Wendy's.

→ Practice Worksheet

How to Figure Your Carbohydrate-to-Insulin Ratio Using the Carbohydrate Gram Method

1. Record the grams (g) carbohydrate that you consistently eat at each meal based on your BG and food records.

    Breakfast _____ g   Lunch _____ g   Supper _____ g

2. Record the Regular (R) insulin meal doses that consistenly meet target BGs. (u = units of insulin)

    Breakfast _____ u   Lunch _____ u   Supper _____ u

3. Determine the carbohydrate g per u insulin for each meal by dividing the total g carbohydrate for each meal by the number of u R.

    Breakfast = B   Lunch = L   Supper = S

    $$\frac{\text{_____ g carbohydrate}}{\text{_____ u R insulin}} = \text{_____ g/u}$$

    $$\text{B} \ \frac{\text{_____ g}}{\text{\_\_\_\_\_ u}} = \text{\_\_\_\_\_ g/u}$$

    $$\text{L} \ \frac{\text{_____ g}}{\text{\_\_\_\_\_ u}} = \text{\_\_\_\_\_ g/u}$$

    $$\text{S} \ \frac{\text{_____ g}}{\text{\_\_\_\_\_ u}} = \text{\_\_\_\_\_ g/u}$$

PRACTICE WORKSHEET *continued*

4. If your answers to step 3 vary from each other by no more than 1 g carbohydrate, add the 3 answerss together and divide by 3 to get the average grams carbohydrate per unit of insulin.

    B _____

    L _____

    + S _____

    _____ total divided by 3 = _____ g/unit

5. If your answers to step 3 vary from each other by no more than 1 g carbohydrate and you and your health-care team agree that your basal insulin doses are well adjusted, then use your answers to step 3 as your carbohydrate-to-insulin ratios for each meal.

    My carbohydrate-to-insulin ratios are
    B _____ g/u   L _____ g/u   S _____ g/u

6. To make insulin adjustments for more or less carbohydrate eaten, add up the total carbohydrate and divide by the appropriate carbohydrate-to-insulin ratio.

    Total carbohydrate _____ g ÷ g/u (ratio) _____ = _____ u R

PRACTICE WORKSHEET *continued*

How to Figure Your Carbohydrate-to-Insulin Ratio Using the Carbohydrate Choice Method

1. Record the Regular (R) insulin meal doses that consistently meet target BGs based on your BG and food records.

   Breakfast _____ u   Lunch _____ u   Supper _____ u

2. Record the number of carbohydrate choices that you consistently eat at each meal.

   Breakfast _____   Lunch _____   Supper _____
   carbohydrate   carbohydrate   carbohydrate
   choices   choices   choices

3. Determine the units of R insulin per carbohydrate choice for each meal by dividing the number of units by the number of carbohydrate choices.

$$\frac{\text{units R}}{\text{carbohydrate choices}} = \underline{\qquad} \text{ units per carbohydrate choice}$$

$$\text{B} \frac{\underline{\quad} \text{ units}}{\underline{\quad} \text{ choices}} = \underline{\quad} \text{ units per carbohydrate choice}$$

$$\text{L} \frac{\underline{\quad} \text{ units}}{\underline{\quad} \text{ choices}} = \underline{\quad} \text{ units per carbohydrate choice}$$

$$\text{S} \frac{\underline{\quad} \text{ units}}{\underline{\quad} \text{ choices}} = \underline{\quad} \text{ units per carbohydrate choice}$$

My carbohydrate/insulin ratio is _____ units per carbohydrate choice.

PRACTICE WORKSHEET *continued*

4. If your answers to step 3 are different for one or more meals, use more than one ratio.

   My carbohydrate/insulin ratios are
   B _____ u/carbohydrate choice

   L _____ u/carbohydrate choice

   S _____ u/carbohydrate choice

5. To make insulin adjustments for more or fewer carbohydrate choices, add up the total number of carbohydrate choices and multiply by your ratio (u/carbohydrate choice).

   Total number of carbohydrate choices _____
   x _____ u/carbohydrate choice
   = _____ u R

➔ How to Calculate Carbohydrate Grams in Your Serving

If you know the serving size for a food product and the grams of carbohydrate in that serving size, you can find the number of grams in a different serving size in two steps:

1. Divide your serving size by the serving size on the label.

2. Multiply the result by the grams of carbohydrate on the label.

Examples

Label information:

Serving size = ½ cup   Carbohydrate: 22 grams

Your serving = ¾ cup

1. **Divide** your serving size by the serving size on the label.

$$\frac{0.75}{0.5} = 1.5$$

2. **Multiply** the result by the grams of carbohydrate on the label.

1.5 × 22 grams = 33 grams

Your serving has 33 grams of carbohydrate.

Sometimes you can estimate the amount without using the formula. In this example, you can see that your serving size is 1½ times as much as the serving size mentioned on the label. You can just add half the carbohydrate (11 grams) to the label amount (22 grams) to get the amount in your serving (33 grams).

continued

HOW TO CALCULATE CARBOHYDRATE GRAMS IN YOUR SERVING *continued*

Label information:

Serving size = 10 oz   Carbohydrate : 15 grams

Your serving = 6 oz

1. **Divide** your serving size by the serving size on the label.

$$\frac{6}{10} = 0.6$$

2. **Multiply** the result by the grams of carbohydrate on the label.

0.6×15 grams = 9 grams

Your serving has 9 grams of carbohydrate.

Note:

- This method works regardless of the serving-size units.

- This method works whether you eat more or less than the serving size on the label.

➜ Tips for Counting Carbohydrate Servings

Grams of carbohydrate	Count as:
0–5 gm	Do not count
6–10 gm	½ carbohydrate serving or ½ starch, fruit, or milk serving
11–20 gm	1 carbohydrate serving or 1 starch, fruit, or milk serving
21–25 gm	1½ carbohydrate servings or 1½ starch, fruit, or milk servings
26–35 gm	2 carbohydrate servings or 2 starch, fruit, or milk servings

Know what you are eating. Measure or weigh your foods to help you learn what carbohydrate servings look like. The foods I will measure are:

_____

The food labels I will check are:

_____

Feel good about what you already do. If you decide to make food changes, choose only one or two changes to make. This is what I will do:

_____

_____

Counting carbohydrate in your food allows you more flexibility in food choices and helps keep your blood glucose levels within target range.

➜ Carbohydrate in My Food

Carbohydrate Grams	Amount	Food Item	Starch	Fruit	Milk	Other	Carbohydrate Servings

| #20 | Diabetes Exchange Lists |

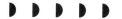

STATEMENT OF PURPOSE

This session provides information about the exchange system. The exchange system builds on the food groups introduced in Outline #4, *Food and Blood Glucose*, and the healthy food choices food guide pyramid approaches discussed in Outline #5, *Planning Meals*. It is a plan to eat a certain amount from each of the six food groups at each meal and snack. This approach addresses all the reasons for meal planning, but its use is not encouraged for participants who do not have access to a dietitian to help them develop a personal meal plan that fits the way they eat.

PREREQUISITES

It is recommended that each participant have attended Session #4, *Food and Blood Glucose*, and Session #5, *Planning Meals*, or have achieved those objectives. This session is intended for individuals who have some experience living and eating with diabetes and who prefer a more calculated meal plan to meet their blood glucose and weight goals. It is recommended that participants who have meal-planning booklets and meal plans bring them to class.

OBJECTIVES

At the end of this session, participants will be able to:

1. state the purpose of the food exchange system;

2. name the six food exchange groups;

3. state why foods are placed in certain groups;

4. identify which exchange groups contain carbohydrate;

5. state reasons for using an individualized meal plan;

6. find each food exchange list in the meal-planning booklet, and name several foods on each list;

7. use exchange lists to find exchange amounts;

8. state why moving carbohydrate exchanges will affect blood glucose more than moving meat or fat exchanges.

CONTENT

Nutritional Management.

MATERIALS NEEDED

VISUALS PROVIDED	**ADDITIONAL**

<table>
<tr><td>

1. Reasons for Meal Planning
2. Exchange Groups
3. Nutrients in Food Exchange Groups
4. Fat Exchange Group
5. Sample Meal Plan
6. Starch Exchange Group
7. Fruit Exchange Group
8. Milk Exchange Group
9. Other Carbohydrates Exchange Group
10. Vegetable Exchange Group
11. Meat Exchange Group
12. Free Foods

</td><td>

- Chalkboard and chalk
- Food models or pictures of foods
- *Exchange Lists for Meal Planning* (available from the American Diabetes Association, 800-232-6733)

</td></tr>
</table>

Handouts (one per participant)
1. Uncooked vs. Cooked Portions
2. Standard Weights and Measures

METHOD OF PRESENTATION

Start by introducing yourself and telling what you do. Ask participants to introduce themselves. Explain that the purposes of this session are to understand how an exchange system meal plan can help them manage their blood glucose, to learn the food groups in the exchange system, and to practice identifying foods in each group.

Present materials in a discussion/question format. Family members and/or significant others (especially those who prepare meals for the person with diabetes) are encouraged to attend. Begin by asking how they did with their short-term goal and what they learned from it.

Because this content is complex for some participants, using culturally appropriate food models is particularly important. For each food, ask participants to identify the food group; protein, fat, and carbohydrate content; and impact on blood glucose. After several items in each group are identified, ask participants to identify which foods can be exchanged for each other and to tell why or why not (e.g., impact on blood glucose level is different).

CONTENT OUTLINE

CONCEPT	DETAIL	INSTRUCTOR'S NOTES
1. Introduction to the exchange system	1.1 The food exchange system is a method of meal planning used by people with diabetes.	Ask, "What questions or concerns do you have about the exchange system? What is it? How many of you use it?"
	1.2 Meal plans using the exchange system provide a consistent balance of carbohydrate, protein, and fat to help keep blood glucose stable. Regular timing of meals also helps to keep blood glucose in the target range.	Ask, "What is the purpose of the exchange system?" Blood glucose test results can help determine an individual's response to various foods.
	1.3 Using an exchange plan can help people with diabetes obtain the variety of foods needed for good health and the calories needed to reach or maintain a desirable body weight. It can also help lower blood fats and regulate blood glucose.	Use Visual #1, Reasons for Meal Planning. Note that following the exchange system can help with all the reasons for meal planning.
	1.4 The meal plan is like a food budget with a certain number of food choices to "spend" at each meal.	
	1.5 Food choices are from six basic groups of food. The food or exchange groups are starch, fruit, vegetables, milk, meat, and fat. These are the same food groups used in the food guide pyramid. However, some foods maybe grouped differently in the food guide pyramid.	Ask, "What are the six food groups?" Use Visual #2, Exchange Groups.
	1.6 The food groups are listed so that all of the carbohydrate-containing groups are together: starch, fruit, milk, sweets, desserts and other carbohydrates, and nonstarchy vegetables.	Ask, "Which groups contain carbohydrate?"
	1.7 Remember that carbohydrate affects blood glucose the most. Carbohydrate in liquid form is absorbed more quickly and affects blood glucose levels faster than solids.	Review how nutrients affect blood glucose.
	1.8 The absorption of carbohydrate will be slowed by the presence of protein or fat in a mixed meal.	

401

CONTENT OUTLINE

CONCEPT	DETAIL	INSTRUCTOR'S NOTES
	1.9 Note the major nutrients in each group. The foods in each group contain similar amounts of carbohydrate, protein, fat, and calories. This means that each food in one group will affect blood glucose in a similar way when used in the amount listed.	Use Visual #3, Nutrients in Food Exchange Groups. You may want to note that nutrient values for different foods in a group are similar, not identical. Using food models or the *Exchange Lists for Meal Planning* booklet, review foods from each group.
	1.10 Exchange means that any food in one group can be exchanged for any other food in the same group because foods in the same group affect blood glucose similarly.	Ask, "What is meant by *exchange*?"
	1.11 The exchange system allows for many choices. You'll learn more about each food group later in this session.	Give examples of choices (for 1 fat exchange, you could use 1 tsp margarine, 1 Tbsp cream cheese, or 2 Tbsp sour cream). Use Visual #4, Fat Exchange Group. Or, using food models, set up a dinner plate that includes 1 vegetable exchange. Show how different vegetables can be "exchanged" to provide 1 vegetable exchange. Repeat with other groups until the concept of exchanging is clear. Note that exchanges are for measured amounts.
2. Individual meal plans	2.1 Your meal plan tells you the number of choices or exchanges from each food group and the meal or snack for which they are planned.	Ask, "How do you know how many exchanges to eat?" Use Visual #5, Sample Meal Plan. Refer to participants' meal-planning booklets.
	2.2 A meal plan is calculated by a dietitian, based on your requests, personal eating habits, activity level, and diabetes medication program. You need to help develop a meal plan that you can use in real life. Tell your dietitian about foods that are important to include or omit. Remember, it's your meal plan.	Ideally, insulin programs are adjusted to fit the meal plan and activity level. It takes trial and error to work out the best plan. Also note that some adaptation of this system is needed for those with special dietary needs.

CONTENT OUTLINE

CONCEPT	DETAIL	INSTRUCTOR'S NOTES
	2.3 Whenever food needs, schedule, or activity level changes, the meal plan needs to be revised. Additional dietary changes may be needed during adolescence, pregnancy and breast-feeding, and after surgery.	Ask, "When might a meal plan need to be changed?" Ask for examples of changes in the participants' lives that cause their eating patterns to change.
	2.4 The kind, number, and timing of exchanges will vary from person to person. In general, the fewer the changes to your usual patterns, the more likely you will be able to use the meal plan over time.	Use Visual #5, Sample Meal Plan, to illustrate. Ask, "How many starch exchanges are in your meal plan?" You may note that standard meal plans are available but usually call for more changes from typical food choices than necessary.
3. Foods in the exchange groups	3.1 Most foods belong to an exchange group that sounds logical, but some foods may seem out of place. For example, all fruits are in the fruit group, but starchy vegetables are in the starch group.	Recall that foods are placed in an exchange group according to their effect on blood glucose. Use food models, visuals, and meal-planning books to illustrate each food group. Provide them for class practice.
4. Starch group	4.1 The starch group contains a variety of foods—bread, cereals, grains, legumes, noodles, and starchy vegetables. Legumes are dried peas and beans, including kidney beans, butter beans, chick peas (garbanzo beans), pinto beans, soy beans, black-eyed peas, miso, and lentils.	Use Visual #6, Starch Exchange Group. Have participants find the starch list in their booklets. Ask each to choose 1 starch exchange for breakfast, 2 for lunch, and 2 for dinner. Use food models to reinforce the exchange idea.
	4.2 Starchy vegetables (corn, peas, yams, potatoes, plantain, and winter squash) contain more carbohydrate than most other vegetables and are included in the starch exchange group.	Corn and peas are vegetables. Explain that in terms of blood glucose, they belong in the starch group because the carbohydrate content of a usual serving is closest to that of a starch exchange.
	4.3 Some starch foods contain added fat (e.g., pancakes, biscuits, hummus, taco shells, muffins and cornbread). Omit 1 fat exchange for each high-fat starch to keep fat and calorie intake consistent.	Ask, "Which starch exchanges contain extra fat?" Find the list in the booklet.

CONTENT OUTLINE

CONCEPT	DETAIL	INSTRUCTOR'S NOTES
5. Fruit exchange group	5.1 The fruit group includes all fruits that have no sugar added, whether fresh, dried, cooked, canned, frozen, or juiced.	Fruit naturally contains sugar, even without added sugar.
	5.2 Heavy syrup-packed fruit has added sugar (rinsing does not remove the sugar). Fruit packed in fruit juice, water, or extra-light syrup is recommended. Count the juice from canned fruit as fruit exchange(s).	Use Visual #7, Fruit Exchange Group. Continue as for other food groups. The variability in exchange amount is due to different amounts of fiber, water, and sugar in different fruits. (Optional: 1½ cups of tomato or V8 juice—3 vegetable exchanges—may be used as 1 fruit.)
6. Milk exchange group	6.1 The milk exchange group includes only milk and yogurt.	Sugar-free hot chocolate mixes, kefir, and soy milk fit in this category. Check carbohydrates on the label.
	6.2 The only difference between the kinds of milk is the fat content.	Note that other dairy items are in the meat group. Use Visual #8, Milk Exchange Group. Continue as for other food groups. Note differences in fat content.
	6.3 Six ounces of sugar-free artificially sweetened yogurt or 6 oz of low-fat plain yogurt is about equal to 1 cup of milk. Flavored or fruit yogurt contains three times as much carbohydrate as artifically sweetened yogurt. The fat content of yogurt varies, as does that of milk. Check the label.	Plain yogurt can be flavored with artificial sweetener, cinnamon, or a flavor extract. It may also be combined with a fruit exchange.
	6.4 Frozen yogurts that are sugar- and fat-free are available. These count as a milk exchange because they are made from skim milk. They just have no added sugar.	Their exchange value may be included in one of the books listed in Outline #21, *Using Exchanges to Plan Meals.*

CONTENT OUTLINE

CONCEPT	DETAIL	INSTRUCTOR'S NOTES
7. Other carbohydrates exchange group	7.1 There is one more carbohydrate list. It includes a variety of snacks and desserts that contain carbohydrate but do not fit well in the other groups.	Ask, "What are some snack foods you enjoy?" Use Visual #9, Other Carbohydrates Exchange Group. Note that all foods depicted are 1 carbohydrate exchange. Some people are happy to learn a way to include sweets in their diet; others resist the idea. If someone is more comfortable with a no sweets/snacks approach, he or she does not need to use this group.
	7.2 An item in this list contains about 15 gm of carbohydrate per serving and may be substituted for any other carbohydrate exchange. Calculate how many carbohydrate exchanges are in the food. Eating more or fewer carbohydrate exchanges than usual at any one time can cause high or low blood glucose readings.	
	7.3 These do not have as many vitamins and minerals as other carbohydrates, and many of the portions are small.	
	7.4 Often these foods contain fat as well.	The number of fat exchanges needs to be counted in the meal plan.
8. Vegetable exchange group	8.1 The vegetable group includes most vegetables such as green beans, okra, broccoli, carrots, greens, beets, eggplant, kohlrabi, and asparagus.	Ask, "What vegetables are included in the vegetable group?" Use Visual #10, Vegetable Exchange Group.
	8.2 Vegetables that belong in the vegetable exchange group tend to be more crunchy (unless they are overcooked).	
	8.3 The serving size for cooked vegetables and vegetable juice is ½ cup. The serving size for raw vegetables is 1 cup.	
	8.4 If you eat 1 or 2 vegetable exchanges at a meal or snack, you do not count them, because they contain very little carbohydrate and calories. If you eat 3 or more, you count it as 1 carbohydrate exchange.	These foods will help participants who are trying to decrease calories to feel more full.
	8.5 All of the vegetables in this group are a good source of fiber.	

CONTENT OUTLINE

CONCEPT	DETAIL	INSTRUCTOR'S NOTES
9. Meat and meat substitute group	9.1 The meat exchange group contains meat, poultry, and fish as well as cheese, eggs, tofu, and peanut butter.	
	9.2 This group is divided into four parts: very lean, lean, medium-fat, and high-fat meats.	
	9.3 To reduce fat and calories, choose lean meats and trim visible fat and skin before cooking or eating.	Use Visual #11, Meat Exchange Group. Have participants find the meat exchange list in their booklets. Compare foods and serving sizes. Note differences in fat content. Ask, "What might you choose for 3 meat exchanges at dinner, 2 at lunch, and 1 at breakfast?" Use food models to demonstrate exchanges.
	9.4 The fat in meat is animal fat, which means that it is saturated. Even if the meat does not contain much cholesterol, your body makes cholesterol from the saturated fat in the meat.	
	9.5 Fat used in cooking is not included in the meat group calculation. Use fat exchanges for this.	
	9.6 Any breading must be counted as 1 or more starch exchanges.	
	9.7 Weigh meat after cooking: 4 oz raw meat = 3 oz cooked meat.	Distribute Handout #1, Uncooked vs. Cooked Portions.
10. Fat exchange group	10.1 The fat exchange group includes fats and oils, but also some unexpected items such as avocado, nuts, olives, and bacon.	Use Visual #4, Fat Exchange Group. Continue as for other food groups.
	10.2 One fat exchange equals 5 gm of fat and 45 calories.	Compare the exchange amount of real mayonnaise to that of mayonnaise-type salad dressing. Compare butter to sour cream.
	10.3 Fats used in cooking or added to vegetables are counted as fat exchanges.	

CONTENT OUTLINE

CONCEPT	DETAIL	INSTRUCTOR'S NOTES
	10.4 The fat exchange group is divided into saturated (hard), polyunsaturated, and monounsaturated fats.	Refer to Outline #18, *Eating for a Healthy Heart*, for a discussion of fat types.
	10.5 Different types of fat perform different functions in the body. Saturated fats are stored and used to make cholesterol. Polyunsaturated fats are incorporated into the cell structure. Monounsaturated fats aid in the reduction of total cholesterol and LDL in particular. Hydrogenated fats contain trans fatty acids, which function in a similar manner as saturated fats. Omega-3, -6, and -9 polyunsaturated fats have specific functions that may be beneficial for preventing or treating heart disease.	While some fats are healthier than others, all have the same number of calories per serving.
	10.6 You can use monounsaturated fats such as canola, peanut, or olive oil in cooking to help balance the fats in your diet. However, monounsaturated fats still add calories to your meal plan.	
	10.7 Some foods contain hard-to-measure fat (sauces, gravies, and deep-fat fried foods).	The importance of limiting fat depends on calorie needs and blood lipid levels.
	10.8 Fats help foods taste good, but they concentrate many calories in a small amount.	
	10.9 You will find fat-free salad dressing, mayonnaise, cream cheese, and sour cream on the free foods list. Lite or low-fat products are generally not free foods, but they may help you to lower your fat intake.	Reduced-fat products still contain fat and calories, but they may be more tasty than fat-free products.
	10.10 Be aware that some fat-free foods contain significant amounts of carbohydrate. This carbohydrate may beabsorbed faster when less fat is present.	

CONTENT OUTLINE

CONCEPT	DETAIL	INSTRUCTOR'S NOTES
11. Free foods	11.1 Certain foods can be eaten without being counted in your meal plan. Any food or drink that contains <20 calories or <5 gm of carbohydrate per serving is free. Up to three 20-calorie servings spread throughout the day should not affect blood glucose levels.	Use Visual #12, Free Foods. Locate in the *Exchange Lists for Meal Planning* booklet.
	11.2 Some foods in this group (coffee, tea, certain seasonings, diet soft drinks, and sugar-free gelatin) are free in unlimited amounts. Others (fat-free cream cheese, fat-free salad dressing, reduced-fat mayonnaise, and sugar-free syrup) are free in limited amounts.	Ask for and provide examples of how free foods can enhance meals.
	11.3 If you add fat or sugar to the foods in this group, they are no longer free.	
12. Tips for using the exchange system	12.1 Milk, vegetable, fruit, and starch exchanges contain carbohydrate and affect blood glucose levels.	Ask, "How will omitting bread at lunch to have more spaghetti at dinner affect your blood glucose levels?"
	12.2 Moving 1 or 2 meat and/or fat exchanges to another meal results in smaller blood glucose changes than moving carbohydrate foods.	
	12.3 Generally, foods cannot be exchanged for those in another group. One fat does not have the same nutrient balance as 1 bread, for example, and will affect your blood glucose differently.	To illustrate, you can't buy an item at one store and exchange it at another. You can't use gas to lubricate your car engine instead of oil.
	12.4 Some substitutions can be made: ■ 1 vegetable = ⅓ bread ■ 1 milk (reduced fat [2%]) = about 1 fruit + 1 meat ■ 6 oz sugar-sweetened yogurt = 1 milk + 2 fruits	These substitutions contain a similar amount of carbohydrate and will affect blood glucose in a similar way, but they do not provide the same nutrients. They offer more flexibility, but may be confusing to those participants new to this approach.

CONTENT OUTLINE

CONCEPT	DETAIL	INSTRUCTOR'S NOTES
	12.5 It is helpful to weigh or measure food until you are familiar with portion sizes and how they appear on your plate or in your bowl. Watch for "portion-size creep," which occurs over time as portions gradually get larger and larger.	Ask participants to identify the amount of food or liquid in various containers. Use Handout #2, Standard Weights and Measures.
	12.6 Cooked foods are measured after cooking. Meat portions shrink and starches expand in cooking.	Refer to Handout #1, Uncooked vs. Cooked Portions. Show how to calculate cooked amounts, using the multiplying factor.
	12.7 The exchange system is one guide for meal planning.	The next session will provide practice using the exchange system to plan meals. Most learning comes from trying things at home and seeing how they work.
	12.8 The more closely you eat the number of exchanges planned at each meal, the more likely you will be able to keep your blood glucose in your target range.	Remind participants, however, that food is not the only cause of high blood glucose readings.
	12.9 Monitoring can help you find out how changes from your usual meal plan affect your blood glucose.	Choose a short-term goal to try before the next session.

SKILLS CHECKLIST

Participants will be able to locate exchange groups and correctly identify foods and serving sizes for each exchange group in their meal-planning booklets.

EVALUATION PLAN

Knowledge will be evaluated by achievement of learning objectives and by responses to questions during the session. The ability to apply knowledge will be evaluated by the development of personal meal-planning goals, by the development and implementation of a plan based on the exchange system to achieve those goals, and through program outcome measures.

DOCUMENTATION PLAN

Record class attendance and achieved objectives as appropriate.

SUGGESTED READINGS

The American Dietetic Association and American Diabetes Association. *Exchange Lists for Meal Planning.* Chicago, IL: The American Dietetic Association; Alexandria, VA: American Diabetes Association, 2003.

The American Dietetic Association and American Diabetes Association. *Exchange Lists for Weight Management.* Chicago, IL: The American Dietetic Association; Alexandria, VA: American Diabetes Association, 2003.

➡ Reasons for Meal Planning

- Maintain blood glucose as close to your target range as possible.

- Maintain cholesterol (blood fats) as close to your target range as possible.

- Maintain blood pressure as close to your target level as possible.

- Prevent, delay, or treat diabetes-related complications.

- Improve health through food choices.

- Meet individual nutritional needs.

➡ Exchange Groups

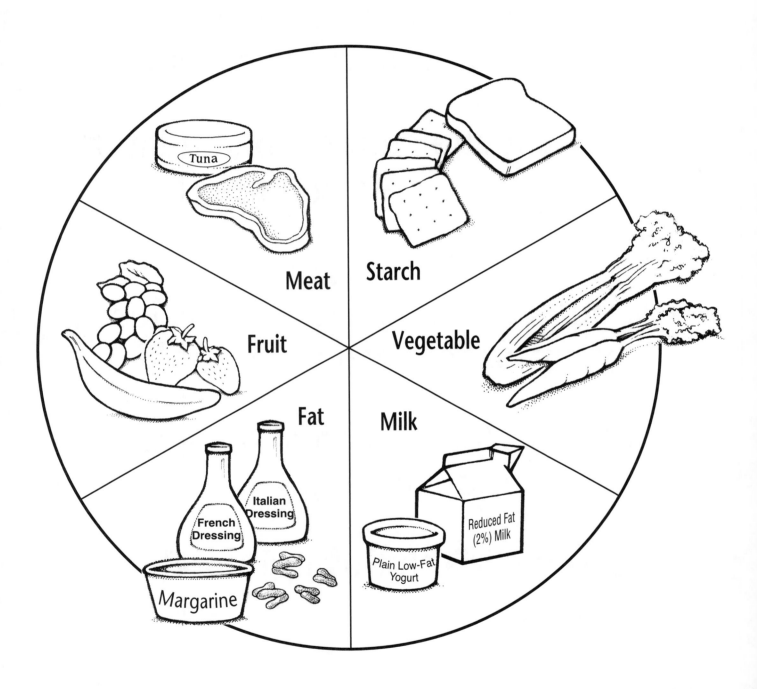

➡ Nutrients in Food Exchange Groups

Group	Carbohydrate (gm)	Protein (gm)	Fat (gm)	Calories
Carbohydrate				
Starch	15	3	1 or less	80
Fruit	15	—	—	60
Milk				
Fat-free (skim)	12	8	0–3	90
Low-fat (1%)	12	8	5	120
Whole	12	8	8	150
Nonstarchy Vegetables	5	2	—	25
Other Carbohydrates	Varies	Varies	Varies	Varies
Meat/Meat Substitute				
Very lean	—	7	0–1	35
Lean	—	7	3	55
Medium fat	—	7	5	75
High fat	—	7	8	100
Fat	—	—	5	45
Monounsaturated	—	—	5	45
Polyunsaturated	—	—	5	45
Saturated	—	—	5	45
Hydrogenated	—	—	5	45

© 2004 American Diabetes Association; The American Dietetic Association

➜ Fat Exchange Group

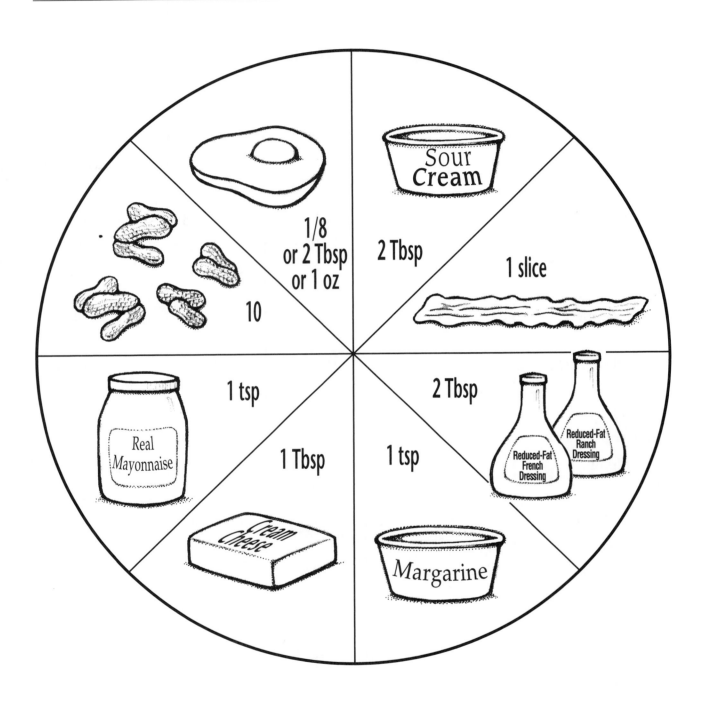

1/8
or 2 Tbsp
or 1 oz

10

Sour
Cream

2 Tbsp

1 slice

1 tsp

Real
Mayonnaise

1 Tbsp

Cream Cheese

1 tsp

Margarine

2 Tbsp

Reduced-Fat
French
Dressing

Reduced-Fat
Ranch
Dressing

➡ Sample Meal Plan

		Grams	Percent
Name	Sally Smith	Carbohydrate 200	51
Date	3/20/04	Protein 81	20
Dietitian	Frank Jones	Fat 50	29
Phone	555-1234	Calories 1600	

Time	Number of Choices	Food Ideas
7:30 A.M. breakfast	3½ Carbohydrate group 　2 Starch 　1 Fruit 　½ Milk 　___ Meat group 　1 Fat group	
12:30 P.M. lunch	4 Carbohydrate group 　2 Starch 　1 Fruit 　1 Milk 　2 Nonstarchy vegetables 　2 Meat group 　2 Fat group	
6:30 P.M. dinner	4 Carbohydrate group 　3 Starch 　1 Fruit 　___ Milk 　1 Nonstarchy vegetables 　3 Meat group 　2 Fat group	
10:30 P.M. snack	1 Starch ½ Milk	

➲ Starch Exchange Group

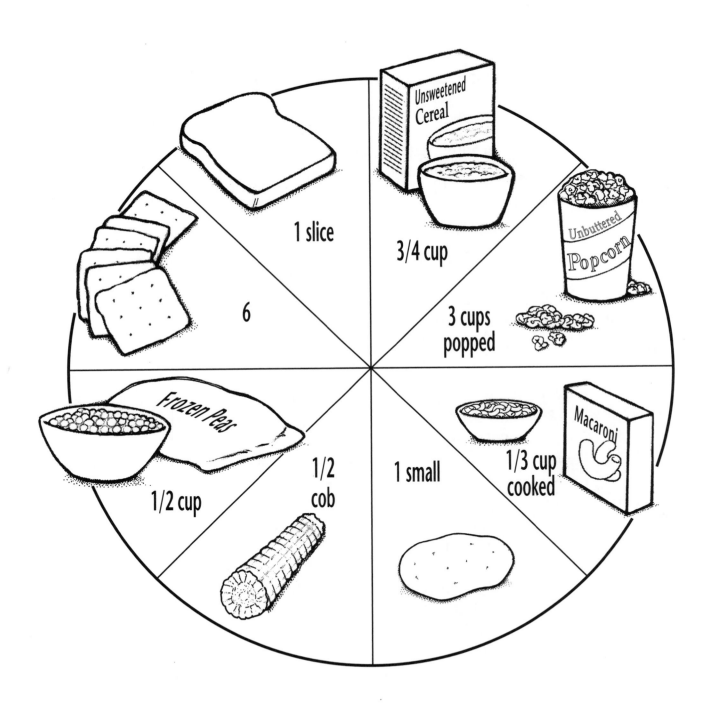

→ Fruit Exchange Group

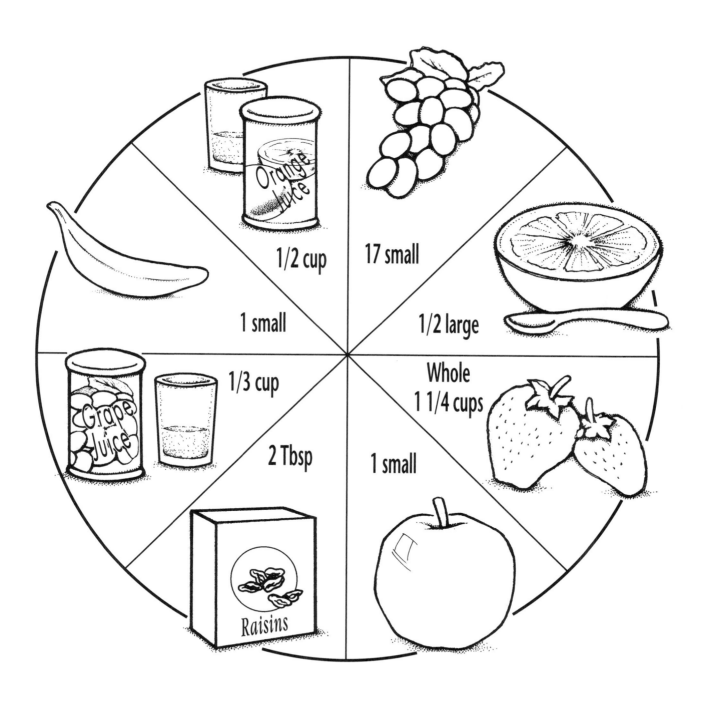

1/2 cup

17 small

1 small

1/2 large

1/3 cup

Whole
1 1/4 cups

2 Tbsp

1 small

➲ Milk Exchange Group

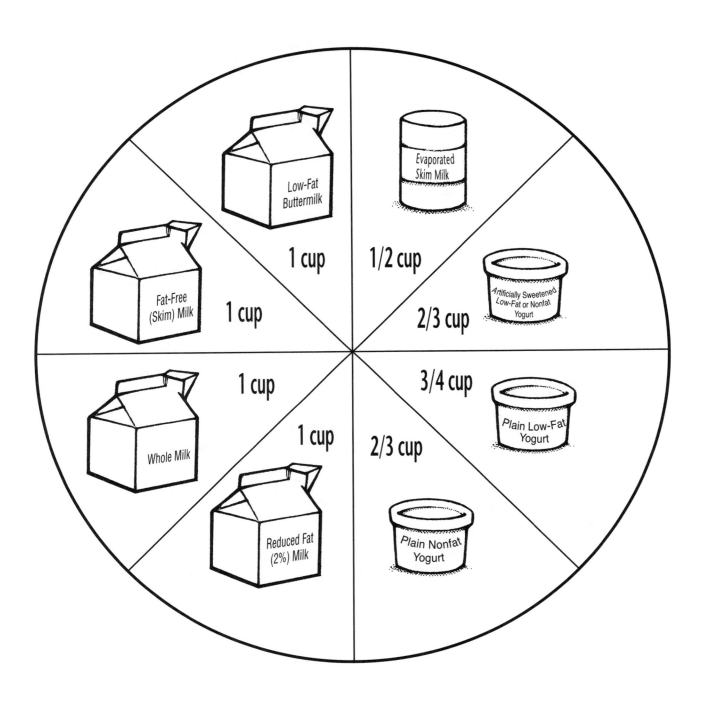

→ Other Carbohydrates Exchange Group

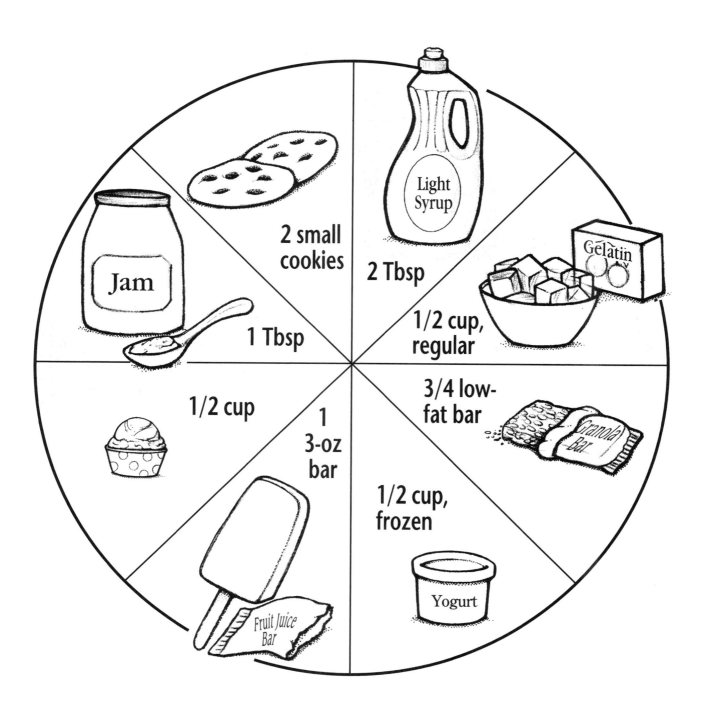

Jam

2 small cookies

Light Syrup

2 Tbsp

Gelatin

1 Tbsp

1/2 cup, regular

1/2 cup

3/4 low-fat bar

Granola Bar

1 3-oz bar

1/2 cup, frozen

Fruit Juice Bar

Yogurt

➡ Vegetable Exchange Group

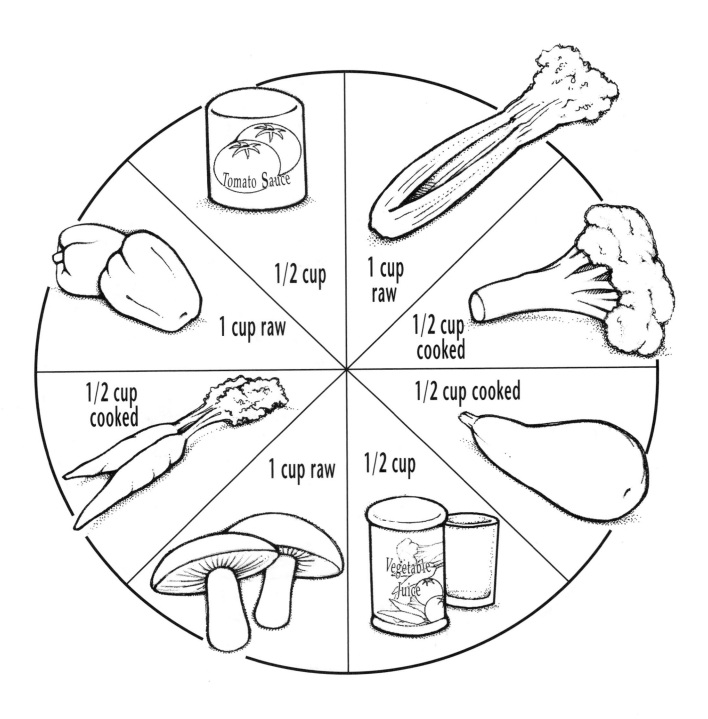

Tomato Sauce

1/2 cup

1 cup raw

1/2 cup cooked

1 cup raw

1/2 cup cooked

1/2 cup cooked

Vegetable Juice

1/2 cup

1 cup raw

➜ Meat Exchange Group

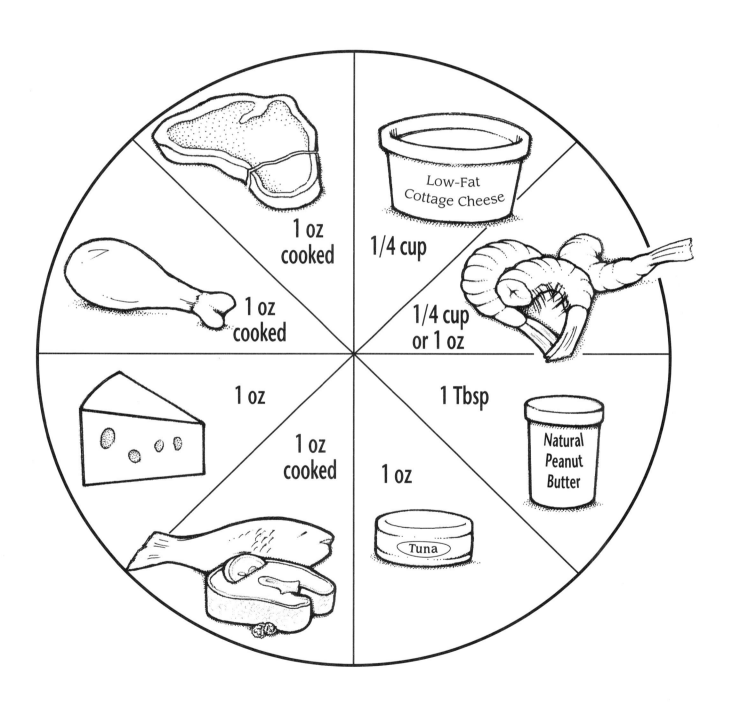

1 oz cooked

1/4 cup

1 oz cooked

1/4 cup or 1 oz

1 oz

1 Tbsp

Low-Fat Cottage Cheese

Natural Peanut Butter

1 oz cooked

1 oz

Tuna

Free Foods

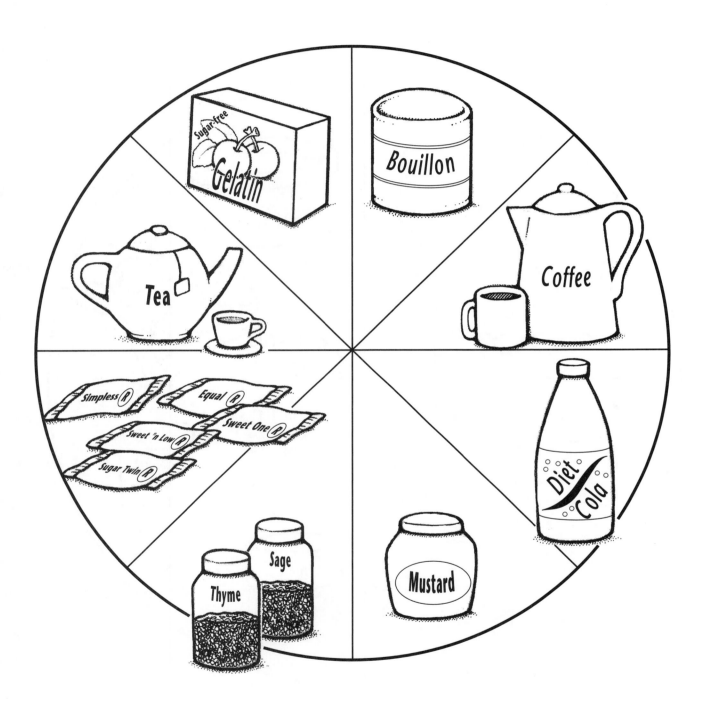

➡ Uncooked vs. Cooked Portions

		Uncooked	**Cooked**
Starches expand when cooked. The following factors can be used to estimate cooked from dry portions.			
Noodles	Dry volume × 1.5 = cooked volume	¾ cup	⅓ cup or 1 exchange
Dried beans, dried peas	Dry volume × 1.8 = cooked volume	¼ cup	½ cup or 1 exchange
Macaroni	Dry volume × 2.0 = cooked volume	¾ oz	⅓ cup or 1 exchange
Oatmeal, grits, lentils	Dry volume × 2.6 = cooked volume	3 Tbsp	⅓ cup or 1 exchange
Cream of Wheat	Dry volume × 4.0 = cooked volume	2 Tbsp	½ cup
Rice	Dry volume × 2.6 = cooked volume	2 Tbsp	⅓ cup or 1 exchange
Pasta measurements are often given in ounces (weight rather than volume). Follow this guideline to estimate the number of cooked exchanges.			
Pasta	Dry weight (oz) × 1.3 = starch exchanges	¾ oz pasta	⅓ cup or 1 starch exchange

continued

UNCOOKED VS. COOKED PORTIONS *continued*

		Uncooked	**Cooked**
Meat shrinks when cooked. Follow this guideline to estimate the weight of cooked meat.			
Meat	Uncooked weight × 0.75 = cooked weight	4 oz hamburger	3 oz hamburger or 3 meat exchanges

➡ Standard Weights and Measures

ABBREVIATIONS—used to indicate food quantities.

Teaspoon	tsp, also t
Tablespoon	Tbsp, also T
Cup	c
Ounce	oz
Fluid ounce	fl oz
Pound	lb, also #

DRY MEASURES—used for measuring solid foods. To measure precisely, level off top with a flat edge. Dry equivalents of measure:

3 tsp	=	1 Tbsp
4 Tbsp	=	¼ cup
5 Tbsp + 1 tsp	=	⅓ cup
8 Tbsp	=	½ cup
10 Tbsp + 2 tsp	=	⅔ cup
12 Tbsp	=	¾ cup
16 Tbsp	=	1 cup

LIQUID MEASURES—used for measuring fluids. To measure precisely, read at eye level.

2 Tbsp	=	1 fl oz
4 Tbsp	=	2 fl oz or ¼ fluid cup
5 Tbsp + 1 tsp	=	2½ fl oz or ⅓ fluid cup
8 Tbsp	=	4 fl oz or ½ fluid cup
10 Tbsp + 2 tsp	=	5½ fl oz or ⅔ fluid cup
12 Tbsp	=	6 fl oz or ¾ fluid cup
16 Tbsp	=	8 fl oz or 1 fluid cup or ½ pint

continued

STANDARD WEIGHTS AND MEASURES *continued*

WEIGHT—used to weigh cooked meats. To measure correctly, read scale at eye level.

4 oz	=	¼ lb
5 oz	=	⅓ lb
8 oz	=	½ lb
10 oz	=	⅔ lb
12 oz	=	¾ lb
16 oz	=	1 lb

#21   Using Exchanges to Plan Meals

▶ ▶ ▶ ▶ ▶

STATEMENT OF PURPOSE

This session focuses on the practical aspects of using the exchange system to plan meals. It includes information on eating out, using alcohol, and including sweets when using an exchange system.

PREREQUISITES

It is recommended that each participant have attended Session #4, *Food and Blood Glucose,* Session #5, *Planning Meals*, and Session #20, *Diabetes Exchange Lists*, or have achieved those objectives. It is also recommended that participants who have meal-planning booklets and meal plans bring them to class.

OBJECTIVES

At the end of this session, participants will be able to:

1. state the calorie level and grams of carbohydrate, protein, and fat in their diets;

2. identify the number of exchanges from each food group planned for each meal;

3. plan meals and snacks using the food exchange system and the daily meal plan;

4. select a meal from a restaurant menu using their exchange plans;

5. state how to include alcohol, if desired, in their exchange plans;

6. state how to include sweets, if desired, in their exchange plans;

7. identify resources that provide exchange values for additional foods;

8. identify cookbooks that provide exchange values.

CONTENT

Nutritional Management.

MATERIALS NEEDED

VISUALS PROVIDED	ADDITIONAL
1. Meal Plan 2. Sample Meal Plan **Handouts** (one per participant) 1. Sample Meal Plan 2. Meal Plan 3. Cookbooks for People with Diabetes 4. Exchange Values of Alcoholic Beverages	■ Chalkboard and chalk ■ Food models or pictures of food ■ Meal-planning books with meal plans ■ Restaurant menus (obtain from restaurants popular with the participants) ■ Examples of diabetes cookbooks and exchange value references, such as *Exchange Lists for Meal Planning, Exchange Lists for Weight Management, ADA Complete Guide and Conveniece Food Counts, Diabetes Meal Planning Made Easy,* and *Guide to Healthy Restaurant Eating* (all available from the American Diabetes Association, 800-232-6733)

METHOD OF PRESENTATION

Start by introducing yourself and telling what you do. Ask participants to introduce themselves. Explain that the purpose of this session is to practice using a meal plan to make food choices.

Present material in a question/discussion format. Some participants may want to understand how an exchange pattern works before they decide if they want an individualized plan. Begin by asking how they did with their short-term goal and what they learned from it.

Family members and/or significant others (especially those who shop or prepare meals for the person with diabetes) are encouraged to attend. Use examples that are culturally relevant for the participants.

CONTENT OUTLINE

CONCEPT	DETAIL	INSTRUCTOR'S NOTES
1. Daily meal plan and sample menu	1.1 Your daily meal plan shows the number and kind of food exchanges you have chosen for each meal and snack.	Ask, "What questions or concerns do you have about using your meal plan?" Briefly review the six exchange groups and have participants name a few foods in each group. List on the board.
	1.2 Ideally, the meal plan is designed by you and your dietitian based on your cultural and other food preferences, lifestyle, treatment, and caloric needs.	Explain that a meal plan that is close to the way you usually eat is easier to use. Offer referral to a dietitian as needed.

CONTENT OUTLINE

CONCEPT	DETAIL	INSTRUCTOR'S NOTES
	1.3 Review key information on the daily meal plan: ■ time of planned meal/snack ■ exchanges for each meal/snack	Use Visual #1, Meal Plan. Diet formats vary. This visual includes commonly used key points. Have participants locate these key points on their own plans. Ask if those with a plan would share with someone who doesn't have one for this activity.
	■ composition of diet—calories, carbohydrate, protein, fat, and other dietary modifications	Note that individuals may have diet modifications other than those listed here.
	■ dietitian's name, telephone number, address, and date that the meal plan was made	Emphasize that participants need to feel free to contact the dietitian with questions, changes, or for more information. It is helpful to update the meal plan as needs change.
2. Planning meals and snacks	2.1 To use the exchange system, you need to know how many exchanges from each food group are planned for each meal.	Ask participants to identify the number of exchanges they will have at each meal. Ask, "How many starch exchanges will you have at breakfast?" Repeat with other food groups and meals until you are confident participants know how to locate their own exchanges.
	2.2 Next you need to look up what foods and amounts to eat for each exchange. Make a check mark next to your favorite foods. Repeat this process until you have chosen a complete meal.	Have participants find the starch list in their meal-planning booklets, and identify what they might eat for 1 starch exchange at breakfast, and then for 2 and 3 starch exchanges. Repeat for fruit and other exchange groups until you are confident that participants can locate foods and prescribed amounts for each group.

CONTENT OUTLINE

CONCEPT	DETAIL	INSTRUCTOR'S NOTES
	2.3 Select one menu to fit a sample meal plan.	Use Visual #2, Sample Meal Plan, and Handout #1, Sample Meal Plan, to identify the number of exchanges and select food items for each until a full-day sample menu is complete. The foods selected may be listed on a chalkboard or overhead transparency of Visual #2 or depicted visually with food models or pictures. Participants can work together in small groups.
	2.4 Choose foods you enjoy eating together for a meal and foods that are available to you.	After a meal has been chosen, review to evaluate if foods go well together (Is there milk for the cereal? Margarine for the toast? Do you really want to eat raisins with potatoes or animal crackers with lunch meat?) Ask participants if the items are available. Some items may be seasonal (strawberries), too (shrimp), or impractical (venison). Note the comfort level of the class with this material. If they seem uncertain, repeat by planning another menu with the same meal plan before going on.
	2.5 Carbohydrate-containing exchanges affect blood glucose levels the most, so they are best left at the meal where planned.	Ask, "Why is it important to eat carbohydrates at the planned meal?"
	2.6 Meat and fat exchanges may be moved from one meal to another.	For example, a meat and a fat from lunch could be saved for dinner. Pose problem-solving situations such as, "How would you have eggs for breakfast?"

CONTENT OUTLINE

CONCEPT	DETAIL	INSTRUCTOR'S NOTES
	2.7 One meal may be totally changed with another meal if the carbohydrate content is the same. (Example: Have Sunday dinner at lunchtime and a lighter meal at dinnertime.)	If the class is interested and able to understand, provide examples of substitutions between exchange groups. For example: 1 vegetable = ⅓ starch 1 meat = reduced fat (2%) milk + 1 fruit
	2.8 If you do not yet have a personalized meal plan, you may want to use a standard exchange plan.	Distribute Handout #2, Standard Exchange Plans.
3. Using the other carbohydrates list	3.1 The other carbohydrates list offers a way to fit sweets and dessert items into your usual meal plan and keep your blood glucose levels in your target range.	Ask participants to find this list in their meal-planning booklets.
	3.2 An item on the other carbohydrates list can be exchanged for any item on the starch, fruit, or milk list. For example, if your lunch plan is 2 starches, 1 milk, 2 meats, and 1 fat: ■ you could have a sandwich with 2 oz of meat and 1 tsp of regular mayonnaise with a glass of milk, or ■ you could have a sandwich with 2 oz of meat, mustard, a diet soft drink, and a small unfrosted brownie	You have exchanged the mayonnaise (fat) and milk for the brownie.
	3.3 Plan a meal including an item from the other carbohydrates list.	Ask, "Would you like to have an item from the other carbohydrates list? How would you include it in your meal plan?"
4. Including combination and fast foods	4.1 Many foods are mixed together so that it is hard to know the amount of starch, meat, or fat included. The combination foods and fast foods lists provide the exchange values of some typical foods.	Ask participants to find the combination foods and fast foods lists in their mealplanning booklets. Using Visual #2, Sample Meal Plan, help participants select a menu that includes a combination or fast food.

CONTENT OUTLINE

CONCEPT	DETAIL	INSTRUCTOR'S NOTES
	4.2 For example, with the same lunch plan shown above, you could have a slice of pizza instead of the sandwich if you borrow a fat from dinner.	One-fourth of a 12″ pizza with meat topping and a thin crust is 2 carbohydrates, 2 meats, and 2 fats.
	4.3 The same process is used to include combination foods from a cookbook that provides exchange values.	If time allows, select a menu that includes recipes from a diabetes cookbook. Refer to Handout #3, Cookbooks for People with Diabetes.
	4.4 If you want to include foods that are not on these lists, there are books that provide the exchange value of many more food items.	Show *ADA Complete Guide to Convinience Food Counts* and *Guide to Healthy Restaurant Eating* Handout #3 lists other books.
	4.5 Many fast-food restaurants provide a pamphlet with the nutrient content and exchange value of their menu items.	Show samples of nutrient information from fast-food restaurants.
5. Including alcohol	5.1 Many people can safely include alcohol in their meal plan.	Review information about alcohol as needed from Outline #5, *Planning Meals*. Show alcohol serving sizes. Participants should consult with their health care teams for specifics related to their individual medications and meal plans.
	5.2 Always eat something if you are drinking alcohol and taking diabetes medications.	
	5.3 Make sure you drink alcohol with a friend who knows you have diabetes and is familiar with hypoglycemic symptoms and treatment.	
	5.4 If you are at your goal weight and use insulin or oral medications, do not omit food to drink an alcoholic beverage. You risk a hypoglycemic reaction.	Alcohol does not require insulin to be metabolized.
	5.5 If you are concerned about your weight, the alcohol calories are best traded for fat calories.	See Handout #4, Exchange Values of Alcoholic Beverages. Review guidelines and note risks.

CONTENT OUTLINE

CONCEPT	DETAIL	INSTRUCTOR'S NOTES
	5.6 Fruit or vegetable juice used as mixers count as their usual exchange value. Mineral water, club soda, and diet soft drinks are free.	
6. Eating out with exchanges	6.1 Using your exchange system when eating out may take some practice.	Review information on eating out in Outline #5, *Planning Meals,* as needed.
	6.2 Become comfortable with the exchange system and familiar with your plan. You may want to carry a copy of your meal plan in your wallet or purse.	If available, distribute wallet cards to use for listing meal plans.
	6.3 Let's select a restaurant dinner based on the exchanges in a sample meal plan.	Distribute the restaurant menus. Use Visual #2 and Handout #1, Sample Meal Plan, to choose a meal that fits the plan.
	6.4 Choose the main dish first. Note the foods that would most easily fit into a meal plan.	Ask, "What items are missing that you might request?"
	6.5 Sometimes you can change your meal plan slightly to accommodate types and preparation of food in restaurants.	Discuss possible changes in the meal plan. If you have time, have participants plan a restaurant meal and make accommodations using their own exchange meal plans. Choose a short-term goal to try before the next session.

SKILLS CHECKLIST

Participants will be able to plan a menu using the exchange system and identify items on a restaurant menu that fit with their meal plans.

EVALUATION PLAN

Knowledge will be evaluated by achievement of learning objectives and by responses to questions during the session. The ability to apply knowledge will be evaluated by using the exchange system to plan meals and through program outcome measures.

DOCUMENTATION PLAN

Record class attendance and achieved objectives as appropriate.

SUGGESTED READINGS

The American Dietetic Association, American Diabetes Association. *Ethnic and Regional Food Practices Series: Food Practices, Customs and Holidays for Jewish, Mexican American, Chinese American, Hmong, Navajo, Alaska Native, Filipino American, Soul and Traditional Southern, Cajun and Creole.* Chicago, IL: The American Dietetic Association; Alexandria, VA: The American Diabetes Association, 1989.

Franz MJ, Bantle JP, Eds. American Diabetes Association Guide to Medical Nutrition Therapy for Diabetes. Alexandria, VA: American Diabetes Association, 1999.

Franz MJ, Reader D, Monk A. *Implementing Group and Individual Medical Nutrition Therapy.* Alexandria, VA: American Diabetes Association, 2002.

Leontos C, Geil P. *Individualized Approaches to Diabetes Nutrition Therapy: Case Studies.* Alexandria, VA: American Diabetes Association, 2002.

Marlett JA, Cheung TF. Dietary fiber guidelines in the exchange lists for menu planning. *Diabetes Care.* 1994;17(12):1534–1541.

Pastors JG, Arnold MS, Daly A, Franz M, Warshaw HS. *Diabetes Nutrition Q&A for Health Professionals.* Alexandria, VA: American Diabetes Association, 2003.

Simkins SW. Lessons from the DCCT: the nutritional challenges of implementing intensive therapy. *Diabetes Spectrum.* 1994;7:294–295.

Wheeler ML. Nutrient database for the 2003 exchange lists for meal planning. *J Am Diet Assoc.* 2003;103(7):894–920.

➲ Meal Plan

	Grams	Percent
Name _____	Carbohydrate _____	_____
Date _____	Protein _____	_____
Dietitian _____	Fat _____	_____
Phone _____	Calories _____	

Time	Number of Choices	Food Ideas

	_____ Carbohydrate group
	    _____ Starch
	    _____ Fruit
	    _____ Milk
	_____ Meat group
	_____ Fat group
	
	_____ _____
	_____ _____	

	_____ Carbohydrate group
	    _____ Starch
	    _____ Fruit
	    _____ Milk
	    _____ Nonstarchy vegetables
	_____ Meat group
	_____ Fat group
	
	_____ _____
	_____ _____	

	_____ Carbohydrate group
	    _____ Starch
	    _____ Fruit
	    _____ Milk
	    _____ Nonstarchy vegetables
	_____ Meat group
	_____ Fat group	

	_____ _____ _____ _____	

➡ Sample Meal Plan

	Grams	Percent
Name __Sally Smith__ Carbohydrate	200	51
Date __3/20/04__ Protein	81	20
Dietitian __Frank Jones__ Fat	50	29
Phone __555-1234__ Calories	1600	

Time	Number of Choices	Food Ideas
7:30 A.M. breakfast	3½ Carbohydrate group 　2　Starch 　1　Fruit 　½　Milk ＿＿ Meat group 　1　Fat group	
12:30 P.M. lunch	4 Carbohydrate group 　2　Starch 　1　Fruit 　1　Milk 　2　Nonstarchy vegetables 　2　Meat group 　2　Fat group	
6:30 P.M. dinner	4 Carbohydrate group 　3　Starch 　1　Fruit ＿＿ Milk 　1　Nonstarchy vegetables 　3　Meat group 　2　Fat group	
10:30 P.M. snack	1　Starch ½　Milk	

➡ Sample Meal Plan

		Grams	Percent
Name _Sally Smith_	Carbohydrate	200	51
Date _3/20/04_	Protein	81	20
Dietitian _Frank Jones_	Fat	50	29
Phone _555–1234_	Calories	1600	

Time	Number of Choices	Food Ideas

7:30 A.M. breakfast	3½ Carbohydrate group
	    2 Starch
	    1 Fruit
	    ½ Milk
	 _____ Meat group
	    1 Fat group	

12:30 P.M. lunch	4 Carbohydrate group
	    2 Starch
	    1 Fruit
	    1 Milk
	    2 Nonstarchy vegetables
	    2 Meat group
	    2 Fat group	

6:30 P.M. dinner	4 Carbohydrate group
	    3 Starch
	    1 Fruit
	 _____ Milk
	    1 Nonstarchy vegetables
	    3 Meat group
	    2 Fat group	

10:30 P.M. snack	1 Starch ½ Milk	

➲ Meal Plan

		Grams	Percent
Name _____	Carbohydrate	_____	_____
Date _____	Protein	_____	_____
Dietitian _____	Fat	_____	_____
Phone _____	Calories	_____	

Time	Number of Choices	Food Ideas
	____ Carbohydrate group ____ Starch ____ Fruit ____ Milk ____ Meat group ____ Fat group ____ _____ ____ _____	
	____ Carbohydrate group ____ Starch ____ Fruit ____ Milk ____ Nonstarchy vegetables ____ Meat group ____ Fat group ____ _____ ____ _____	
	____ Carbohydrate group ____ Starch ____ Fruit ____ Milk ____ Nonstarchy vegetables ____ Meat group ____ Fat group	
	____ _____ ____ _____	

© 2004 American Diabetes Association, The American Dietetic Association

➜ Cookbooks for People with Diabetes

Cookbooks written for people with diabetes may add variety to your meal planning. Choose a cookbook that:

- lists the serving size and number of servings per recipe
- lists the carbohydrate content and food exchange value for each serving
- contains recipes with acceptable ingredients (evaluate each recipe before you use it)

Many diabetes cookbooks are available. Check your local bookstore or library. The following cookbooks can be obtained from the American Diabetes Association by calling 800-232-6733 or by visiting http://store.diabetes.org.

At Home with Gladys Knight: Her Personal Recipe for Living Well, Eating Right, and Loving Life.
by Gladys Knight

Cooking with the Diabetic Chef
by Chris Smith

Diabetes Meal Planning Made Easy, 2nd Edition
by Hope Warshaw

Diabetes Quickflip Cookbook
by Eileen Faughey

Diabetic Cooking for Latinos
by Olga V. Fuste

Diabetic Cooking for Seniors
by Kathleen Stanley

Diabetic Meals in 30 Minutes—or Less!
by Robyn Webb

Express Lane Diabetic Cooking
by Robyn Webb

Forbidden Foods Diabetic Cooking
by Maggie Powers and Joyce Hendley

Last Minute Meals for People with Diabetes
by Nancy Hughes

COOKBOOKS FOR PEOPLE WITH DIABETES *continued*

More Diabetic Meals in 30 Minutes—or Less!
by Robyn Webb

One Pot Meals for People with Diabetes
by Ruth Glick and Nancy Baggett

Quick & Easy Diabetic Recipes for One
by Kathleen Stanley and Connie Crawley

Quick & Easy Low-Carb Cooking for People with Diabetes
by Nancy S. Hughes

The Diabetes Food & Nutrition Bible
by Hope S. Warshaw and Robyn Webb

The Diabetes Snack Munch Nibble Nosh Book, 2nd Edition
by Ruth Glick

The Healthy HomeStyle Cookbook
by Ruth W. McGary

The New Soul Food Cookbook for People with Diabetes
by Fabiola Demps Gaines and Roniece Weaver

Also by the American Diabetes Association:

Brand-Name Diabetic Meals in Minutes
Cook'n for Diabetes (recipe software)
Guide to Health Restaurant Eating, 2nd Edition
How to Cook for People with Diabetes
Magic Menus for People with Diabetes
Mix 'n Match Meals in Minutes for People with Diabetes
Month of Meals: All-American Fare
Month of Meals: Classic Cooking
Month of Meals: Festive Latin Flavors
Month of Meals: Meals in Minutes
Month of Meals: Old-Time Favorites
Month of Meals: Soul Food Selections
Month of Meals: Vegetarian Pleasures
Mr. Food's Every Day's a Holiday Diabetic Cookbook
Mr. Food's Quick & Easy Diabetic Cooking
The Complete Quick & Hearty Diabetic Cookbook
The NEW Family Cookbook for People with Diabetes

→ Exchange Values of Alcoholic Beverages

Beverage	Serving Size	Exchange Value
Beer		
Regular	12 oz	1 starch + 2 fats
Light	12 oz	2 fats
Nonalcoholic	12 oz	1 starch
Liquor (80 proof, or 40%)		
Gin, rum, scotch, vodka, and whiskey	1½ oz	2 fats
100 proof or 50%	1½ oz	3 fats
Wine		
Dry white, red, and rose	4 oz	2 fats
Champagne	4 oz	2 fats
Light wine	4 oz	1 fat
Sweet wine	4 oz	½ fruit + 1½ fats
Wine cooler	4 oz	2 fruits + 2 fats

Free Mixers
- Water
- Mineral water
- Club soda
- Seltzer
- Diet soft drinks
- Diet tonic water

Fruit/Vegetable Exchange
- Unsweetened fruit juice
- Tomato juice
- V8 juice

Adapted from *Exchanges for All Occasions.* Franz M. Minneapolis, MN: Chronimed Publishing, 1993.

#22	**Calculating Exchange Values**

STATEMENT OF PURPOSE

This session is intended to provide information about calculating exchange values for convenience foods and personal recipes.

PREREQUISITES

This is an advanced-level class for those who routinely use the exchange system and want to incorporate foods with unpublished exchange values and personal recipes. It is recommended that each participant have attended Session #4, *Food and Blood Glucose,* Session #20, *Diabetes Exchange Lists,* and Session #21, *Using Exchanges to Plan Meals,* or have achieved those objectives, and have some experience using the exchange system. It is also recommended that participants bring their meal-planning booklets, meal plans, a favorite recipe, the label from a convenience food, and a calculator.

OBJECTIVES

At the end of this session, participants will be able to:

1. calculate exchange values for convenience foods and/or personal recipes;

2. incorporate these convenience foods and/or personal recipes into their own meal plans.

CONTENT

Nutritional Management.

MATERIALS NEEDED

VISUALS PROVIDED

None.

Handouts (one per participant)
1. Nutrients in Food Exchange Groups
2. Calculating Food Exchanges from a Product Label
3. Calculating Food Exchanges for a Recipe

ADDITIONAL

- Chalkboard and chalk
- Paper and pencil for each participant
- Convenience-food product containers or labels
- Calculator for instructor and each participant
- Commercial product information nutrient lists (from companies)
- Recipes (to practice calculations)
- *Exchange Lists for Meal Planning* (available from the American Diabetes Association, 800-232-6733)

METHOD OF PRESENTATION

Start by introducing yourself and telling what you do. Ask participants to introduce themselves. Explain that the purpose of this session is to learn how to calculate the exchange value of convenience foods and personal recipes so that they may be used in their meal plans.

Present material in a question/discussion format, working through each sample calculation. Allow time for participants to practice the calculations. Use examples that are culturally relevant for the participants. Begin by asking how they did with their short-term goal and what they learned from it.

CONTENT OUTLINE

CONCEPT	DETAIL	INSTRUCTOR'S NOTES
1. Using combination foods	1.1 It is possible to include a variety of combination foods in your meal plan.	Ask, "What questions or concerns do you have about calculating exchange values?"
	1.2 The exchange values of many combination foods are published in reference articles and books and in cookbooks.	Refer to Outline #21, *Using Exchanges to Plan Meals*. Many people also use the exchange system for weight loss.
	1.3 It is possible to calculate the exchange value of favorite foods if you know the nutrients (carbohydrate, protein, and fat) they contain or have the recipe.	By law, nutrient and ingredient information is available on all but a few food labels. Nutrient information not available on a package label can often be obtained by writing to the manufacturer.

CALCULATING EXCHANGES FROM NUTRIENT INFORMATION

2. Identify ingredients in product	2.1 Read the ingredient list to determine what foods are in the product.	
	2.2 Identify all possible exchange groups represented. For example, flour or noodles = starch group, and green beans = vegetable group.	
	2.3 Note that ingredients are listed in order by weight. If milk is listed first, it contributes the most to the product weight.	
	2.4 If sugar is a primary ingredient, then the product is recommended for occasional use only because it is of limited nutritional value. Count sugar as part of the fruit group.	Other names for sugar are corn syrup, dextrose, sucrose, and fructose.

CONTENT OUTLINE

CONCEPT	DETAIL	INSTRUCTOR'S NOTES
3. Translating nutrient information into food exchanges	3.1 Label information can be used to figure exchange values. To do this: ■ identify grams of carbohydrate, protein, and fat from the label ■ translate grams of carbohydrate into equivalent food exchanges ■ determine protein exchange values ■ calculate any fat exchanges	Distribute Handout #1, Nutrients in Food Exchange Groups.

EXAMPLE

Beef Pot Pie

INGREDIENT LIST

Beef, flour, peas, shortening, salt, preservatives

NUTRITION INFORMATION

# of servings in container	1
# of calories per serving	445
Carbohydrate	30 gm
Protein	25 gm
Fat	25 gm

3.2 Figure carbohydrate exchanges first. The nutrition panel shows 30 gm of carbohydrate. The ingredients include flour and peas, which are in the starch group (15 gm of carbohydrate and 3 gm of protein per exchange). Thus, 30 gm of carbohydrate in the pot pie = 2 starch exchanges.

3.3 Figure the protein exchanges next. Twenty-five grams of protein are present. The starch exchanges have 6 gm of protein, which we have subtracted. The ingredients include beef, which is in the medium-fat meat group (7 gm of protein and 5 gm of fat per exchange). Thus, 19 gm of protein = about 3 meat exchanges.

Use the chalkboard to demonstrate. Calculations:

	Carbo-hydrate	Protein	Fat
	30	25	25
2 starch	− 30	− 6	− 0
	0	19	25
3 meat		− 21	− 15
		0	10
2 fat			− 10
			0

CONTENT OUTLINE

CONCEPT	DETAIL	INSTRUCTOR'S NOTES

3.4 Figure the fat exchanges last. Twenty-five grams of fat are in the pot pie. Subtract the 15 gm of fat from the meat exchanges, which leaves 10 gm of fat. Shortening is listed in the ingredients, which is from the fat group (5 gm per exchange). Thus, 10 gm of fat = 2 fat exchanges.

Total for the beef pot pie:
2 starch exchanges
3 meat exchanges
2 fat exchanges

Have participants practice with other convenience foods that they routinely use. Use foods that include a variety of exchange groups and those that may contain partial exchanges. Round partial exchanges to the nearest half or full exchange.

3.5 Some package labels provide the exchange values for the product. As discussed in an earlier class, books are also available that give this information.

Show sample food labels that provide exchange values for the product.

4. Fitting into meal plan

4.1 Check your meal plan to see if the meal contains enough exchanges to equal the convenience food.

4.2 If not, determine if a smaller portion could fit into the meal plan. For example, if exchanges are as follows:

pot pie	your lunch
2 starch	1 starch
3 meat	1 fruit
2 fat	2 meat
	1 fat

You could eat the whole pie using the fruit as a starch and reduce dinner by 1 meat and 1 fat; or eat half the pie, keep the fruit at lunch, and add 1 meat to dinner.

Point out that 2 starches or 1 starch plus 1 fruit equals 30 gm of carbohydrate. The grams of carbohydrate need to remain consistent at each meal for glycemic control.

Ask, "Would the beef pot pie fit into your meal plan? What would happen if you ate both the pot pie and the fruit?"

CONTENT OUTLINE

CONCEPT	DETAIL	INSTRUCTOR'S NOTES

4.3 Low-calorie frozen pot pies are now available. The nutrition information might look like this:

# of servings	1
# of calories/serving	280
Carbohydrate	32 gm
Protein	18 gm
Fat	10 gm

With the same meal plan, you could eat the whole low-calorie pot pie. For your fruit exchange, substitute the extra starch exchange; for the fat exchange, use salad dressing on a free vegetable salad or save it for another meal.

Calculations:

	Carbo-hydrate	Protein	Fat
2 starch	30 − 30	18 − 6	10 − 0
	0	12	10
2 meat		− 14	− 10
		0	0

5. Practice: evaluating convenience foods

5.1 Activity: calculate the exchange values of veal parmesan:

Distribute Handout #2, Calculating Food Exchanges from a Product Label. Ask participants to use Handout #1, Nutrients in Food Exchange Groups, to calculate the exchange values of veal parmesan. Refer to sections 2 and 3 in this outline as needed.

■ Identify ingredients and the possible exchange groups represented.

Ask "What foods are on the ingredient list? To which food groups do they belong?"

■ Subtract the number of starch exchanges in 12 gm of carbohydrate.

(Or two vegetables.)

■ Then subtract the meat exchanges in 21 gm of protein.

In this case there are no additional fat exchanges.

5.2 Determine the portion size of veal parmesan that will fit into your meal plan.

Encourage participants to help each other. Be available to help individuals as needed.

5.3 Calculate the exchange values of a food of your choice, using the label.

Answer questions as needed. Provide the opportunity to share food label calculations.

CONTENT OUTLINE

CONCEPT	DETAIL	INSTRUCTOR'S NOTES

CALCULATING EXCHANGES FROM A RECIPE

CONCEPT	DETAIL	INSTRUCTOR'S NOTES
6. Recipe exchange values	6.1 To determine the exchange value of a recipe: ■ list all the ingredients and amounts called for in each recipe	Distribute Handout #3, Calculating Food Exchanges for a Recipe. Work through the example to illustrate steps.
	■ determine the exchange value of each ingredient ■ total the number of exchanges ■ divide each total exchange by the number of servings in the recipe ■ determine portion size by measuring the total volume of the recipe and dividing by the number of servings	Refer to *Exchange Lists for Meal Planning* to determine the exchange value of each ingredient. Notice whether the recipe calls for cooked or uncooked meats and starches (see Outline #20, *Diabetes Exchange Lists*).
	■ determine portion size by measuring the total volume of the recipe and dividing by the number of servings	Use Handout #3, pages 3–4. Provide the opportunity to share recipe calculations. Choose a short-term goal to try before the next session.
	6.2 Calculate the exchange values for a recipe of your choice.	

SKILLS CHECKLIST

Each participant will be able to calculate the exchange value of a food item from a food label or recipe and fit these items into his or her personal meal plan.

EVALUATION PLAN

Knowledge will be evaluated by achievement of learning objectives and by responses to questions during the session. The ability to apply knowledge will be evaluated by calculating exchange values of various foods and through program outcome measures.

DOCUMENTATION PLAN

Record class attendance and achieved objectives as appropriate.

SUGGESTED READINGS

Daly A, Franz M, Holzmeister LA, Kulkarni K, O'Connell B, Wheeler M. New diabetes nutrition resources. *J Am Diet Assoc.* 2003;103(7):832-834.

Wheeler ML. Nutrient database for the 2003 exchange lists for meal planning. *J Am Diet Assoc.* 2003;103(7):894–920.

➜ Nutrients in Food Exchange Groups

Group	Carbohydrate (gm)	Protein (gm)	Fat (gm)	Calories
Carbohydrate				
Starch	15	3	1 or less	80
Fruit	15	—	—	60
Milk				
Fat-free (skim)	12	8	0–3	90
Low-fat (1%)	12	8	5	120
Whole	12	8	8	150
Nonstarchy vegetables	5	2	—	25
Other carbohydrates	Varies	Varies	Varies	Varies
Meat/Meat Substitutes				
Very lean	—	7	0–1	35
Lean	—	7	3	55
Medium fat	—	7	5	75
High fat	—	7	8	100
Fat	—	—	5	45
Monounsaturated	—	—	5	45
Polyunsaturated	—	—	5	45
Saturated	—	—	5	45
Hydrogenated	—	—	5	45

➡ Calculating Food Exchanges from a Product Label

Using the nutrition information and ingredient list given below, Handout #1, and your own diet plan:

1. Calculate exchange values for this product.
2. Determine what portion of this food you can eat for dinner.

Veal Parmesan

Nutritional Information
1 serving (1 package) contains:

Calories	243
Fat	11 gm
Carbohydrate	12 gm
Protein	24 gm

Ingredients
Tomato puree, veal, bread crumbs, zucchini, part-skim mozzarella cheese, vegetable oil, garlic, onion, salt, spices, guar gum.

The exchange values for one serving of veal parmesan are:

_____

_____

_____

_____

The portion that will fit my planned dinner exchanges is:

_____

_____

➡ Calculating Food Exchanges for a Recipe

BEEF GOULASH

3 cups cooked noodles   ¾ cup sliced mushrooms
1 lb uncooked ground beef   1½ cups canned tomatoes
3 Tbsp chopped onion   2 tsp salt
¾ cup sliced celery   ¼ tsp pepper
¾ cup tomato puree   1 Tbsp vinegar

Cook and stir the ground beef and chopped onion in a large skillet until the meat is brown and the onion is tender. Drain off fat. Stir in the celery, tomato puree, mushrooms, tomatoes, salt, pepper, and vinegar. Cover and simmer for 30–45 minutes. Add the drained noodles and stir until warm. Makes 4 servings.

Ingredient	Amount	Starch	Meat	Vegetable	Fruit	Milk	Fat
Cooked noodles	3 cups	9					
Uncooked ground beef	1 lb		(after cooking) 12				
Onion	3 Tbsp						
Celery	¾ cup						
Tomato puree	¾ cup			3			
Mushrooms	¾ cup						
Tomatoes	1½ cups			3			
Salt	1 tsp						
Pepper	¼ tsp						
Vinegar	1 Tbsp						
Divide by 4 to get per-serving amount	Totals	9	12	6			
	Per serving	2	3	1½			

continued

CALCULATING FOOD EXCHANGES FOR A RECIPE *continued*

To determine exchanges per serving:

1. Make a grid, or use the grids on the following page.

2. List all the ingredients and the amount called for in each recipe.

3. Determine the exchange value of each ingredient.

4. Total the number of exchanges.

5. Divide each total exchange by the number of servings in the recipe.

To determine serving size:

1. Measure the total volume of the recipe.

2. Divide by the number of servings.

continued

CALCULATING FOOD EXCHANGES FOR A RECIPE *continued*

Recipe Name _____

Ingredient	Amount	Starch	Meat	Vegetable	Fruit	Milk	Fat
	Totals						
	Per serving						

continued

CALCULATING FOOD EXCHANGES FOR A RECIPE *continued*

Recipe Name _____

Ingredient	Amount	Starch	Meat	Vegetable	Fruit	Milk	Fat
	Totals						
	Per serving						

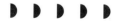

#23	Sexual Health and Diabetes

STATEMENT OF PURPOSE

This session is intended to provide information about sexual health and sexual function and how they can be affected by diabetes.

PREREQUISITES

It is recommended that participants have basic knowledge about diabetes and its complications, either from personal experience or from attending previous sessions.

OBJECTIVES

At the end of this session, participants will be able to:

1. express greater insight about their own sexuality;

2. state ways to initiate discussion about sexual concerns with people who are important to them and with members of the health care team;

3. identify effective methods of contraception;

4. describe sexual functioning in either men or women that can be affected by diabetes;

5. state therapies available for sexual dysfunction.

CONTENT

Preconception Care; Chronic Complications; Psychosocial Adjustment.

MATERIALS NEEDED

VISUALS PROVIDED

1. Sexual Response Cycle—Physical Changes
2. Changes in Sexual Function with Aging
3. Normal Menstrual Cycle
4. Contraceptive Methods
5. Penile Prostheses—Semirigid
6. Penile Prostheses—Inflatable

ADDITIONAL

- Chalkboard and chalk
- Samples of products available for use in treating sexual dysfunction

METHOD OF PRESENTATION

Start by introducing yourself and telling what you do. Ask participants to introduce themselves. Explain that the purpose of this session is to present information about diabetes and sexual health for men and women throughout their lifespan.

Present material in a question/discussion format. Begin by asking how they did with their short-term goal and what they learned from it. To initiate discussion, ask participants what thoughts they have when they first hear the word sexuality. Ask them to call out their ideas as you write them on a chalkboard. Facilitate a brief discussion about the items.

This outline is only a guide. It does not need to be presented in its entirety, but should be tailored to meet the needs of each group. Participants may feel most comfortable in groups of either all men or all women, with only pertinent content presented. The content can also be provided on an individual basis. As an instructor, you need to be knowledgeable and feel comfortable talking about sexual health issues before leading this session.

CONTENT OUTLINE

CONCEPT	DETAIL	INSTRUCTOR'S NOTES
1. Meaning of human sexuality	1.1 Sexuality is an important dimension of our lives.	Incorporate ideas that the participants listed in the opening activity. Ask, "What questions or concerns do you have about sexual health and diabetes?"
	1.2 It is present from birth to death.	
	1.3 It involves integrating ideas and emotions with actions.	
	1.4 It involves the giving and receiving of sensual pleasure.	
	1.5 It is involved in all human relationships and is part of having effective, satisfying interpersonal relationships with others, including being able to give and receive.	
2. Components of sexual health	2.1 Sexual health involves an awareness and appreciation of your feelings and attitudes about your sexuality.	
	2.2 Male and female roles in relationships, the family, and society play a part as well.	

CONTENT OUTLINE

CONCEPT	DETAIL	INSTRUCTOR'S NOTES
	2.3 Sexual function fulfills two basic purposes: reproduction and recreation (the giving and receiving of physical and psychological pleasure).	Point out differences between sexuality/sexual role and sexual functioning. The capacity for engaging in satisfying relationships need not be altered because of diabetes.
	2.4 There are four phases of sexual response: ■ excitement ■ plateau ■ orgasm ■ resolution	Review the four phases of sexual response. Use Visual #1, Sexual Response Cycle—Physical Changes.
	2.5 Sexual function changes as a normal part of the aging process.	Use Visual #2, Changes in Sexual Function with Aging.
3. Impact of diabetes on sexual health	3.1 You need to decide who to tell you have diabetes and how and when to tell them.	Ask, "How can diabetes affect sexual health?" Discuss why it's important to tell certain people, how and when this can be best accomplished, and any fears about how it will affect relationships.
	3.2 It may be hard to tell others that you have diabetes because you may fear losing a friendship or close relationship. If someone ends a relationship for this reason, it may help to know that the person probably didn't have your best interests in mind.	It may be helpful for partners to attend an education program or diabetes support group together.
	3.3 Diabetes can affect sexual roles. For example, if men or women are physically unable to work or to prepare certain foods the family enjoys, they may feel like they are no longer fulfilling their obligations as husbands or wives.	
	3.4 Diabetes can also influence decisions about having children for both men and women. Concerns include: Will my children inherit diabetes? What are the risks involved in pregnancy for a person with diabetes?	Risk if one parent has: ■ type 1: 1–6% ■ type 2: 10–15% ■ MODY (maturity-onset diabetes of the young): 50% See Outline #24, *Pregnancy and Diabetes.*

CONTENT OUTLINE

CONCEPT	DETAIL	INSTRUCTOR'S NOTES
	3.5 Diabetes can also affect sexual functioning in both men and women.	
4. Sexual health issues for women— Menstruation	4.1 Some women experience delayed onset of menses or irregular menstrual cycles. This is often relieved by better blood glucose control.	Ask, "What questions or concerns do you have about menstruation?"
	4.2 Some women experience elevated blood glucose levels before and during their menstrual period that can lead to ketosis and/or diabetic ketoacidosis. This can be treated with a planned increase in insulin dose or a planned decrease in food intake.	An increase in estrogen and progesterone levels before menses can cause some insulin resistance. Use Visual #3, Normal Menstrual Cycle. Food cravings associated with the menstrual cycle may also affect blood glucose levels.
	4.3 Some women experience a decrease in blood glucose levels during menstruation, when estrogen and progesterone levels decrease. A smaller insulin dosage may be needed during this time.	Suggest that women seek advice from their provider if this is a problem.
Planning for pregnancy	4.4 Fertility is not generally affected by diabetes.	Ask, "What questions or concerns do you have about pregrancy?"
	4.5 More women with diabetes are having healthy babies now than ever before. However, women with high blood glucose levels are at risk for premature births, high-birth-weight babies, infants with birth defects, and infant deaths.	
	4.6 For the best possible pregnancy outcome, women should achieve near-normal blood glucose regulation before conception and during pregnancy by paying close attention to diet, medicines, exercise, and monitoring.	Regulation of blood glucose before and during pregnancy is a critical factor in promoting a successful pregnancy.

CONTENT OUTLINE

CONCEPT	DETAIL	INSTRUCTOR'S NOTES
	4.7 Along with your partner, talk with your provider about the many factors that will need to be considered with a pregnancy: ■ increased care demands ■ increased financial costs ■ presence and severity of complications	Preconception care and counseling are important first steps in pregnancy for women with diabetes. See Outline #24, *Pregnancy and Diabetes.*
Contraception	4.8 All of the current methods of birth control are available for people with diabetes. No one method is recommended.	Ask, "What questions or concerns do you have about contraception?"
	4.9 Choose the method that will work best for you. An unplanned pregnancy generally does not allow for the needed blood glucose regulation before conception.	Use Visual #4, Contraceptive Methods. Discuss each method, how it works, side effects, and effectiveness.
Menopause	4.10 Changes in estrogen and other hormone levels can cause widely varying blood glucose levels.	The current recommendation for hormone replacement therapy (HRT) is the lowest possible dose for the shortest time to manage symptoms.
	4.11 Mood swings are common with the changes in hormone levels.	
	4.12 A decrease in estrogen can also cause hot flashes, fast heartbeat, and flushed skin. It is important not to treat these hot flashes as an insulin reaction.	
	4.13 Taking estrogen may reduce these symptoms but may increase your risk for other health problems. Talk with your provider about the risks and benefits of hormone replacement therapy for you. Estrogen acts against insulin, so changes in your treatment plan may be needed if you take HRT.	Menopause increases risk for heart disease, and calcium is depleted from the bones. The risk of vaginal infections increases with changes in vaginal tissue secretions. Encourage women to have frequent visits with both a gynecologist and diabetes provider during menopause.

CONTENT OUTLINE

CONCEPT	DETAIL	INSTRUCTOR'S NOTES
Vaginitis	4.14 Vaginitis, especially caused by yeast infections, is more common in women with diabetes.	Recurring vaginal infections can decrease interest in sexual intercourse. Ask, "What questions or concerns do you have about infections?"
	4.15 This occurs because high blood glucose levels provide an excellent medium for growth of these organisms. These infections are not related to sexual activity, age, or personal hygiene.	
	4.16 Treat promptly at first sign of symptoms: itching, foul-smelling discharge, or pain.	
	4.17 Antifungal preparations are the treatment of choice for yeast infections and are available without a prescription. If the infection is not gone after a week, contact your provider.	Infections that are not responsive may need a more potent prescriptive preparation or may be trichomonas or bacterial vaginosis. These generally respond to metroniadazole.
5. Sexual dysfunction in women with diabetes	5.1 Not much is known about sexual dysfunction in women with diabetes. It seems to develop slowly; sexual desire is usually not affected.	Ask, "What questions or concerns do you have about sexual function?"
	5.2 Damage to the autonomic nerves from neuropathy may make a woman unable to experience orgasm, or it may take longer for a woman to reach high levels of arousal and require more intense stimulation.	
	5.3 Painful intercourse is related to vaginitis or a lack of lubrication. Inadequate lubrication is often a problem in women with decreased estrogen production after menopause. Preparations to relieve vaginal dryness are available without a prescription.	

CONTENT OUTLINE

CONCEPT	DETAIL	INSTRUCTOR'S NOTES
6. Treatment of sexual dysfunction in women	6.1 Evaluation is the first step of treatment. Tell your health care professional the nature of your concerns and when you first noticed the problem. A pelvic exam may be needed as part of the evaluation.	
	6.2 Regulation of blood glucose should receive key attention. Often, high or low blood glucose levels may detract from overall well-being and sexual functioning.	
	6.3 Specific types of treatment may include: ■ medications for vaginitis ■ use of water-soluble lubricating gels ■ use of estrogen-based lubricating gels ■ postmenopausal hormone replacement therapy	
7. Sexual health issues for men—Puberty	7.1 Some men experience delayed onset of puberty and sexual maturation.	Ask, "What questions or concerns do you have about sexual function?"
Parenthood	7.2 Fertility is generally not affected by diabetes, except in retrograde ejaculation.	Retrograde ejaculation occurs rarely.
	7.3 Retrograde ejaculation is the flow of liquid and sperm back into the bladder, rather than forward out of the penis. Orgasm is experienced, but less fluid is released in a forward direction. This does not affect sexual enjoyment, but may affect fertility because few sperm are deposited during intercourse.	Neuropathy may affect the valve that normally closes off the bladder during ejaculation.
	7.4 Treatment for infertility caused by retrograde ejaculation includes harvesting sperm from urine.	

CONTENT OUTLINE

CONCEPT	DETAIL	INSTRUCTOR'S NOTES
	7.5 Several methods of birth control are available for people with diabetes. No one method is recommended.	Use Visual #4, Contraceptive Methods. Discuss each method, how it works, side effects, and effectiveness.
	7.6 Hypoglycemia may occur during sexual activity.	One carbohydrate exchange before sexual activity is usually adequate to prevent a reaction.
8. Sexual dysfunction in men with diabetes	8.1 Erectile dysfunction (impotence) occurs in 40–60% of all men who have diabetes. It is often caused by damage to autonomic nerves from neuropathy. Changes in blood vessels are also common.	"Erectile dysfunction" is the preferred term because of negative connotations associated with the term "impotence."
	8.2 Erectile dysfunction can also be caused by: ■ drugs, including some blood pressure medicines and tranquilizers ■ decreased testosterone levels ■ alcohol ■ hardening of arteries in the pelvis ■ psychological factors ■ smoking	Many drugs can affect sexual functioning. Men taking any of these drugs should bring this to the attention of the health care team for evaluation.
9. Treatment of sexual dysfunction	9.1 Tell your health care professionals about your concerns and when you first noticed a problem. You may be referred to a urologist for further evaluation.	Encourage participants to discuss sexual problems—problems cannot be treated if health care professionals are unaware of them.
	9.2 A blood sample may be taken for male hormone measurement, and a nocturnal penile tumescence study may be done (this involves the placement of a device around your penis while you sleep to measure the number of erections that occur with deep sleep). This test is not painful.	The presence of three to six erections during two to three nights of sleep generally indicates that the impotence is not organic.
	9.3 High or low or fluctuating blood glucose levels may affect sexual functioning and overall well-being. Regulating blood glucose levels is the first step in treatment.	

CONTENT OUTLINE

CONCEPT	DETAIL	INSTRUCTOR'S NOTES

9.4 In spite of recent publicity about erectile dysfunction and its treatment, no one therapy is effective for everyone. Some current treatment options include:

- avoidance of alcohol

- change in drug therapy

- psychological counseling

- hormonal treatment

  Hormonal treatment is effective in 3–4% of men.

- drug therapies

  New medications for the treatment of sexual dysfunction for men and women are under development.

- devices to assist with erection

  These devices are effective in 90% of patients.

- surgery

  Surgery has high success rates.

9.5 Medications include:
- Caverject and Edex: prostaglandin injections

  Medications are effective in 70% of men. Drugs are injected near the base of the penis. Using an injection device makes the process easier.

- Muse: prostaglandin urethral suppository

- Sildenafil (Viagra), vardenafil (Levitra), and tadalafil (Cialis): oral medications that will cause or improve erections.

  A total of 82% of men had improved erections, and intercourse was successful in 66% of attempts. Caution is needed among men with cardiovascular disease.

9.6 Devices to assist with erection are available.
- Erection and rigidity are achieved by creating a vacuum around the penis. Once the penis is engorged with blood, an entrapment band is placed around the base of the penis to maintain rigidity.

  This is the most common type of device used. Units include the Osbon ErecAid, Response II Unit, VED unit, Touch II, Rejoyn, Pos-T-Vac System, Encore, Vet-Co, and the Piston II.

CONTENT OUTLINE

CONCEPT	DETAIL	INSTRUCTOR'S NOTES

■ Entrapment bands are worn around the penis to increase rigidity for the man who can achieve but not maintain an erection.

The unit is called Restore. All of these devices are contraindicated in men using anticoagulants, with bleeding disorders, or with a history of priapism.

■ Penile orthoses (to support the penis) or external penile prostheses substitute for a dysfunctional penis.

The unit is called Rejoyn support sleeve.

9.7 Surgical intervention includes placement of a prosthesis into the penis. The three types of prostheses are semirigid, inflatable, and hydraulic. All are implanted into both sides of the penis, just above the urethra.

Stress the need for a thorough evaluation by a urologist and counseling for both partners.

■ **Semirigid.** This method involves two semirigid rods inserted beside each other into the penis. The man then has a constantly erect penis that can be bent down.

Use Visual #5, Penile Prostheses—Semirigid.

■ **Inflatable.** There are two types. Both have two chambers placed inside the penis.

In one, a fluid reservoir is implanted in the groin area. The man can inflate the chambers to have an erection and collapse the chambers when an erection is no longer wanted.

Inflatable prostheses are more complicated and expensive, but allow for more familiar functioning.

In the other, each chamber contains a pump, fluid, and a release valve. Squeezing the head of the penis forces the fluid to move into the other chamber, causing an erection. Bending the penis causes fluid to flow back into the storage area, ending the erection.

The units are called HydroFlex and Flexi-flate. Use Visual #6, Penile Prostheses—Inflatable.

■ **Hydraulic.** This is a self-contained unit. The rods are activated by bending to cause an erection.

Microvascular surgery for impotence is appropriate for only 1% of men.

CONTENT OUTLINE

CONCEPT	DETAIL	INSTRUCTOR'S NOTES
10. Treatment resources for men and women	10.1 Difficulties with sexual functioning can lead to many behaviors, such as: ■ anxiety ■ sexual avoidance ■ poor communication ■ anger ■ feelings of hopelessness or rejection ■ loss of self-esteem ■ searching for explanation (myths) ■ partner dissatisfaction	Suggestive comments and acting out may also occur in people who are experiencing sexual dysfunction.
	10.2 One of the keys to success in treatment is being able to have good communication with your partner.	
	10.3 A health professional, counselor, or sexual therapist in whom you have confidence, and to whom you can relate, will be invaluable.	Counseling is often recommended as treatment for sexual dysfunction and may also be beneficial for patients with physiologically based problems.
	10.4 Other avenues of treatment are available, such as support groups, couples retreats (often sponsored by church groups), and sexual counselors.	There are national support and information sources. Have a list of community resources available Note: Sex therapists and marriage counselors do not have standard education requirements—participants need to be careful to find a reputable therapist.
	10.5 There is help available, and the first step is to talk with a health care professional about your concerns.	The Impotency Information Line is 800-221-5517 and the Impotency Information Center is at 800-843-4315.

SKILLS CHECKLIST

None.

EVALUATION PLAN

Knowledge will be evaluated by achievement of learning objectives and by responses to questions during the session. The ability to apply knowledge will be evaluated through program outcome measures.

DOCUMENTATION PLAN

Record class attendance and achieved objectives as appropriate.

SUGGESTED READINGS

Beckman TJ, Cuddihy RM, Scheitel SM, Naessens JM, Killian JM, Pankratz VS. Screening mammogram utilization in women with diabetes. *Diabetes Care*. 2001;24:2049–2053.

Betschart J. Oral contraception and adolescent women with insulin-dependent diabetes mellitus: risks, benefits and implications for practice. *The Diabetes Educator*. 1996; 22:374–378.

Boyko EJ, Fihn DS, Scholes D, Chen CL, Normand EH, Yarbro P. Diabetes and the risk of acute urinary tract infection among postmenopausal women. *Diabetes Care*. 2002;25:1778–1783.

Chasan-Taber L, Willett WC, Stampfer MJ, Hunter DJ, Colditz GA, Spiegelman D, Manson JE. A propective study of oral contraceptives and NIDDM among US women. *Diabetes Care*. 1997;20:330–335.

Chau DL, Goldstein-Fuchs J, Edelman SV. Osteoporosis among patients with diabetes: an overlooked disease. *Diabetes Spectrum*. 2003;16:176–183.

Crespo CJ, Smit E, Snelling A, Sempos CT, Andersen RE. Hormone replacement therapy and its relationship to lipid and glucose metabolism in diabetic and nondiabetic postmenopausal women. *Diabetes Care*. 2002;25:1675–1680.

De Berardis G, Franciosi M, Belfiglio M, Di Nardo B, Greenfield S, Kaplan SH, Pellegrini F, Sacco M, Tognoni G, Valentini M, Nicolucci A. Erectile dysfunction and quality of life in type 2 diabetic patients. *Diabetes Care*. 2002;25:284–291.

De Tejada IS, Anglin G, Knight JR, Emmick JT. Effects of tadalafil on erectile dysfunction in men with diabetes. *Diabetes Care*. 2002; 25:2159–2164.

Enzlin P, Mathieu C, Denmytteanere K. Diabetes and female sexual functioning: a state of the art. *Diabetes Spectrum*. 2003;16:256–259.

Enzlin P, Mathieu C, Van den Bruel A, Bosteels J, Vanderschuren D, Demyttenaere K. Sexual dysfunction in women with type 1 diabetes. *Diabetes Care*. 2002;25:672–677.

Enzlin P, Mathieu C, Van den Bruel A, Vanderschuren D, Demyttenaere K. Prevalence and predictors of sexual dysfunction in patients with type 1 diabetes. *Diabetes Care*. 2003;26:409–414.

Goldstein I, Lue TF, Padma-Nathan H, Rosen RC, Steers WD, Wicker PA. Oral sildenafil in the treatment of erectile dysfunction. *The New England Journal of Medicine*. 1998; 338:1397–1404.

Jayagopal V, Alvertazzi P, Kilpatric ES, Howarth EM, Hennings PE, Hepburn DA, Atkins SL. Beneficial effects of soy phytoestrogen intake in postmenopausal women with type 2 diabetes. *Diabetes Care*. 2002; 25:1709–1714.

Owens MD. Diabetes and women's health issues. *Diabetes Spectrum*. 2003;16:146–173.

Paty B, Hirsch I. Erectile dysfunction in diabetes. *Practical Diabetology*. 2000;18(2):16–20.

Penson DF, Latini DM, Lubeck DP, Wallace KL, Henning JM, Lue TF. Do impotent men with diabetes have more severe erectile dysfunction and worse quality of life than the general population of impotent patients? *Diabetes Care*. 2003;26:1093–1099.

Poirier-Solomon L. Contraception. *Diabetes Forecast*. 2001;54(8):32–34.

Poirer-Solomon L. HRT. *Diabetes Forecast*. 2002;55(2):34–36.

Poirer-Solomon L. PMS, periods and problematic blood sugars. *Diabetes Forecast*. 2001;54:7:28–31.

Poirer-Solomon L. UTIs. *Diabetes Forecast*. 2002;55(8):28–30.

Poirer-Solomon L. Vaginitis. *Diabetes Forecast*. 2002;55(7):35–37.

Raffel LJ. The genetics of diabetes. *Practical Diabetology*. 1992;11(3):6–11.

Spollett GR. Assessment and management of erectile dysfunction in men with diabetes. *The Diabetes Educator*. 1999; 25:65–73.

➜ Sexual Response Cycle—Physical Changes

Phase	Woman	Man
Excitement	▪ Vaginal lubrication ▪ Expansion and lengthening of the inner ⅔ of the vagina ▪ Increase in size of clitoris ▪ Erection of nipples	▪ Erection of penis ▪ Smoothing out of skin ridges of scrotum ▪ Rising of testes toward the pelvis ▪ Erection of nipples (in some men)
Plateau	▪ Blood vessels filled with more blood than usual in the outer ⅓ of the vagina ▪ Opening of vagina narrows, "gripping" action occurs ▪ Rash may appear on chest or elsewhere	▪ Blood vessels filled with more blood than usual cause further increase in size of testes ▪ Deepening in color of penis ▪ Small amounts of fluid may appear from urethra at end of penis ▪ Rash may appear on chest or elsewhere

continued

SEXUAL RESPONSE CYCLE—PHYSICAL CHANGES *continued*

Phase	Woman	Man
Orgasm	■ Rhythmic contractions of uterus, outer ⅓ of the vagina, and rectal sphincter ■ Total-body response ■ May have more than one orgasm before resolution	■ Rhythmic contractions of testes and penis cause movement of fluid into the urethra and then suddenly out of the penis (ejaculation) ■ Total-body response ■ Has only one orgasm, requires period of resolution before another erection and orgasm are possible
Resolution	■ Orgasm disappears as muscle contractions move blood away from genital area ■ Uterus, vagina, and clitoris return to normal position and size	■ Blood leaves penis, which becomes limp ■ Testes and scrotum return to normal position and size

Adapted from Masters WH, Johnson VE. *Human Sexual Response*. Boston, MA: Little, Brown and Co., 1966.

➔ Changes in Sexual Function with Aging

	Younger Women	Older Women
Breasts	■ Nipple erection ■ Increase in size, areolar engorgement, flush	■ Same ■ Intensity of reactions may diminish
Sex flush	■ Vasocongestive skin response to tension	■ Diminishes
Clitoris	■ High degree of responsivity	■ Same
Major labia	■ Flatten, separate, and elevate with increased sexual tension	■ Response diminishes
Minor labia	■ Vasocongestive thickening; color change from cardinal red to burgundy before orgasm	■ Color change and thickening diminish
Bartholin's glands	■ Small amount of mucoid secretion during plateau	■ Response diminishes
Vagina	■ Walls thickened; vaginal lubrication within 10–30 seconds of stimulation ■ During resolution, slow collapse of expanded portion of vagina	■ Walls thin; vagina shortens; expansibility decreases; lubrication may take ≥1–3 minutes
Uterus	■ Expulsive contractions (3–5 with orgasm)	■ Decrease in number

continued

CHANGES IN SEXUAL FUNCTION WITH AGING *continued*

	Younger Men	**Older Men**
Breasts	■ Nipple erection	■ Diminishes
Penis	■ Erection develops within 3–5 seconds of stimulation, full erection early in cycle	■ Erection takes 2–3 times longer after 50 years of age; full erection not attained until just before orgasm
	■ Ejaculatory control varies	■ Maintain erection longer without ejaculation
	■ May attain and partially lose full erection several times	■ When erection partially lost, difficulty in returning to full erection
	■ Forceful ejaculation; expulsive contractions during orgasm	■ Force diminishes; sensual experience may be reduced
	■ Refractory phase variable	■ Prolonged refractory period after orgasm; rapid penile detumescence
Ejaculation	■ Two-stage, well-differentiated process	■ Single-stage expulsion of seminal fluid
	■ Awareness of fluid emission and pressure	■ May experience seepage rather than expulsion; fewer, less visible sperm
Testes	■ Testicular elevation in late excitement or early plateau; increase in size	■ Diminished response
	■ Testicular descent during resolution	■ Rapid descent

Adapted from Masters WH, Johnson VE. *Human Sexual Response*. Boston, MA: Little, Brown and Co., 1966.

→ Normal Menstrual Cycle

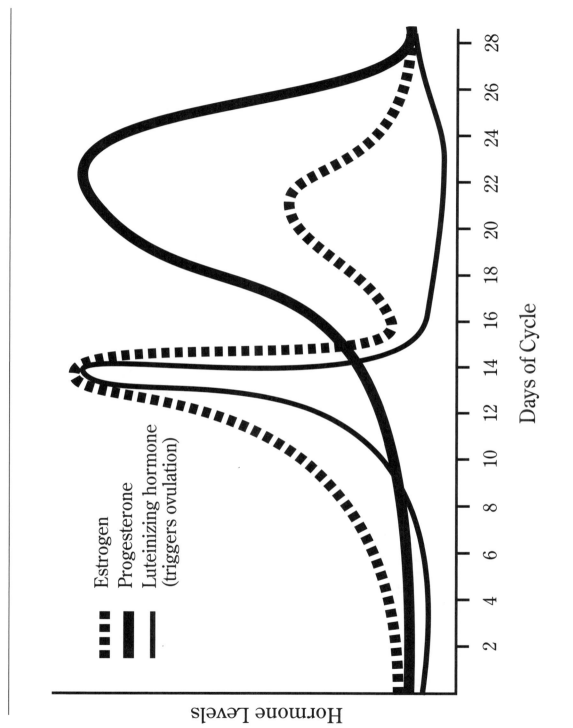

Estrogen

Progesterone

Luteinizing hormone
(triggers ovulation)

Hormone Levels

Days of Cycle

2 4 6 8 10 12 14 16 18 20 22 24 26 28

➔ Contraceptive Methods

Method	How It Works	Side Effects	Effectiveness in Preventing Pregnancy
None	It doesn't	Worry	20% (luck!)
Biological (rhythm)	Intercourse avoided 3 days before and 3 days after ovulation	Worry	60–80%
Breast-feeding	Delays ovulation after birth; not dependable	Insecurity about when ovulation returns	0–84%
Withdrawal	Penis pulled out of vagina before ejaculation	Difficult to stop and do	75–80%
Contraceptive vaginal creams, jellies, foams, and suppositories	Placed in vagina, kills sperm	Interruption of lovemaking to place; may cause burning or itching	72–90%
Diaphragm*	Fits over mouth of uterus to block sperm entry	Interruption of lovemaking to place	70–85%
Diaphragm plus spermicidal cream or jelly	Fits over cervix to block sperm entry; spermicidal barrier to sperm and kills sperm	Interruption of lovemaking to place; may cause burning or itching	85–97%
Cervical cap plus spermicidal cream or jelly	Fits over cervix to block sperm entry; held in place by suction; spermicidal barrier to sperm and kills sperm	Interruption of lovemaking to place; may cause burning or itching	60–90%
Male condom*	Placed over penis, prevents sperm from entering vagina	Interruption of lovemaking to place; some decrease in sensation; some people allergic to latex	85–90%

*A diaphragm or condom should be used with spermicidal cream or jelly. Make sure your cream or jelly is not one just for lubrication. Be sure the expiration date of the product has not passed.

© 2004 American Diabetes Association

CONTRACEPTIVE METHODS *continued*

Method	How It Works	Side Effects	Effectiveness in Preventing Pregnancy
Female condom	Inserted into vagina; blocks entry of sperm	Interruption of lovemaking to place; some reduction of sensation; awkward to insert correctly	74–79%
Condom plus spermicidal cream or jelly	Barrier to sperm and kills sperm	Interruption of lovemaking to place; some decrease in sensation; some people allergic to latex	95–97%
Contraceptive ring	Placed in the vagina every 28 days; left in place for 21 days; provides low dose combination hormones	Estrogen may decrease effectiveness of insulin although doses of estrogen low; headache, breast tenderness	95–99%
Intrauterine device (IUD)	Placed in uterus by doctor, prevents planting of egg	Heavier menstrual periods and cramping; possible infection	95–98%
Birth control pill or patch (combined estrogen and progestin, and progestin only [mini-pill] available)	Blocks ovulation, thickens mucus of uterine lining to block sperm	Estrogen may decrease effectiveness of insulin; increased vascular disease; mood changes; weight gain	95–99%
Long-acting progestin (available by injection every 3 months, or subdermal implants [NorPlant])	Blocks ovulation, thickens mucus of uterine lining to block sperm	Has not been tested with women who have diabetes; irregular and longer menstrual periods and spotting; decreased libido	Nearly 100%
Sterilization (vasectomy for men; tubal ligation for women)	Blocks passage of sperm or egg	Requires surgery; usually permanent (hard to reverse surgically)	Nearly 100%

*A diaphragm or condom should be used with spermicidal cream or jelly. Make sure your cream or jelly is not one just for lubrication. Be sure the expiration date of the product has not passed.

© 2004 American Diabetes Association

473

➲ Penile Prostheses——Semirigid

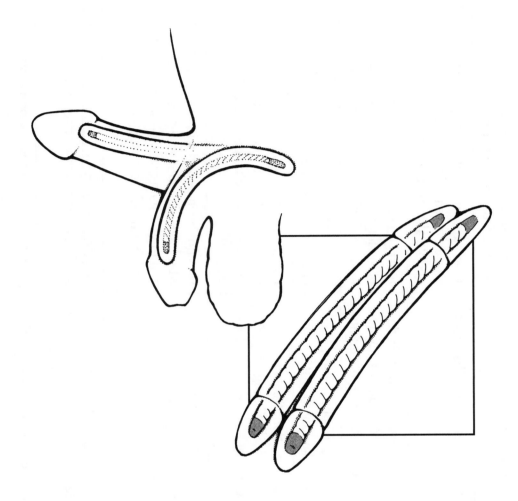

➡ Penile Prostheses—Inflatable

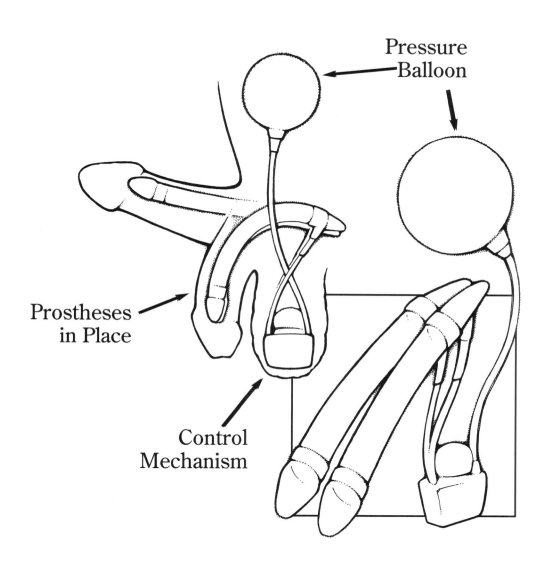

Pressure
Balloon

Prostheses
in Place

Control
Mechanism

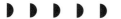

#24	Pregnancy and Diabetes

STATEMENT OF PURPOSE

This session is intended to provide information about preconception care for women with existing diabetes, care of diabetes during pregnancy, gestational diabetes, and the effect diabetes has on pregnancy and its outcomes.

PREREQUISITES

It is recommended that participants have a basic understanding of both diabetes and pregnancy.

OBJECTIVES

At the end of this session, participants will be able to:

For Preconception Counseling:

1. identify the need for normal blood glucose levels before pregnancy;

2. identify that blood glucose control has an effect on the outcome of pregnancy;

3. identify one risk of pregnancy for the woman with diabetes;

4. list tests for diabetes complications that need to be done before pregnancy.

For Gestational Diabetes:

5. define gestational diabetes;

6. state the purpose of a meal plan during pregnancy;

7. identify the effect that blood glucose control has on birth weight;

8. identify the value of monitoring blood glucose levels;

9. describe the correct treatment for hypoglycemia during pregnancy;

10. identify two emergency situations in which a doctor should be notified;

11. define one specialized test that the pregnant woman with diabetes may undergo;

12. define areas of special care that her baby might receive.

For Preexisting Diabetes and Pregnancy:

13. identify that blood glucose control has an effect on the outcome of pregnancy;

14. state the value of intensification of insulin therapy during pregnancy;

477

15. identify the value of monitoring blood glucose levels;

16. identify the effects insulin, different types of food, and exercise have on blood glucose levels;

17. describe the correct treatment for hypoglycemia during pregnancy;

18. identify two emergency situations in which a doctor should be notified;

19. define one specialized test that the pregnant woman with diabetes may undergo;

20. define areas of special care that her baby might receive.

CONTENT

Pregnancy; Preconception Care.

MATERIALS NEEDED

VISUALS PROVIDED	ADDITIONAL
1. Insulin Action Times 2. Where Weight Goes During Pregnancy 3. Insulin Needs During Pregnancy **Handouts** (one per participant): 1. Menstrual Chart 2. Treatment of Low Blood Glucose During Pregnancy	■ Samples of prenatal vitamins ■ Samples of glucose products ■ Insulin pump and tubing ■ Information about childbirth options, high-risk clinics or medical centers, local hospital policies and tours, childbirth classes, La Leche League, child care classes, and smoking cessation programs

METHOD OF PRESENTATION

Start by introducing yourself and telling what you do. Ask participants to introduce themselves and their partners, if present. If most of the participants are pregnant, ask that they tell their due dates, if they have other children, and any other information they wish. Explain the purposes of this session and that although some of the information may be frightening, it is important to know so that they can be alert for early signs of problems, seek help promptly when needed, and understand the purpose of recommended therapy.

Present the material in a question/discussion format.

This topic is divided into three main sections: Preconception Counseling, Gestational Diabetes, and Preexisting Diabetes and Pregnancy. Present only the sections appropriate for the participants. It is probably most reasonable to present preconception information and pregnancy information in separate sessions. Preconception information should be provided to all women of child-bearing age who have diabetes.

CONTENT OUTLINE

CONCEPT	DETAIL	INSTRUCTOR'S NOTES
PRECONCEPTION COUNSELING		
1. Overview	1.1 Pregnancy is often an exciting time of joy and anticipation.	Ask, "What feelings do you have about becoming or being pregnant? What questions or concerns do you have?"
	1.2 It may also be a time when you are more concerned about your health.	
	1.3 In the past, some women with diabetes experienced unsuccessful pregnancies.	Ask, "What is diabetes?" Review the basic pathophysiology of diabetes.
	1.4 Today, the chances are better than ever that a woman with diabetes will have a healthy baby.	
	1.5 Keeping blood glucose levels near the target range before and during pregnancy helps to ensure a positive outcome.	Ask, "What are target plasma blood glucose values for the non-pregnant person with diabetes?" (Before meals: 90–130 mg/dl; after meals: <180 mg/dl)
	1.6 A careful balance of your meal plan, activity, and insulin needs to be achieved and maintained before and during pregnancy. Blood glucose monitoring and frequent medical care are also important.	Ask, "What are target blood glucose levels for pregnant women with diabetes?" (Before meals: 60–90 mg/dl; after meals: <120 mg/dl). Recommended target values may vary. Provide information appropriate for your participants.
2. Need for care	2.1 It is true that having diabetes increases the risk of problems for you and your baby.	
	2.2 During pregnancy, some of the glucose in the mother's bloodstream goes to the baby so that it can grow and develop.	The glucose provides nourishment to the baby.
	2.3 However, blood glucose levels that are too high are harmful. They can cause birth defects and other problems.	If most women in the group are already pregnant, present information about preconception care with sensitivity to their situation.

CONTENT OUTLINE

CONCEPT	DETAIL	INSTRUCTOR'S NOTES
	2.4 Because the baby's organs are formed during the first 6 weeks of pregnancy, the risk for birth defects is greatest if blood glucose values are poorly controlled during that time. (This may be before you know you're pregnant.)	Incidence is 6–10% for women with diabetes, compared to 2% in the general population. However, with near-normal glucose control in the first trimester, incidence decreases to that of the general population.
	2.5 You can reduce the risks by having a normal A1C level at or near the upper limit of normal and blood glucose levels consistently in your target range before you become pregnant.	Ask, "What is a normal A1C level? What does this number tell you?" Note that individual targets may vary.
	2.6 You will need to continue to use contraception until your blood glucose levels are in the preconception target range.	Preconception premeal plasma glucose targets: 80–110 mg/dl; 2 h after the start of the meal: <155 mg/dl.
3. Caring for your diabetes	3.1 It is a good idea to begin working before pregnancy with the health care team who will provide your prenatal care. The team includes an obstetrician, pediatrician, nurse educator, dietitian, and perhaps a social worker.	Ask, "Do you have a care team to help you manage your pregnancy?" Define team members' roles. Encourage women to seek care at a high-risk clinic or tertiary care center.
	3.2 If you take oral agents, you will stop taking them and begin taking insulin. Talk with your provider about all medications you take.	Oral agents may be harmful to the developing fetus. Angiotensin-converting enzyme inhibitors will be replaced. Other drugs may be stopped or changed as well.
	3.3 Your insulin needs may increase, and you may take more than one type of insulin to keep your blood glucose level more consistent throughout the day.	Use Visual #1, Insulin Action Times.
	3.4 Most insulin programs will include two to four insulin injections a day before and during pregnancy. Some women use an insulin pump.	Show an insulin pump, if available.
	3.5 Your meals, activity, and insulin program need to be carefully balanced.	

CONTENT OUTLINE

CONCEPT	DETAIL	INSTRUCTOR'S NOTES
	3.6 You will meet with the dietitian to develop a meal plan.	
	3.7 If you have a regular exercise program, you can continue it. You will need to test more often when you exercise. You may need an exercise snack with a more intensive insulin program.	
	3.8 If you plan to start an exercise program, choose something less strenuous, such as walking or swimming, that you can continue throughout your pregnancy.	
	3.9 You will need to test and record your blood glucose at least four times a day to be sure that the balance is working.	Review recommended times and the information provided.
	3.10 Because your blood glucose levels are lower, you are more likely to experience hypoglycemic reactions.	Ask, "How do you treat an insulin reaction?" Review treatment.
	3.11 You need to carry a quick-acting source of sugar with you at all times, such as glucose tablets or gels.	Show sample products. Stress the value of wearing diabetes identification.
4. Health considerations	4.1 Cigarette smoking and alcohol are harmful to your unborn child. If you smoke, now is a good time to stop. Alcohol should be avoided during pregnancy.	Provide information about smoking cessation programs in your area.
	4.2 Pregnancy can negatively affect some of the long-term complications of diabetes. You need a thorough medical and diabetes checkup before you become pregnant.	Blood pressure, including orthostatic measures, and heart, vascular, thyroid, and kidney function need to be evaluated. It is also important to test for signs of autonomic and peripheral neuropathy.
	4.3 Retinopathy can become worse during pregnancy. You need to see an eye specialist for a dilated eye exam before pregnancy and receive treatment for any retinal damage.	Define *retinopathy* and *eye specialist*. Laser therapy can be done safely during pregnancy.

CONTENT OUTLINE

CONCEPT	DETAIL	INSTRUCTOR'S NOTES
	4.4 After this exam, you, your partner, and your health care team should discuss any risks of pregnancy.	
	4.5 A vitamin supplement that includes folic acid is needed.	Sufficient vitamins, iron, calcium, and supplemental folic acid are needed.
5. Other considerations	5.1 There is very little chance your baby will be born with diabetes. If you have type 1 diabetes, there is a 1–2% chance your child will ever get diabetes. If you have type 2 diabetes, there is a 10–15% chance your child will get diabetes as an adult and up to a 33% chance for glucose intolerance.	Men with type 1 diabetes have a 6% chance of having a child with diabetes. The risks are higher if both parents have diabetes. Risks for both types decrease the older parents are at the time of diagnosis.
	5.2 There is no best age to be pregnant. Women who have their children between 20 and 40 years of age have fewer health risks.	A pelvic exam and pap smear are needed before pregnancy. It may be harder to become pregnant as you get older.
	5.3 A pregnancy is very demanding when you have diabetes. It takes knowledge, time, effort, and money for the extra health care costs. You may need to take time off from work or have help caring for other children or with housework.	Point out that this can be a stressful time. Encourage participants to talk with their partners and other supporting people about the demands of pregnancy.
6. Becoming pregnant	6.1 Once your A1C and your blood glucose levels are in your target range, you can safely become pregnant.	Encourage participants to talk with their providers before becoming pregnant.
	6.2 You can become pregnant 1–2 h after you ovulate. Ovulation occurs 12–16 days before your period starts.	Ask, "What is ovulation? When does it occur?"
	6.3 Your basal temperature goes up slightly just before you ovulate. Your basal temperature is your temperature first thing in the morning, before you get out of bed.	

CONTENT OUTLINE

CONCEPT	DETAIL	INSTRUCTOR'S NOTES
	6.4 Keeping track of your basal temperature and menstrual cycle or using home prediction kits will help you know when you ovulate.	Distribute and review Handout #1, Menstrual Chart. Participants may want to use the commercial ovulation predictor test kits.
	6.5 Diabetes does not affect fertility for women. You may get pregnant right away, or it can take 6–12 months. If it takes longer than that, talk with your health care team.	Remind participants that they need to maintain target blood glucose levels during this time. PCOS does affect fertility.
7. Conclusion	7.1 Pregnancy can be a very happy time and a time to look forward to good things ahead.	
	7.2 Planning your pregnancy helps to ensure the best outcome for you and your baby.	

GESTATIONAL DIABETES

CONCEPT	DETAIL	INSTRUCTOR'S NOTES
8. Why does it occur?	8.1 This type of diabetes appears for the first time during pregnancy. It occurs in approximately 7% (range 1–14%) of all pregnant women.	Ask, "What questions or concerns do you have about gestational diabetes? What is diabetes?" Review normal food metabolism and the role of insulin. Refer to Outline #1, *What Is Diabetes?*
	8.2 Women who are older, have had babies weighing 9 lb or more, have a family history of diabetes, are from certain ethnic groups, or are overweight are at risk.	
	8.3 Gestational diabetes may occur because hormones produced by the placenta in all pregnant women may make insulin less effective (insulin resistance).	Ask, "What is the placenta?" Review insulin resistance.
	8.4 These hormones increase as pregnancy progresses. More insulin is needed to maintain normal glucose levels. If the pancreas is unable to produce enough insulin, gestational diabetes occurs.	Use Visual #3, Insulin Needs During Pregnancy.

CONTENT OUTLINE

CONCEPT	DETAIL	INSTRUCTOR'S NOTES
	8.5 Gestational diabetes is usually found in the 5th to 6th month (24–28 weeks) of pregnancy. A special screening blood test is done at that time.	Ask, "How did you find out you had diabetes?" Review the value and results of the glucose challenge tests used during pregnancy in your setting.
9. Caring for gestational diabetes	9.1 The purpose of the treatment is to keep the blood glucose near the target range. The target plasma blood glucose levels for pregnancy are as follows: fasting, ≤95 mg/dl; 1 hour after a meal, <140 mg/dl; and 2 hours after a meal, ≤120 mg/dl.	The actual recommended target blood glucose values may vary. Provide information appropriate for your setting and the participant's situation.
	9.2 The first treatment is a meal plan. This is not a diet to lose weight, but a plan to spread your food out over the day so that your blood glucose levels are more even. You will work with a dietitian to develop this meal plan.	Provide participants with the name of a dietitian. Explain the rationale for frequent, small meals. For obese women (BMI >30), a moderate calorie restriction of 30–33% (≥1800 kcal/day) may reduce hyperglycemia and triglyceride levels with no ketonuria.
	9.3 Exercise helps to lower blood glucose levels by decreasing insulin resistance. Appropriate exercises are those that use the upper-body muscles. Talk to your provider about the safety of upper-body exercise.	When the lower body is kept from an excessive weight-bearing load, the load can be increased safely without fear of fetal distress.
	9.4 Test and record your blood glucose levels. Use this information to see how food, activity, and insulin (if taken) affect your blood glucose. Bring this record with you to each of your appointments.	Refer to Outline #10, *Monitoring Your Diabetes*. Ask, "How does food affect your blood glucose? Exercise? Insulin?" Ketone testing may be recommended for women using caloric restriction meal plans.
	9.5 Insulin injections may be needed for blood glucose control.	Refer to Outline #9, *All About Insulin.* Oral hypoglycemic agents are contraindicated during pregnancy.

CONTENT OUTLINE

CONCEPT	DETAIL	INSTRUCTOR'S NOTES
	9.6 You will be asked to visit your obstetrician more often than women without gestational diabetes. It is very important that you do so. You may be referred to a specialist in diabetes or high-risk pregnancies.	
10. Risks related to gestational diabetes	10.1 Gestational diabetes does increase the risks of certain problems for the mother and baby. The risks are greatest in the last trimester and if the blood glucose levels are too high.	Ask, "What is meant by trimester?" Birth defects generally occur early in pregnancy and are not thought to be related to gestational diabetes that develops later in pregnancy.
	10.2 Although it is frightening to hear about these possible problems, it is important to understand why glucose control is so important in pregnancy.	A pregnant woman who has experienced any of these problems in the past should be referred to a perinatologist or high-risk pregnancy clinic.
	10.3 Some of the problems are: ■ large babies at birth (more than 9 lb)	Birth weight is closely related to the mother's blood glucose level in the last trimester. The baby's pancreas becomes functional at 13 weeks. If the mother is hyperglycemic, the baby also becomes hyperglycemic and produces excessive amounts of insulin, which is a growth factor for fetal tissue. Large babies can cause difficult deliveries.
	■ low blood glucose (hypoglycemia) and breathing problems for the baby after birth ■ jaundice or yellowish skin in the baby 2–3 days after birth	Hypoglycemia occurs because the baby has been producing insulin in response to the mother's elevated blood glucose levels. After birth, the baby's glucose drops.
	■ preeclampsia (a combination of high blood pressure, protein in the urine, and swelling in the mother's hands, face, and feet)	Ask, "What is normal blood pressure?" Remind participants to tell their provider of any excessive edema.

CONTENT OUTLINE

CONCEPT	DETAIL	INSTRUCTOR'S NOTES
	■ hydramnios (too much amniotic fluid around the baby), which may cause the uterus to stretch and may lead to early delivery	Hydramnios occurs in 25% of diabetic pregnancies. Bed rest and glucose control is recommended.
	■ urinary tract infections	Ask, "What are symptoms of a urinary tract infection?" Remind participants to inform their providers of any symptoms.
	■ stillbirth or neonatal death	
10.4	After pregnancy, the symptoms of diabetes usually disappear. Only 2% still have diabetes after delivery. You need to have your blood glucose tested after delivery to be sure you no longer have diabetes.	Define type 2 diabetes. Explain the importance of a 2-hour glucose tolerance test 6 weeks postpartum or after stopping nursing. Encourage women who have a history of gestational diabetes to seek preconception care.
10.5	Type 2 diabetes may return later in your life. If you are at your ideal body weight, you have a 25% chance of developing type 2 diabetes. If overweight, your chances increase to 75%.	Review the symptoms and diagnostic criteria for type 2 diabetes and the results of the Diabetes Prevention Program. Stress the need to lose weight after delivery as one way to prevent subsequent type 2 diabetes. Maintaining a regular exercise program also helps prevent type 2.
10.6	If you no longer have diabetes, you will need to be screened for diabetes at least every 3 years. If you plan to become pregnant again, ask for a screening glucose test before becoming pregnant. Once you become pregnant again, ask to have your blood glucose tested early in the pregnancy.	Women with impaired fasting glucose or impaired glucose tolerance in the postpartum period should be screened annually. If there are women in the class who had diabetes before becoming pregnant, continue with Concept 11. If not, go on to Concept 14.

CONTENT OUTLINE

CONCEPT	DETAIL	INSTRUCTOR'S NOTES
	10.7 If you continue to have diabetes after delivery, you need to be sure that you seek care and get your blood glucose levels near to normal before becoming pregnant again.	

PREEXISTING DIABETES AND PREGNANCY

CONCEPT	DETAIL	INSTRUCTOR'S NOTES
11. Changes during pregnancy	11.1 Women with diabetes are affected by all of the normal changes that occur during a pregnancy. Some of these changes can cause problems with blood glucose control.	Ask, "What questions or concerns do you have about diabetes and pregnancy?"
	11.2 The amount of glucose lost into the urine increases. Therefore, glycosuria can occur with normal blood glucose levels.	Define *glycosuria*. Stress that blood glucose testing is essential during pregnancy.
	11.3 All women produce ketones more easily during pregnancy. Thus, ketosis and diabetic ketoacidosis (DKA) can occur more rapidly.	Ask, "What are ketones?" Remind participants that ketones result when body fats are broken down for energy. In type 1 diabetes, this usually happens because there is not enough insulin to use the glucose in the bloodstream for energy. Ketones cross the placental barrier and may affect fetal cognitive development.
	11.4 The placenta produces hormones that counteract insulin action. These hormones increase as pregnancy progresses. This leads to an increase in insulin needs during pregnancy.	The hormones "act against" or "block" insulin. Show Visual #3, Insulin Needs During Pregnancy. You'll need more insulin as the weeks go by.
	11.5 When you have an infection such as a cold, the need for insulin increases and the risk of DKA increases.	If you have an infection, test your urine for ketones. Provide guidelines for when to contact a health professional.

487

CONTENT OUTLINE

CONCEPT	DETAIL	INSTRUCTOR'S NOTES
12. Diabetes-related risks in pregnancy	12.1 Diabetes increases the risk for certain problems in the mother and baby:	A pregnant woman who has experienced any of these problems in the past should be referred to a perinatologist or high-risk pregnancy clinic.
	■ preeclampsia (a combination of high blood pressure, protein in the urine, and swelling in the hands, face, and feet)	Ask, "What is normal blood pressure?" Remind participants to tell their doctor about any excessive edema. Bed rest and hospitalization are usual treatments.
	■ urinary tract infections	Ask, "What are symptoms of a urinary tract infection?" Remind patients to inform doctors of any symptoms.
	■ hydramnios (too much amniotic fluid around the baby), which may cause the uterus to stretch and may lead to early delivery	Hydramnios occurs in 25% of diabetic pregnancies. Bed rest and glucose control is recommended.
	■ large babies at birth (more than 9 lb)	Birth weight is closely related to the mother's blood glucose level in the last trimester. If the mother is hyperglycemic, the baby also becomes hyperglycemic and produces excessive amounts of insulin, which is a growth factor for fetal tissue. The baby's pancreas becomes functional at 13 weeks. Large babies can cause difficult deliveries.
	■ low blood glucose and breathing problems in the baby	Hypoglycemia occurs because the baby has been producing insulin in response to the mother's elevated blood glucose levels.
	■ physical defects of the baby	The incidence is 6–10% for women with diabetes who have elevated blood glucose levels, compared with 2% in the general population.
	■ stillbirth or neonatal death	

CONTENT OUTLINE

CONCEPT	DETAIL	INSTRUCTOR'S NOTES
	12.2 While it is frightening to hear about these possible problems, it is important to know why blood glucose control is so important. Keeping your blood glucose in the target range will help prevent these problems.	Ask, "What are your usual target blood glucose levels? What are target blood glucose values during pregnancy?" Point out that these may be lower than their usual targets.
13. Caring for diabetes during pregnancy	13.1 The purpose of the treatment is to keep blood glucose in the target range. The target blood glucose level for pregnancy is 60–90 mg/dl before meals and <120 mg/dl after meals.	Ask, "What questions or concerns do you have about the care you need during pregnancy?" The actual recommended target blood glucose values may vary. Provide information appropriate for your setting and the participants' situations.
	13.2 Your prenatal care will probably be provided by a team of health professionals. The team includes an obstetrician, endocrinologist/diabetologist, nurse educator, dietitian, and perhaps a social worker.	Define team members' roles.
	13.3 You need to visit your doctor every other week during the first and second trimesters, and then every week until delivery.	Provide information according to the participant's situation.
	13.4 Test and record your blood glucose levels frequently. Use this information to see how the food you eat, your activity, and your insulin affect your blood glucose levels. Bring your record with you to each of your appointments.	
	13.5 Do not take any medicine (including medicines you buy without a prescription) until you talk with your health care team.	Remind participants of the risks of alcohol and smoking. Provide information about smoking cessation programs in your area.
	13.6 You may already be taking insulin, using a meal plan, exercising, and testing your blood glucose levels. Your treatment plan will probably change during your pregnancy.	Monitoring ketone levels on arising may also be recommended.

CONTENT OUTLINE

CONCEPT	DETAIL	INSTRUCTOR'S NOTES
14. More about managing your blood glucose— meal plan	14.1 Your meal plan will change during pregnancy. Eating the meals and snacks as recommended throughout the day and at bedtime will help to keep your blood glucose levels in the target range and prevent hypoglycemia.	Ask, "What questions or concerns do you have about self-care during pregnancy? Do you currently use a meal plan or count carbohydrates?" Refer participants to a dietitian for an individualized meal plan. A decrease in carbohydrate may be recommended.
	14.2 Do **NOT** go on a weight-reduction diet during pregnancy. More calories are needed to meet the energy needs of the growing baby.	Starvation ketosis can occur and may be dangerous to the developing baby.
	14.3 You can expect to gain about 25 pounds. Talk with your health care team about your recommended weight gain.	Use Visual #2, Where Weight Goes During Pregnancy.
	14.4 Prenatal vitamins with iron and folic acid are recommended.	Show samples of prenatal vitamins. If you feel nauseated in the morning, you can take the vitamin at dinner.
Exercise	14.5 Exercise burns calories, decreases blood glucose levels, and increases feelings of well-being.	Ask, "What are the benefits of exercise?"
	14.6 If you have a regular exercise program, such as aerobics or swimming, check with your health care team about continuing with it.	Bicycling is generally not recommended late in pregnancy because of the risk for falls.
	14.7 Walking is a safe activity if started early in pregnancy; otherwise, upper-body exercise is recommended during pregnancy. Check with your doctor before starting any exercise, including walking.	Ask, "What would be an exercise you would consider during pregnancy?"
	14.8 Monitor your blood glucose levels more often when you exercise. If exercise-induced hypoglycemia occurs often, your meal plan or insulin dose will need to be adjusted, or an exercise snack included.	

CONTENT OUTLINE

CONCEPT	DETAIL	INSTRUCTOR'S NOTES
	14.9 Your insulin dosage will change often, especially during the last half of pregnancy.	Use Visual #3, Insulin Needs During Pregnancy.
Insulin	14.10 Most women take two or more injections of insulin per day. This helps to keep the blood glucose levels in the target range.	Refer to Visual #1, Insulin Action Times. Oral medications are not recommended during pregnancy. Refer to Outline #9, *All About Insulin*.
	14.11 The technique for injecting insulin doesn't change. Site rotation is still important. There is no reason to stop using abdominal sites, unless you have trouble pinching up your skin.	
	14.12 You can learn to adjust your insulin dose based on your blood glucose tests.	
	14.13 Some women prefer to use an insulin pump.	Show an insulin pump, if available. See Outline #25, *Insulin Pump Therapy*.
15. Hyperglycemia	15.1 High blood glucose may lead to or go along with ketoacidosis.	Ask, "What is high blood glucose during pregnancy?"
	15.2 Signs and symptoms of hyperglycemia are: ■ elevated blood glucose ■ ketones ■ more urine output than usual ■ increased thirst ■ dry skin and mouth ■ decreased appetite, nausea, and vomiting ■ fatigue, drowsiness, or no energy ■ fever	Ask, "What are symptoms of high blood glucose?" Stress the importance of ketone testing if blood glucose levels are elevated (>200 mg/dl).
	15.3 Hyperglycemia usually develops slowly, over several hours or days.	
	15.4 Call your doctor right away if you have these symptoms. Do **NOT** skip your insulin dose.	If not nauseated, drink extra sugar-free liquids.

CONTENT OUTLINE

CONCEPT	DETAIL	INSTRUCTOR'S NOTES
16. Hypoglycemia	16.1 Hypoglycemia in pregnancy is defined as blood glucose levels below 60 mg/dl. It may occur more often during pregnancy, because of the intensification of therapy.	Ask, "What is hypoglycemia in pregnancy?" A blood glucose level of 60 mg/dl is low. Hypoglycemia is not harmful to the baby, but can be to the mother if untreated.
	16.2 Signs and symptoms of hypoglycemia are: ■ low blood glucose (<60 mg/dl) ■ sweating ■ weakness, trembling, and fast heartbeat ■ hunger ■ anxiety ■ nausea ■ inability to think straight ■ irritability or grouchiness ■ headache ■ confusion, coma, or convulsions	Ask, "What are symptoms of a low blood glucose reaction?"
	16.3 Hypoglycemia occurs suddenly and without warning. You need to carry something with you to treat it at all times.	Show examples of glucose products. Stress the need for diabetes identification.
	16.4 Skim milk is the preferred treatment during pregnancy.	Distribute and review Handout #2, Treatment of Low Blood Glucose During Pregnancy. Stress the need to retest and retreat if needed.
	16.5 Treat hypoglycemia promptly. Always carry something with you to treat low blood glucose reactions when you are away from home.	Glucagon injection technique should be taught to families of patients prone to severe hypoglycemia, who have asymptomatic hypoglycemia, or are using intensive insulin therapy. Refer to Outline #11, *Managing Blood Glucose.*
17. Team care	17.1 At each visit to your obstetrician, your weight, blood pressure, general health, and growth of the baby will be evaluated.	Ask, "Do you have any questions or concerns about the care you will receive?" A urine culture is needed if significant pyuria is present.

CONTENT OUTLINE

CONCEPT	DETAIL	INSTRUCTOR'S NOTES

17.2 Your urine will be checked each time for glucose, ketones, protein, and bacteria.

17.3 At each visit to your diabetologist, your meal plan, insulin needs, and blood glucose levels will be evaluated. Your A1C level will be measured every 4–6 weeks. Be sure to bring your blood glucose monitoring records and meter.

17.4 You may meet with a dietitian to learn more about your meal plan or with a nurse to learn more about diabetes during pregnancy.

17.5 All team members are available to answer any questions you might have. Between visits, write down any questions or concerns you have so that you remember to ask them.

17.6 You may be referred to a medical center in your area for specialized care.

Have information available on centers in your area.

17.7 If you take insulin, you may be hospitalized at any time, if needed for better blood glucose control.

Pregnant women with diabetes may need to be hospitalized for blood glucose control to ensure the birth of a healthy baby.

17.8 Contact your doctor right away if you notice:
- more than trace ketones in your urine
- two glucose levels >200 mg/dl
- decreased movement of your baby
- any infection or illness (fever, nausea, or vomiting)
- lower abdominal (stomach) cramps
- vaginal bleeding
- sharp back pain or abdominal pain
- burning or pain when passing urine

Provide specific guidelines for your setting as appropriate.

CONTENT OUTLINE

CONCEPT	DETAIL	INSTRUCTOR'S NOTES

- dizziness, fainting, blurred vision, or spots before your eyes
- rapid weight gain
- swelling of your hands, face, or feet
- hypoglycemia that someone else had to treat, or so severe that you passed out
- severe nausea or vomiting with hyperglycemia and ketonuria

18. Special tests and procedures

18.1 Special tests may be carried out during your pregnancy. The results of these tests are used to monitor your health and your baby's development.

18.2 An ultrasound test is used to determine the size, growth, and position of the baby and placenta. It may be done several times during your pregnancy.

This is often first done at 8 weeks to date the pregnancy.

- This test is safe for your baby and causes no discomfort. It uses sound waves, not radiation.

- A full bladder is needed to push the uterus into position so the baby can be visualized better. You will be asked to drink water before the test.
- You will lie on your back as the ultrasound instrument is passed over your abdomen. Pulses of light appear on a screen and form a picture of the baby and placenta. Ask for a copy of the picture.
- The test lasts for 15–60 minutes.
- A more comprehensive ultrasound is done at 18–22 weeks.
- A fetal echogram in midpregnancy (20–22 weeks) is used to screen for congenital heart defects.

CONTENT OUTLINE

CONCEPT	DETAIL	INSTRUCTOR'S NOTES

18.3 A 24-hour urine test will be done every trimester. You will be asked to save all your urine for 24 hours so it can be tested for protein and creatinine. A blood sample will be drawn when you bring in the urine. These tests give an indication of kidney function.

Remind patients of the importance of saving all urine on ice during the test.

18.4 Starting at 28 weeks, a nonstress test (NST) will be done once. Starting at 32 weeks an NST will be done twice a week. An external fetal monitor is used to record your baby's movements and the changes in the fetal heart rate. This test indicates how the baby is adjusting to his or her environment.

This is the primary test of fetal well-being. If there are complications, this test will be done twice a week starting at 28 weeks.

18.5 The triple test (or alpha-fetoprotein [AFP] profile) is a blood test done at 15–18 weeks gestation. This is a screening test to give information about whether your baby is in a high-risk category for defects of the brain and spinal cord (neural tube defects) or genetic syndromes. A high or low level indicates only that further tests are needed. This test is offered to all women, but babies of women with diabetes are at higher risk.

The triple test (or AFP profile) measures:
- alpha-fetoprotein (believed to be low in a Down's syndrome pregnancy because the fetus is immature; it is high in a fetus with neural tube defects)
- unconjugated estriol (believed to be low in a Down's syndrome pregnancy because of isolated defects in the endocrine fetoplacental system—immature placenta)
- human chorionic gonadotropin (believed to be higher in a Down's syndrome pregnancy because normally this chemical declines appreciably between 10 and 20 weeks' gestation; if placenta is immature, this decline would not occur on schedule)

CONTENT OUTLINE

CONCEPT	DETAIL	INSTRUCTOR'S NOTES
	18.6 Starting at 26–32 weeks, you may be asked to monitor and record your baby's movements (kick counting). You will choose an hour each day to lie on your left side and count and record movements you feel.	A baby is usually very active, including kicks, stretches, and rollovers.
	18.7 Starting at 28–32 weeks, biophysical profiles may be done if additional information is needed after an NST. This consists of an additional NST combined with an ultrasound viewing of the baby. The obstetrician will directly observe fetal movements, amount of amniotic fluid, fetal breathing motions, and condition of the placenta.	
19. Labor and delivery	19.1 Your baby will be delivered as close to your due date as is safe. Normal gestation is 40 weeks. The decision about when to deliver the baby is based on how you and your baby are doing.	Ask, "What questions or concerns do you have about your labor and delivery?" Some of the factors considered are insulin needs, blood pressure, kidney functioning, results of the biophysical profiles, daily fetal movement counts, NSTs, and results of the amniocentesis.
	19.2 Your baby can be born vaginally, even if you had a low-transverse cesarean section in the past.	A low-transverse cesarean section is also called a "bikini cut."
	19.3 If early delivery is needed and the baby is to be delivered vaginally, labor will be induced by medication. A cesarean delivery may be needed in some cases.	The indicators for a cesarean delivery are the same as for women without diabetes.
	19.4 During labor, you will receive any needed insulin intravenously, and your blood glucose levels will be monitored every 1–2 hours.	
	19.5 Most hospitals encourage your partner to be present for either a vaginal or cesarean delivery.	Have a list of area hospitals and their policies available.

CONTENT OUTLINE

CONCEPT	DETAIL	INSTRUCTOR'S NOTES
	19.6 There are classes in your area on childbirth, including the Lamaze method and cesarean delivery.	Have a list of classes in your area available.
	19.7 Tours of the delivery and nursery area are available at many hospitals.	
20. Care after delivery	20.1 After delivery, your insulin needs drop dramatically.	Ask, "What questions or concerns do you have about your care after delivery?" Refer to Visual #3, Insulin Needs During Pregnancy.
	20.2 Your blood glucose will be monitored very closely.	
	20.3 If you continue taking insulin, your insulin needs will go back to your prepregnancy level in 2–6 weeks.	
21. Care of your baby	21.1 A pediatrician may be present during delivery to care for your newborn.	Ask, "What questions or concerns do you have about your baby's care?"
	21.2 Your baby may need to stay in an intensive care nursery so that any problems can be dealt with quickly.	
	21.3 Blood will be obtained through a small prick in your baby's heel to test for blood glucose levels.	Hypoglycemia is often a problem in babies who have mothers with diabetes.
	21.4 Your baby may have an intravenous (IV) line to provide fluids and glucose. The IV line will be placed in a blood vessel in the baby's scalp, hand, foot, or umbilical cord.	
	21.5 Your baby may be placed in a crib with radiant heaters to keep him or her warm. Respiration and heart rate may be monitored by special machines.	
	21.6 The babies are kept without clothing under the warmer so that the doctors and nurses can observe them easily.	

CONTENT OUTLINE

CONCEPT	DETAIL	INSTRUCTOR'S NOTES
	21.7 You can visit, hold, and feed your baby in the special care nursery. The doctors and nurses are available to care for your baby and answer any questions you may have.	Review standard practices in your setting.
	21.8 Your baby will be transferred to the regular nursery as soon as less intensive care is needed. Some babies require intensive care for only a few hours, or not at all.	
22. Postpartum care	22.1 While you are in the hospital, you will develop a plan for glucose monitoring patterns, activity levels, and insulin dosages for home.	Ask, "What questions or concerns do you have about your care after delivery?" The risk for hypoglycemia increases in the first few weeks postpartum.
	22.2 The dietitian can help you adjust your diet for breast-feeding or weight loss.	
	22.3 Coping with a newborn and the demands of diabetes can be overwhelming. It can be hard to balance your health needs with those of your new baby. Some women become depressed.	Review the signs and symptoms of postpardum depression.
	22.4 The doctors and nurses are available to answer any questions about post-delivery care, including sexual activity and contraception.	
	22.5 Many hospital or community groups offer child care classes.	Have a list of resources available.
	22.6 Before discharge, you will find out when you need to return for a visit. At that time, your weight, blood pressure, blood glucose levels, and any incision will be examined.	
23. Breast-feeding	23.1 Mothers with diabetes are able and encouraged to breast-feed their babies if they want to do so.	Ask, "What are some advantages of breast-feeding?"

CONTENT OUTLINE

CONCEPT	DETAIL	INSTRUCTOR'S NOTES
	23.2 About 300 calories per day should be added to the prepregnancy diet to cover the extra needs of milk production. A decrease in your nighttime insulin dose may be needed to prevent hypoglycemia.	Point out the need to work with a dietitian after delivery.
	23.3 Breast-feeding may be postponed for a short time until the mother and baby are more fully recovered. Breast pumps are available to use until the baby is able to nurse. You will be able to hold and feed your baby using a bottle of milk you have expressed.	Because of the initial low blood glucose level, some infants may not suck well at first. Also, if they are getting IV fluids and glucose, they may not be hungry.
	23.4 Support groups, such as the La Leche League, are available in many communities.	Have a list of resources available.
24. Summary	24.1 Diabetes increases the risks associated with pregnancy and requires more work on the part of the expectant parents.	
	24.2 Keeping blood glucose levels in the target range increases the chances for a healthy mother and baby.	Risk for birth defects is the same for women with well-controlled diabetes as for women without diabetes.

SKILLS CHECKLIST

None.

EVALUATION PLAN

Knowledge will be evaluated by achievement of learning objectives and by responses to questions during the session. The ability to apply knowledge will be evaluated through program outcome measures.

DOCUMENTATION PLAN

Record class attendance and achieved objectives as appropriate.

SUGGESTED READINGS

American Diabetes Association. Position statement: gestational diabetes. *Diabetes Care.* 2004;27(Suppl 1):S88–S91.

American Diabetes Association. Position statement: preconception care of women with diabetes. *Diabetes Care.* 2004;27 (Suppl 1):S76–S78.

Batholomew S. Managing type 1 diabetes during pregnancy. *The Diabetes Educator.* 2001;27:76–08.

El-Hashimy M, Angelico MC, Martin BC, Krolewski AS, Warren JH. Factors modifying the risk of IDDM in offspring of IDDM parents. *Diabetes.* 1995;44:295–299.

Garcia-Patterson, Martin E, Ubeda J, Maria MA, et al. Nurse-based management in patients with gestational diabetes. *Diabetes Care.* 2003;26:998–1001.

Jornsay D. Pumps for pregnancy. *Diabetes Forecast.* 2000;53(9):69–71.

Jovanovic L, Ilic S, Pettitt DJ, Hugo K, Gutierrez M, Bowsher RR, Bastyr EJ. Metabolic and immunologic effects of insulin lispro in gestational diabetes. *Diabetes Care.* 1999; 22:1422–1427.

Jovanovic-Peterson L. *Medical Management of Pregnancy Complicated by Diabetes.* 2nd Edition. Alexandria, VA: American Diabetes Association, 1995.

Kim C, Newton KM, Knopp RH. Gestational diabetes and the incidence of type 2 diabetes: a systematic review. *Diabetes Care.* 2002; 25:1862–68.

Kitzmiller JL, Buchanan TA, Kjos S, Combs CA, Ratner RE. Preconception care of diabetes, congenital malformations, and spontaneous abortions: a technical review. *Diabetes Care.* 1996;19:514–541.

Lauenborg J, Mathiesen E, Ovesen P, Westergaard JG, Ekbom P,

Molsted-Pedersen L, Damm P. Audit on stillbirths in women with pregestational type 1 diabetes. *Diabetes Care.* 2003; 26:1385–1389.

Metzger BE, Coustan DR, The Organizing Committee: Summary and recommendations of the Fourth International Workshop-Conference on Gestational Diabetes Mellitus. *Diabetes Care.* 1998;21(Suppl 2):B161–B167.

Moses RG, Knights AJ, Lucas EM, Moses M, Russell KG, Coleman KJ, Davis WS. Gestational diabetes: is a higher cesarean section rate inevitable? *Diabetes Care.* 2000;23:15–17.

Moses RG. The recurrence rate of gestational diabetes in subsequent pregnancies. *Diabetes Care.* 1996;19:1348–1350.

Poirier-Solomon L. Bringing up baby: pregnancy and diabetes. *Diabetes Forecast.* 2002; 55(9):42–45.

Poirier-Solomon L. Contraception. *Diabetes Forecast.* 2001;54(8):32–34.

Reader D, Sipe M. Key components of care for women with gestational diabetes. *Diabetes Spectrum.* 2001;14:188–191.

Sharma M, Ratner R. Gestational diabetes mellitus: Controversies in screening and diagnosis. *Practical Diabetology.* 2002; 21(1):7–13.

Simon ER. Gestational diabetes mellitus: diagnosis, treatment and beyond. *The Diabetes Educator.* 2001;27:69–74.

Simmons D, Thompson CF, Contoy C, Scott DJ. Use of insulin pumps in pregnancies complicated by type 2 diabetes and gestational diabetes in a multiethnic community. *Diabetes Care.* 2001;24:2078–2081.

Wood SL, Sauve R, Ross S, Brant R, Love EJ. Prediabetes and perinatal mortality. *Diabetes Care.* 2000;23:1752–1754.

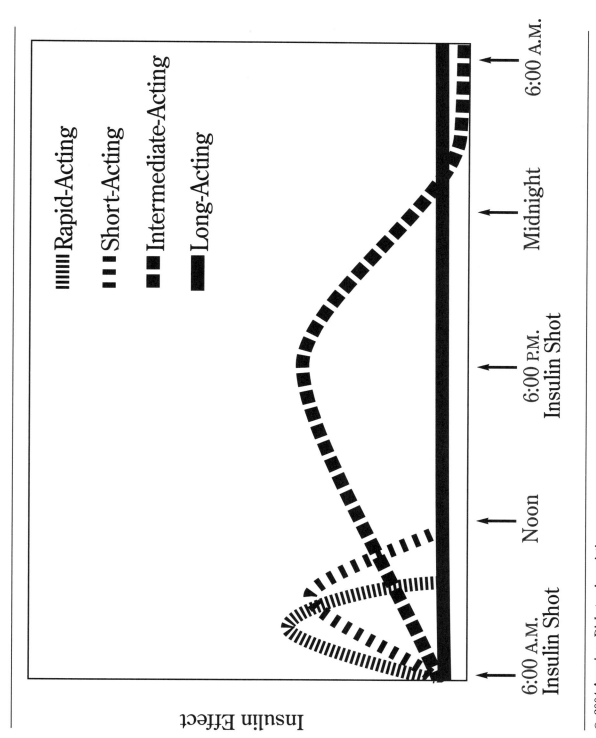

➲ Where Weight Goes During Pregnancy

Developing unborn baby	=	7 – 8 lb
Placenta	=	1½ – 2 lb
Amniotic fluid	=	2 – 2½ lb
Increased uterine size	=	2½ – 3 lb
Breasts	=	2 – 3 lb
Increased blood volume	=	3 – 3½ lb
Normal water retention	=	3 – 3½ lb

Total   = 21 – 25½ lb

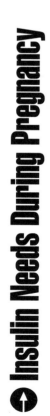

Insulin Needs During Pregnancy

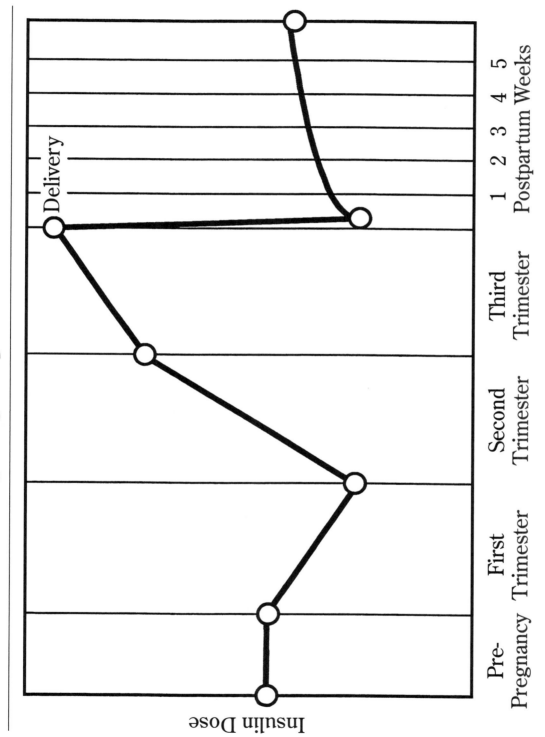

Insulin Dose

Delivery

Pre-Pregnancy | First Trimester | Second Trimester | Third Trimester | 1 2 3 4 5 Postpartum Weeks

➔ Menstrual Chart

Put an X in each box for each day of your period. This will help you determine when your next period will occur. By knowing this, you can count 12–16 days ahead to determine your time of ovulation.

Month:

Days of cycle	1	2	3	4	5	6	7	8	9	10	11	12	13	14	15	16	17	18	19	20	21	22	23	24	25	26	27	28	29	30	31	32	33	34	35	36	37	38	39	40
Date																																								
Period																																								
Temperature																																								

Month:

Days of cycle	1	2	3	4	5	6	7	8	9	10	11	12	13	14	15	16	17	18	19	20	21	22	23	24	25	26	27	28	29	30	31	32	33	34	35	36	37	38	39	40
Date																																								
Period																																								
Temperature																																								

Month:

Days of cycle	1	2	3	4	5	6	7	8	9	10	11	12	13	14	15	16	17	18	19	20	21	22	23	24	25	26	27	28	29	30	31	32	33	34	35	36	37	38	39	40
Date																																								
Period																																								
Temperature																																								

➡ Treatment of Low Blood Glucose During Pregnancy

Low blood glucose (hypoglycemia) can happen to anyone with diabetes who uses insulin—even if diabetes has only occurred during pregnancy. Hypoglycemia is also called an insulin reaction or low blood glucose. A low blood glucose reaction is easily treated. If it is not treated, a reaction usually will become more serious, and you may pass out.

The symptoms and signs of a reaction are caused by the body's response to a low level of glucose in the blood. This is most likely to happen:

- at the time insulin has its peak effect
- during exercise, or up to 24 hours after hard exercise
- if too much insulin has been taken
- if a meal or snack is late or has been missed
- if you are more active than usual
- between 2:00 and 4:00 a.m., when your body is most sensitive to insulin

How Can You Tell If You Are Having A Low Blood Glucose Reaction?

You can learn to notice the early signs and symptoms of a low blood glucose reaction. Some signs are:

- sudden mood changes
- nervousness
- anxiousness
- heart beating rapidly or forcefully

- excess hunger
- sweating
- irritability
- nausea (symptoms of morning sickness will worsen)

If a reaction is more severe, you may notice other symptoms:

- blurred vision
- nightmares
- tingling or numbness around your mouth or your tongue

- headaches
- impaired thinking
- slurred speech

Not everyone has the same symptoms. Sometimes you may have no symptoms at all. When your blood glucose is low, you may feel signs other than those listed here.

continued

TREATMENT OF LOW BLOOD GLUCOSE DURING PREGNANCY *continued*

Whatever your symptoms are, you will usually have the same ones each time you have a reaction. Remember that you may not notice these signs yourself. Instead, others may notice sudden mood changes or confusion.

How Do You Treat A Mild Low Blood Glucose Reaction?

The treatment for a low blood glucose reaction during pregnancy is slightly different than for a person with diabetes who is not pregnant. Skim or low-fat milk is used instead of juice or another sugar, unless you are lactose intolerant. Milk is used because it contains both carbohydrate and protein. This raises the blood glucose level and then keeps it at a level so that another reaction does not occur. If you think that you are having a reaction:

1. Test your blood glucose level. If you are not able to do this, yet you feel you are having a reaction, begin with step 2.
2. Treat the reaction if your blood glucose level is less than 60 mg/dl. Take 3–4 glucose tablets or drink 8 oz of fat-free (skim) or low-fat (1%) milk.
3. Wait 15 minutes, then test your blood glucose level again. If it is still less than 60 mg/dl, treat the reaction again.
4. Wait 15 minutes, then test your blood glucose level again.
5. If your blood glucose level is still less than 60 mg/dl, drink 8 oz of fat-free (skim) or low-fat (1%) milk, and eat 15 gm carbohydrate (1 serving).
6. After your blood glucose level is above 60 mg/dl, test it again in 1 hour to be sure it has stayed above 60 mg/dl.
7. If the reaction happens after exercise or at night, eat 30 gm (2 servings) carbohydrate AFTER your blood glucose level has risen above 60 mg/dl.
8. Write down the steps you took to treat the reaction. Think about and write down what may have caused it to happen. This will help you learn how to avoid low blood glucose reactions in the future.

You may show no signs of low blood glucose until it is so bad that you pass out. If this happens, you will need to rely on a relative or friend to treat you with the drug glucagon. Ask your health care provider for information about glucagon.

If no glucagon is available and you are not conscious, **your family should call an ambulance or paramedic immediately!**

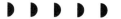

| #25 | Insulin Pump Therapy |

STATEMENT OF PURPOSE

This session is intended to provide information about what continuous subcutaneous insulin infusion therapy is, what can be expected from it, and how to operate and care for a pump.

PREREQUISITES

It is recommended that participants have an understanding of diabetes, insulin therapy, intensive insulin therapy, carbohydrate counting, and self-care and have a desire to explore insulin pump therapy as a treatment option.

OBJECTIVES

At the end of this session, participants will be able to:

1. define insulin pump therapy (continuous subcutaneous insulin infusion);

2. state the purpose of pump therapy;

3. state three personal advantages of pump therapy versus conventional and intensive therapy;

4. define basal rate and bolus dose;

5. state that the infusion site and tubing should be changed every 48 hours;

6. define both high and low blood glucose and the corrective action to take for each;

7. state two ways in which activities of daily living can be modified to accomodate wearing a pump;

8. demonstrate how to prepare the syringe or cartridge and tubing for use in the pump;

9. demonstrate how to adjust the basal rate and bolus dose;

10. demonstrate how to insert the needle into the subcutaneous tissue;

11. demonstrate how to disconnect and reconnect the syringe or cartridge and tubing;

12. state three symptoms of infection at the infusion site and corrective actions to take;

13. state three steps to take if the pump is not working correctly;

14. verbalize confidence in own ability to perform each of the skills learned and successfully live with pump therapy.

CONTENT

Medications.

MATERIALS NEEDED

VISUALS PROVIDED	ADDITIONAL
1. Normal Blood Glucose and Insulin Levels 2. Insulin Action Times	■ Instruction booklet prepared by pump manufacturer ■ Insulin pump (type patient will use) ■ Reservoir, cartridge, or syringe (appropriate for pump)
Handouts (one per participant) 1. Insulin Program for Infusion Pump 2. Blood Glucose Profile 3. Treatment of Low Blood Glucose 4. How to Use Glucagon	■ Tubing with different types of needles ■ Battery or batteries (appropriate for pump) ■ Occlusive dressing (if needed) ■ Alcohol wipes ■ Insulin (appropriate for pump) ■ Glucagon kit ■ Samples of glucose products ■ Videotape produced by pump manufacturer

METHOD OF PRESENTATION

Start by introducing yourself and telling what you do. Ask participants to introduce themselves. Explain the purpose for this session.

Present the material in a question/discussion format, with demonstration of the necessary skills. One of the most important determinants of successful pump therapy is the ability of the individual to adapt to its use. It is therefore important to provide time for the participants to discuss their concerns and feelings. The instructor can facilitate this by initiating the session with asking questions, listening reflectively, and assisting participants in problem-solving. It is also helpful if someone who is successfully using a pump can attend and discuss some personal experiences with the participants. One way to begin is to ask participants to identify why they chose pump therapy, their fears and concerns, and the benefits they believe they will receive.

This outline can be used for individual teaching or in a classroom setting. It contains information needed before selecting pump therapy (Concepts 1–5), the necessary information to live with a pump (Concepts 6–13), and the skills to successfully operate a pump (Concepts 14–22). Present only the concepts appropriate for the audience. Because operating a pump is somewhat complex, this material will need to be reviewed with the individual more than once. Provide copies of the manufacturer's videotapes for home use; this gives participants additional information and opportunities to practice. It is important that the participants have an adequate opportunity to practice each skill and receive feedback from the instructor within a short time after it is presented.

CONTENT OUTLINE

CONCEPT	DETAIL	INSTRUCTOR'S NOTES
CHOOSING PUMP THERAPY		
1. Review definition and action of insulin	1.1 Insulin is a hormone, a protein substance, produced in the pancreas.	Ask, "What questions or concerns do you have about pump therapy? How does insulin work?"
	1.2 Insulin is secreted continuously in people who do not have diabetes.	Use Visual #1, Normal Blood Glucose and Insulin Levels.
	1.3 In diabetes, there is not enough insulin action.	
2. Purpose of intensive insulin therapy	2.1 Intensive therapy usually consists of combining types of insulin and taking multiple injections.	Ask, "What do you know about intensive insulin programs?" This information is provided in Outline #9, *All About Insulin*.
	2.2 The goal is to maintain near-normal glucose levels.	
	2.3 Insulin pumps also provide intensive therapy without multiple shots and types of insulins.	
3. Definition of pump therapy	3.1 Pump therapy uses a battery-operated device called an insulin infusion pump.	Show participants an actual pump and tubing.
	3.2 The pump gives very small, repeated pulses of short-acting insulin under the skin (basal rate).	Pumps are manufactured by several companies: ■ Animas Corporation 877-YES-PUMP www.animascorp.com ■ Dana 866-342-2322 www.theinsulinpump.com ■ Deltec 800-826-9703 www.delteccozmo.com ■ Disetronic Medical Systems* 800-280-7801 www.disetronic.com ■ MiniMed, Inc. 800-646-4633 www.minimed.com *Not currently available in the U.S. and Canada.
	3.3 This occurs so often that the pump provides an almost continuous flow of insulin under the skin.	

CONTENT OUTLINE

CONCEPT	DETAIL	INSTRUCTOR'S NOTES
	3.4 Larger amounts of insulin are given before meals (bolus dose) by programming the pump.	
	3.5 The pump is worn outside the body, usually attached to a belt or another article of clothing.	
	3.6 Rapid- and short-acting insulins are approved for pumps.	Aspart is currently the only insulin specifically approved for use in pumps.
	3.7 You need to insert a needle only every 72 hours.	
4. Goal of pump therapy	4.1 The goal of pump therapy is to improve blood glucose levels.	Ask, "What are the advantages of pump therapy for you?" Clarify any misconceptions. Review results from the Diabetes Control and Complications Trial.
	4.2 Most individuals have improved or more even blood glucose levels. They feel better and feel their quality of life has improved.	
	4.3 Because of improved blood glucose levels, the risk for the long-term complications of diabetes is decreased.	
	4.4 Pump therapy affords greater flexibility for timing and content of meals and daily scheduling.	Use of carbohydrate counting may further increase flexibility.
	4.5 Pump therapy can make managing sick days or other acute complications easier.	
	4.6 Fractional doses are easier and more accurate to administer.	
	4.7 Pump therapy can help to manage the "dawn phenomenon."	The dawn phenomenon is fasting hyperglycemia.

CONTENT OUTLINE

CONCEPT	DETAIL	INSTRUCTOR'S NOTES
5. Things to consider when choosing pump therapy	5.1 If delivery of insulin is interrupted, ketoacidosis develops very quickly (within 4–5 hours).	Ask, "What are the disadvantages of pump therapy for you?" Draw out participants' feelings about these problems and ideas for handling.
	5.2 There is a potential increase in hypoglycemia as control improves. On the other hand, severe recurrent hypoglycemia and post-exercise hypoglycemia may occur less often.	Checking blood glucose levels before giving a bolus dose will help prevent this.
	5.3 The cost of therapy, monitoring, and frequent medical care may be greater.	Participants need to determine insurance coverage before choosing this therapy.
	5.4 Pump therapy gives the person with diabetes greater responsibility for his or her daily care.	Ask, "How do you feel about making many decisions each day about your diabetes care?"
	5.5 The pump is visible to others and can be a constant reminder of diabetes.	Ask, "Are you comfortable explaining diabetes to others?"
	5.6 It takes more time to care for a pump.	
	5.7 There is a potential for infusion site discomfort and infections.	
	5.8 You must be willing to monitor and record blood glucose many four to eight times a day and test for ketones when needed.	
	5.9 Pump therapy is not for everyone, and it will not cure diabetes.	Ask, "Do you have concerns about pump therapy? Do you think that a pump is a good choice for you? Why? Why not?" Participants should not feel bad or like failures if they discontinue or choose not to start pump therapy.
MECHANICS OF PUMP THERAPY		
6. Basal rate	6.1 Basal rate is the amount of insulin that is infused throughout the day and night.	Use Visual #1, Normal Blood Glucose and Insulin Levels, to illustrate the need for continuous infusion.
	6.2 It is designed to meet your insulin needs between meals (fasting state) and at night.	

CONTENT OUTLINE

CONCEPT	DETAIL	INSTRUCTOR'S NOTES
	6.3 If basal insulin needs vary over 24 hours, different basal rates can be programmed into the pump.	Pumps offer multiple basal rates.
	6.4 Blood glucose levels during fasting periods (e.g., midnight to 6:00 a.m.) are used to determine the basal rate. The basal rate replaces your intermediate- or long-acting insulin doses.	Distribute Handout #1, Insulin Program for Infusion Pump.
7. Bolus dose	7.1 A bolus dose of insulin is delivered by the pump. It is given to keep postmeal blood glucose near normal.	Use Visual #1, Normal Blood Glucose and Insulin Levels, to illustrate the need for insulin at mealtimes.
	7.2 This is similar to getting an injection of rapid- or short-acting insulin.	Bolus doses can also be used to correct a high blood glucose level. Use Visual #2, Insulin Action Times, to illustrate.
	7.3 It is given before each meal and usually before each snack. When your mealtime changes, the time of the bolus dose changes, too. You can vary your mealtime without becoming hypoglycemic.	
	7.4 The dose is determined on the basis of glucose monitoring at the time the bolus is to be given or on carbohydrate intake.	Some pumps can be programmed to provide the bolus dose over a longer time period.
8. Equipment needed to operate pump	8.1 Review the equipment needed: ■ pump	Pass around each item. Demonstrate the type of pump the patient will be using.
	■ battery	Use a battery suitable for that pump.
	■ pump reservoir, cartridge, or syringe to hold insulin	This device is different from syringes used for insulin injections.
	■ tubing	
	■ short-acting insulin	
	■ occlusive dressing (if not included with tubing)	"Op-site" is a common brand name.
	■ alcohol wipes	

CONTENT OUTLINE

CONCEPT	DETAIL	INSTRUCTOR'S NOTES
9. Wearing a pump	9.1 The pump can be hooked on a belt, carried in a pocket, or attached to other clothing.	Ask, "What questions or concerns do you have about wearing a pump?" Demonstrate how a pump can be worn comfortably. If the pump is worn hooked onto a belt, be careful that it stays connected when you adjust clothing or go to the bathroom.
	9.2 Modifications in clothing may need to be made to accommodate the pump.	Demonstrate modifications. Have a person who wears a pump share successful ideas.
	9.3 Other people may be curious about the pump and ask questions.	Discuss possible statements or questions and have individuals tell how they might respond.
	9.4 Some pumps can be worn in the water. If your pump is not waterproof, remove it for bathing or swimming. The tubing can be worn or removed.	Demonstrate the procedure for bathing or swimming with and without the tubing in place. If tubing is left in place, Op-site or waterproof tape should be placed over the infusion site.
	9.5 Generally, a pump can be worn during exercise. During strenuous exercise, a pump is more likely to be damaged.	If the pump is removed for exercise, a bolus dose is generally not necessary before removing it.
	9.6 A pump can be worn during sexual activity or removed, according to personal preference.	
	9.7 During sleep, the pump can be placed beside you, under a pillow, or attached to your pajamas. Be sure there is enough tubing to allow for movement without disconnecting the pump.	Electric blankets may be too warm and overheat the insulin in the tubing, decreasing its potency.
	9.8 When you are traveling, carry enough syringes, tubing, and insulin for the trip, plus extras.	It should not be necessary to change doses when changing time zones.
	9.9 When you are ill and unable to eat, continue the basal rate and do not give bolus doses, unless blood glucose rises.	Stress the need to establish a plan before illness occurs.

CONTENT OUTLINE

CONCEPT	DETAIL	INSTRUCTOR'S NOTES
10. Review of monitoring	10.1 It's important to monitor your blood glucose levels.	Ask, "How do you monitor your diabetes now?"
	10.2 Test your blood glucose before meals and at bedtime, at a minimum. Testing after meals and at 3:00 a.m. on occasion gives you an overall picture of your control.	Monitoring provides information for daily decision-making. Blood glucose levels are often used to determine bolus dose.
	10.3 Other times to test include whenever you are feeling as if your blood glucose is low or high, or if you feel nauseated.	
	10.4 Keeping records of blood glucose levels is important to: ■ learn the effect of factors such as food, activity, and stress on your blood glucose level ■ make effective decisions ■ serve as the basis to model and remodel the treatment program ■ provide information to your health care team	Some centers use monthly blood glucose profiles. These involve checking blood glucose levels before and 2 hours after eating, at bedtime, midnight, 3:00 a.m., and 6:00 a.m. See Handout #2, Blood Glucose Profile, as an example.
	10.5 It is important to check ketones routinely and whenever blood glucose is greater than 300 mg/dl.	Trace ketones on arising may indicate nocturnal hypoglycemia.
11. Hypoglycemia and hyperglycemia	11.1 Review the signs and symptoms of hypoglycemia.	Ask, "What symptoms do you usually have?"
	11.2 Hypoglycemia should be treated according to a standard plan. You need to carry something with you to treat it at all times. Talk to your health care team about removing the pump if hypoglycemia is severe.	Ask, "How do you treat low blood glucose now?" Show examples of glucose products. Distribute Handout #3, Treatment of Low Blood Glucose. Stress the need for diabetes identification.
	11.3 A family member or friend needs to know how to give glucagon.	Distribute Handout #4, How to Use Glucagon. Demonstrate use.
	11.4 Review the signs and symptoms of hyperglycemia.	Ask, "What are the symptoms of high blood glucose?"

CONTENT OUTLINE

CONCEPT	DETAIL	INSTRUCTOR'S NOTES
	11.5 If you are hyperglycemic for two readings for no apparent reason, change the tubing and site.	Insulin may aggregate and clog the needle or catheter. For people with type 1 diabetes, blood glucose levels typically rise about 45 mg/dl for every hour without insulin.
	11.6 Hyperglycemia should be treated according to a standard plan. Urine should also be checked for ketones.	
	11.7 If moderate to large ketones are present, assume a lack of insulin.	Corrective actions include taking an insulin injection, determining if the pump is mal-functioning, and changing the infusion set and site. Provide guidelines for contacting the health care team.
12. Determining insulin dose	12.1 Individual guidelines are used to determine basal rates.	A variety of approaches can be used. Provide guidelines for your site and demonstrate correct use.
	12.2 Individual guidelines are used to determine the bolus doses, based on blood glucose levels, carbohydrate intake, and activity.	Give examples of different blood glucose readings and times of day, including high and low glucose readings and modifications.
	12.3 The bolus requirements will be different for different meals.	Have participants determine correct bolus doses using the information in the examples.
13. Living with a pump	13.1 Care of the pump is time-consuming and may mean changes in daily routine.	Have participants talk with someone who wears a pump. Help participants plan time to care for the pump and do necessary monitoring.
	13.2 The pump will be a constant reminder of diabetes and may prompt questions from others.	Encourage participants to discuss their feelings about having diabetes and using pump therapy.
	13.3 People who wear pumps are very much in control of their diabetes and their lives. The pump does not control them.	Review the advantages of pump therapy that the participants identified.

CONTENT OUTLINE

CONCEPT	DETAIL	INSTRUCTOR'S NOTES
	13.4 Meal planning, exercising, and blood and urine testing are part of an effective pump therapy plan.	
PUMP OPERATION **14. Preparing the pump for use**	14.1 Insert the battery into the correct position.	Demonstrate, then observe patient inserting battery and confirming its status.
	14.2 Prepare the syringe or insulin cartridge with the correct insulin using the aseptic technique.	Use the same technique as drawing up for injection. You need enough insulin to fill the syringe or cartridge, flush the tubing, and last at least 24 hours.
	14.3 Prime the tubing with a minimal amount of wasted insulin, and free all air bubbles.	Demonstrate, then observe the patient preparing the syringe or cartridge and tubing correctly. Review the rationale for removal of all air bubbles.
	14.4 Insert the syringe or cartridge into the correct position in the pump. It is **essential** that these be inserted correctly to ensure infusion.	Demonstrate, then observe the patient inserting the syringe or cartridge correctly.
15. Operating the pump	15.1 Set the prescribed basal rate by following the pump programming instructions.	Demonstrate, then observe the patient adjusting the basal rate. Demonstrate the procedure for confirming the basal rate.
	15.2 Review the rationale and timing of a bolus dose.	Say, "Tell me in your own words when and why you need bolus doses of insulin."
	15.3 Deliver a bolus dose according to the pump instructions.	Demonstrate, then observe the patient delivering a bolus dose correctly.
	15.4 Check to determine if the bolus dose was given correctly.	Demonstrate the procedure for confirming the bolus dose.
16. Preparation of the site	16.1 Locate the appropriate site for needle insertion.	Assess the site for lipodystrophy or scars.
	16.2 Appropriate sites can include the abdomen, arms, thighs, and lateral buttocks.	Choice of site depends on personal preference and wearing style.

CONTENT OUTLINE

CONCEPT	DETAIL	INSTRUCTOR'S NOTES
	16.3 Wash your hands.	Give the rationale for clean technique.
	16.4 Prepare the skin with alcohol, cleansing in a circular motion from the inside out. Let the skin dry.	Demonstrate, then observe the patient preparing the skin correctly.
	16.5 Pinch 3 inches of skin between your fingers and insert the needle.	Demonstrate, then observe the patient inserting the needle correctly. Remove the needle if using a catheter-type infusion set.
	16.6 Place occlusive dressing over the needle or catheter, if needed.	Demonstrate the proper technique for placement of the dressing. Occlusive dressings decrease risk of infection.
17. Disconnecting procedure	17.1 You may disconnect the pump safely for up to 1 hour, depending on blood glucose levels.	A bolus may be needed before disconnecting if pump is to be off for more than 1 hour.
	17.2 Most people use tubing that can be easily disconnected. If not, disconnect tubing	Demonstrate, then observe individual disconnecting the pump from the tubing correctly.
	17.3 Place a clean cap on the tubing and a sterile needle with the cover on the end of the reservoir, cartridge, or syringe.	You may use the cap from the infusion set and the needle and cover you saved when you opened your supplies.
	17.4 Leave the reservoir, cartridge, or syringe in the pump while disconnected.	If the syringe is taped to the skin, you may inadvertently administer a bolus dose.
18. Reconnecting procedure	18.1 Before reconnecting, uncap the tubing and fill the top of the tubing with insulin.	This will decrease the risk of air bubbles.
	18.2 Keep the tubing below the level of the needle site so that insulin will not infuse inadvertently because of gravity.	Tubing is available with a connect/disconnect mechanism, but it tends to be more expensive.
	18.3 Reconnect the tubing.	

CONTENT OUTLINE

CONCEPT	DETAIL	INSTRUCTOR'S NOTES
19. Syringes and tubing	19.1 Reservoirs, cartridges, or syringes and infusion tubing need to be ordered from the pump company or from a diabetes supply company.	Provide the telephone number of the pump company's customer service department to place orders for new supplies.
	19.2 There are a variety of tubing and needle sets available. Needle options include non-needle, straight, and bent. Tubing is available in different lengths.	Show infusion set options. Point out that participants may need to try different types to see which they prefer.
	19.3 Keep at least a 1-week supply of reservoirs, cartridges, or syringes and tubing on hand.	In case of an emergency or shipping delay, the patient will still be able to use the pump.
20. Care of the infusion site	20.1 The tubing should be changed every 72 hours, unless the manufacturer indicates otherwise.	The risk of needle plugging and infection is greater when the infusion site and tubing are changed less often.
	20.2 Sites should also be rotated when the tubing is changed.	
	20.3 Look for signs and symptoms of irritation, inflammation, and infection.	Assess for signs and symptoms daily.
	20.4 Measures to prevent irritation, inflammation, and infection include: ■ cleanliness and aseptic technique ■ proper placement of the needle	Irritation is often caused when the needle tip is placed too close to the surface or at the wrong angle. Catheter-type tubing may be less irritating.
	20.5 Corrective measures for signs and symptoms of infection are: ■ change the site and tubing ■ wash the area with soap ■ apply sterile dressing ■ if infection is still present in 24–48 hours, call your health care team	Prompt care can prevent serious problems.
21. Battery care	21.1 Change the battery according to the procedure for the specific type of pump.	Review the manufacturer's guidelines. Demonstrate the procedure for inserting a fresh battery and observe the patient doing this.
	21.2 Batteries need to be changed at appropriate intervals.	Advise patients to have extra batteries available.
	21.3 Store batteries in a cool place.	

CONTENT OUTLINE

CONCEPT	DETAIL	INSTRUCTOR'S NOTES
22. Pump maintenance and repair	22.1 You need to know the purpose and sound of each alarm.	Refer to the manufacturer's guidelines. Demonstrate each alarm system.
	22.2 Understand what corrective action to take for each alarm.	Demonstrate correct action and observe patient doing this.
	22.3 Monitor your pump often for signs of malfunction.	
	22.4 If your pump malfunctions, check your blood glucose level, then call your provider and the pump manufacturer immediately. Ask your treatment team for an injection therapy plan in case of pump failure.	Remind participants of the appropriate 800 numbers.
	22.5 If your pump becomes very wet, assume it has malfunctioned (unless your pump is waterproof).	Check your blood glucose level, then call your physician and the pump manufacturer.
	22.6 A loaner pump may be available from the manufacturer if repairs are needed.	Participants should not try to make repairs.

SKILLS CHECKLIST

Each participant beginning pump therapy will be able to:

1. Gather all equipment needed.

2. Insert the battery into correct position and confirm its status.

3. Fill a syringe or cartridge using aseptic technique.

4. Prime the tubing without introducing air bubbles.

5. Place the syringe or cartridge into the pump, making sure that it is in the correct position and attached securely to the tubing.

6. Set the prescribed basal program and confirm.

7. Deliver the prescribed bolus dose and confirm.

8. Locate appropriate sites for needle insertion.

9. Prepare the skin.

10. Insert the needle and place occlusive dressing over the needle, if needed.

11. Disconnect the tubing from the syringe while maintaining a closed system, if needed.

12. Reconnect the tubing and syringe with no air in the line.

13. Attach the pump to an appropriate article of clothing (e.g., a belt).

EVALUATION PLAN

Knowledge will be evaluated by achievement of learning objectives and by responses to questions during the session. Skills will be evaluated by observing return demonstration of techniques. The ability to apply knowledge will be evaluated by the choice to use or not use pump therapy, by the appropriate implementation of this therapy, and through program outcome measures.

DOCUMENTATION PLAN

Record class attendance and achieved objectives as appropriate.

SUGGESTED READINGS

AADE Position Statement. Education for continuous subcutaneous insulin infusion pump users. *The Diabetes Educator.* 1997; 23:397–398.

AADE Position Statement. Education for continuous subcutaneous insulin infusion pump users. *The Diabetes Educator.* 2003;29:97–99.

Ahern JA. Are you ready for the pump? *Diabetes Forecast.* 2002;55(11):60–62

American Diabetes Association. Position statement: continuous subcutaneous insulin infusion. *Diabetes Care.* 2004;27(Suppl 1):S110.

Boland EA, Ahern J. Use of continuous subcutaneous insulin infusion in young adolescents with diabetes mellitus: a case study. *The Diabetes Educator.* 1997;23:52–54.

Colberg S. Exercising with an insulin pump. *Diabetes Self-Management.* 2002;19(1):63–70.

Edelman SV. Pumps and type 2 diabetes. *Diabetes Forecast.* 2002;55(6):62–65.

Frazzitta-Luerssen M, Taylor M. Basal rates. *Diabetes Forecast.* 1997;50(10);45.

Kordella T. 5 things you should know before you pump. *Diabetes Forecast.* 2004; 57(5):56–57.

Pickup J, Keen H. Continuous subcutaneous insulin infusion at 25 years. *Diabetes Care.* 2002;25:593–598.

Sanfield JA, Hegstad M, Hanna RS. Protocol for outpatient screening and initiation of continuous subcutaneous insulin infusion therapy: impact on cost and quality. *The Diabetes Educator.* 2002;28:599–607.

Sheiner G. An insider's look at insulin pump therapy. *Diabetes Self-Management.* 2000;17(2):28–33.

Weissberg-Benchell J, Antisdel-Lomaglio J, Seshadri R. Insulin pump therapy. *Diabetes Care.* 2003;26:1079–1087.

➲ Normal Blood Glucose and Insulin Levels

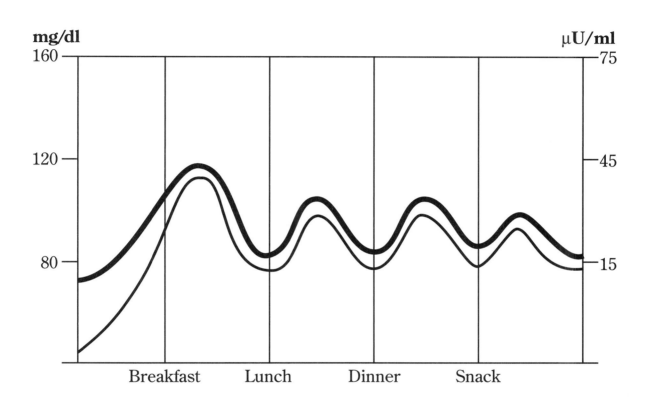

mg/dl

μU/ml

Breakfast   Lunch   Dinner   Snack

▬▬▬ Blood Glucose Level

─── Plasma Insulin Level

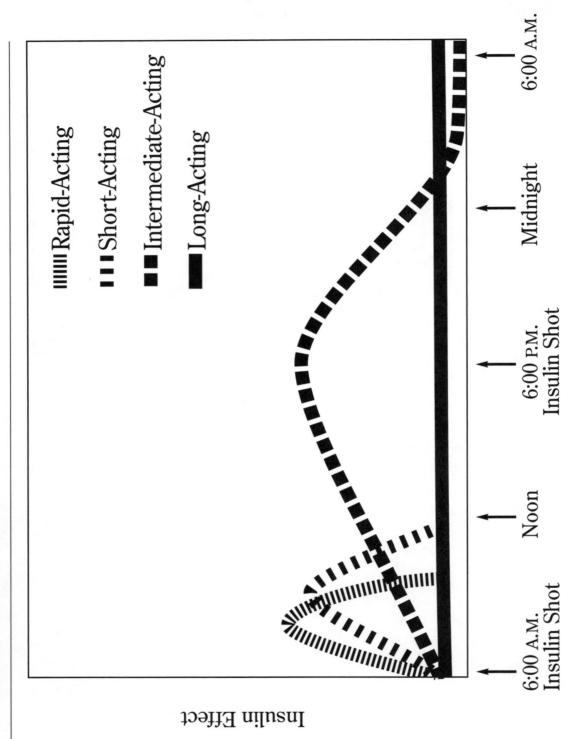

Insulin Action Times

Insulin Effect

Rapid-Acting
Short-Acting
Intermediate-Acting
Long-Acting

6:00 A.M.
Insulin Shot

Noon

6:00 P.M.
Insulin Shot

Midnight

6:00 A.M.

6:00 A.M.
Insulin Shot

➜ Insulin Program for Infusion Pump

Name _____ Date _____

BASAL INFUSION OF REGULAR INSULIN

Please set your pump to give the following basal doses of insulin.

Infusion Periods (clock time)				
Infusion Rates (units per hour)				
Amount Infused (units per period)				

Total Amount Infused as Basal Dose _____ units per day

continued

INSULIN PROGRAM FOR INFUSION PUMP *continued*

BOLUS INJECTIONS

Please use the scale below to give the premeal bolus dose of insulin, according to your blood glucose level at that time.

Blood Glucose Ranges (mg/dl)	Breakfast	Lunch	Dinner	Bedtime Snack

For each additional 15 grams of carbohydrate, add _____ unit(s) to the designated dose.

For each 15 grams of carbohydrate not eaten, subtract _____ unit(s) from the designated dose.

For exercise, subtract _____ unit(s) from the pre-exercise dose.

For stress, add _____ unit(s) to the designated dose.

➡ Blood Glucose Profile

A blood glucose profile is a "snapshot" of your blood glucose fluctuations throughout the day and can tell you how well your basal and bolus doses are working for you.

To do a blood glucose profile, check your blood glucose at the following times of the day:

> Before breakfast
> 2 hours after breakfast
> Before lunch
> 2 hours after lunch
> Before dinner
> 2 hours after dinner
> Bedtime
> Midnight
> 3:00 a.m.
> 6:00 a.m.

Do the profile when you are first starting on the pump and then before each clinic visit.

➲ Treatment of Low Blood Glucose

If your blood glucose test is:	The amount of food or drink to take is:
Between 50 and 69 mg/dl	15 gm carbohydrate (1 carbohydrate serving **or** 1 cup fat-free [skim] milk)
Less than 50 mg/dl	30 gm carbohydrate (2 carbohydrate servings)

You should feel better in 10–15 minutes after you treat yourself. If your blood glucose is still less than 70 mg/dl or you don't feel better 10–15 minutes after the treatment, take 1 more carbohydrate serving. Test your blood glucose an hour after the reaction to make sure that your blood glucose has gone above 70 mg/dl and stayed there.

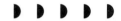

EXAMPLES OF TREATMENTS FOR LOW BLOOD GLUCOSE
(All equal about 15 gm carbohydrate or 1 fruit serving)

If your blood glucose is between 50 and 69 mg/dl, take the amount listed. If your blood glucose is less than 50 mg/dl, take twice the amount listed.

Foods	Amount
Orange or apple juice	½ cup
Grape or cranberry juice	⅓ cup
Non-diet soft drink	½ cup
Honey or corn syrup	1 Tbsp
Sugar packets	3
Life Savers	3–8 pieces
Glucose tablets	3–4 tablets

An additional carbohydrate snack may be needed at night or after exercise to keep your blood glucose above 70 mg/dl.

➡ How to Use Glucagon

Glucagon is an emergency drug that is given as a shot to raise the blood glucose level. It should be given when the person is unable to swallow or is at risk for choking, or in case of a severe insulin reaction or coma.

A prescription is needed to buy glucagon. It comes in two ways: in a kit or in a box to be mixed. If you use the kit, follow the package instructions.

To prepare glucagon for injection if you do not use a kit:

1. Remove the flip-off seals on bottles 1 and 2. Bottle 1 holds a diluting liquid and bottle 2 holds a white powder.

2. Draw the plunger of an insulin syringe (U-100) back to the 50-unit mark.

3. Steady the smaller bottle with the liquid in it (bottle 1) on the table. Push the needle through the stopper.

4. Inject the air from the syringe into the bottle and then turn the bottle upside down.

5. Withdraw as much of the liquid as possible into the syringe.

6. Remove the needle and syringe from bottle 1 and insert this same needle into bottle 2, the bottle with the powder. Inject all of the liquid from the syringe into bottle 2.

7. Remove the needle and syringe. Shake the bottle **gently** until the glucagon powder dissolves and the liquid becomes clear.

8. Withdraw the entire contents of bottle 2 (the mixed glucagon) into the syringe.

9. Inject the glucagon in the same way you would insulin, using the buttock, thigh, or arm.

10. Turn the person onto one side or stomach. (Vomiting is common after glucagon.)

11. As soon as the person is alert and not feeling sick, he or she should eat something, because glucagon acts for only a short period of time. First, give some juice or a non-diet soft drink, and then additional carbohydrate.

HOW TO USE GLUCAGON *continued*

12. If the person does not wake up within 15 minutes, the dose may be repeated. Call an ambulance.

13. Always call the doctor after an insulin reaction when coma or seizure occurs.

14. Check the package of glucagon periodically to be sure that it hasn't passed the expiration date. It's a good idea to keep an insulin syringe taped to the box so it will be ready.

Support Materials

Resources for Health Professionals

▶ ▶ ▶ ▶ ▶

AUDIOVISUAL AND PRINT MATERIALS

Abott Laboratories, Inc.
Medisense Products
4A Crosby Dr.
Bedford, MA 01730
800-527-3339

Amylin Pharmaceuticals
9360 Town Center Drive
San Diego, CA 92121

Altschul Group Corporation
1560 Sherman Avenue, #100
Evanston, IL 60201
800-421-2363; 708-328-6706

Aventis Pharmaceutical
PO Box 6977
Bridgewater, NJ 08807
800-633-1610

Bayer Corporation
400 Morgan Lane
West Haven, CT 06516
800-348-8100

Becton-Dickinson
Franklin Lakes, NJ 07417
888-232-2737

Roche Diagnostics
Diabetes Customer Service
9115 Hague Road
P.O. Box 50100
Indianapolis, IN 46250-0100
800-858-8072

Bristol-Meyers-Squibb Company
1350 Liberty Ave.
Hillside, NJ 07207
800-468-7746

Diabetes Control Network
Pratt Pfizer
1800 DCN 5554 Blvd.
600 Penn Center
Pittsburgh, PA 15235-9838
800-326-5554

Eli Lilly and Company
Pharmaceutical Division
Lilly Corporate Center
Indianapolis, IN 46285
800-545-5979

Glaxo Smith Kline
1 Franklin Plaza
PO Box 7929
Philadelphia, PA 19101
888-825-5249

Health Literacy Project
311 South Jupiter Street, #308
Philadelphia, PA 19107-5803
215-731-6154

Home Diagnostics, Inc.
2400 NW 55th Court
Fort Lauderdale, FL 33309
800-342-7226

IDC Publishing
3800 Park Nicollet Blvd.
Minneapolis, MN 55416
888-637-3874

Leap Program
4350 Bethel Road, Suite 208
Bethesda, MD 20814
301-594-4424

LifeScan
Johnson & Johnson
Milpitas, CA 95035
800-524-7226

continued

Media Library
University of Michigan Medical Center
1327 Jones Drive, #104
Ann Arbor, MI 48109
734-998-6140

Milner-Fenwick
2125 Greenspring Drive
Timonium, MD 21093
800-432-8433

National Oral Health Information Clearinghouse
1 NOHC Way
Bethesda, MD 20892
301-402-7364

Novartis Pharm. Corp.
1 Health Plaza
East Hanover, NJ 07936
888-669-6682

Novo Nordisk
211 Carnegie Center
Princeton, NJ 08540-7810
800-727-6500

Oracle Film & Video
3309 Pico Blvd.
Santa Monica, CA 90405
310-450-6637

Pfizer Inc.
235 E 42nd St.
NY, NY 10017
212-573-2323

Takeda Pharmaceuticals America, Inc.
Millbrook Business Center
475 Half Day Road, Suite 500
Lincolnshire, IL 60069
877-825-3327

TheraSense, Inc.
1360 South Loop Road
Alameda, CA 94502
888-522-5226

FOOD MODELS

National Dairy Council
10255 W. Higgens Rd., Suite 900
Rosemont, IL 60018

Nasco
P.O. Box 901
901 Janesville Avenue
Ft. Atkinson, WI 53538-0901
800-558-9595

Wisconsin Dairy Council
8418 Exelsior Dr.
Madison, WI 53717
608-836-8820

DIABETES ORGANIZATIONS

American Association of Diabetes Educators
100 W. Monroe St., Suite 400
Chicago, IL 60603
800-338-3633 or 312-644-4411

American Diabetes Association
1701 N. Beauregard Street
Alexandria, VA 22311
800-806-7801 (membership information)
800-232-6733 (to order publications)

American Dietetic Association
120 S. Riverside Plaza, Suite 2000
Chicago, IL 60606-6995
800-877-1600

American Heart Association
7272 Greenville Avenue
Dallas, TX 75231
214-373-6300

Canadian Diabetes Association
15 Toronto Street
Toronto, Ontario, M5C 2E3
Canada
416-363-3373

continued

International Diabetes Center
5000 West 39th Street
Minneapolis, MN 55416
888-825-6315

Joslin Diabetes Center
One Joslin Place
Boston, MA 02215
617-732-2400

**National Diabetes Information
   Clearinghouse**
1 Information Way
Bethesda, MD 20892
800-860-8747

DIABETES RESEARCH AND TRAINING CENTERS

Albert Einstein College of Medicine
Belfer, 705A
1300 Morris Park Avenue
Bronx, NY 10461
718-430-3242

Indiana University
Regenstrief Institute for Health Care
1001 West Tenth Street
Indianapolis, IN 46202-2859
317-630-6375

University of Chicago
Center for Research in Medical
   Education/Health Care
5801 S. Ellis Ave.
Chicago, IL 60637
312-753-1310

University of Michigan Medical Center
1331 E. Ann St.
Box 0580, Room 5111
Ann Arbor, MI 48109-0580
734-763-5730

Vanderbilt University
315 Medical Arts Building
1211 21st Avenue South
Nashville, TN 37212-2701
615-936-1149

Washington University Medical Center
Center for Health Behavior Research
4444 Forest Park Avenue, #6700
St. Louis, MO 63108
314-286-1900

INTERNET RESOURCES FOR PROFESSIONALS

A variety of diabetes resources are available on the Internet, primarily through the World Wide Web. Patient and professional information on diabetes and its complications, chat rooms, and support groups can be found under "health and diabetes" through a variety of on-line services and search engines. Not all information found on the Internet is accurate or useful—be sure to verify information and warn patients to check before making any changes in their care.

Other on-line resources include:

American Diabetes Association (ADA)
http://www.diabetes.org
Listing of ADA-recognized education programs, Association events, general background on diabetes, patient and professional publications, selected articles from *Diabetes Forecast*, selected text from the medical journal *Diabetes Care*, comprehensive review of and links to other sites, and more.

**American Diabetes Association
Professional Section Councils**
http://www.diabetes.org/councils
Listing of professional education meetings, bulletin boards for employment postings and available fellowships, links to related diabetes sites, and council announcements.

**American Association of Diabetes
Educators**
http://www.aadenet.org
Listing of Association events, member services, publications, and continuing education.

continued

American Dietetic Association

http://www.eatright.org

Listing of Association events, member services, publications, and continuing education.

Braille Translations

http://www.rfbd.org

Offers translations to Braille.

Canadian Diabetes Association

http://www.diabetes.ca

Information about activities and an educational section.

Centers for Disease Control

http://www.cdc.gov/diabetes

Current diabetes statistics, links to state diabetes control programs, information, and articles.

Centerwatch

http://www.centerwatch.com/

Listing of clinical trials and information on FDA drug approvals. See the section on endocrinology.

Children with Diabetes

http://www.childrenwithdiabetes.com

Online community for kids, families, and adults with type 1 diabetes.

National Guideline Clearinghouse

http://www.guideline.gov

A public resource for evidence-based clinical practice guidelines.

National Institute of Diabetes and Digestive and Kidney Diseases

http://www.niddk.nih.gov

Information about DCCT results, diabetic eye disease, statistics, questions to ask your doctor, a directory of diabetes organizations, and the National Diabetes Information Clearinghouse.

National Library of Medicine (NLM)

http://www.nlm.nih.gov

Access to diabetes literature at the NLM. You need to sign up and pay for an account.

National Lipid Education Council

http://www.lipidhealth.org

Provides guidance on recommendations and treatment of lipid disorders.

Online Resources for Diabetes

http://www.mendosa.com

Listing of and direct links to mailing lists and online resources and frequently asked questions about diabetes.

PUBLICATIONS FOR HEALTH PROFESSIONALS

Diabetes, Diabetes Care, Diabetes Spectrum, Clinical Diabetes
American Diabetes Association

The Diabetes Educator
American Association of Diabetes Educators

Journal of the American Dietetic Association
The American Dietetic Association

Diabetes Dateline
National Diabetes Information Clearinghouse

Practical Diabetology
Pharmaceutical Communications, Inc.
42-15 Crescent Street
Long Island City, NY 11101

Resources for People with Diabetes

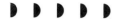

DIABETES ORGANIZATIONS

American Diabetes Association
1701 N. Beauregard Street
Alexandria, Virginia 22311
800-232-3472 (membership information)
800-232-6733 (to order publications)
703-549-1500 (National Center)

For information on local chapters and their activities, consult your local white pages.

For information about diabetes, call
800-DIABETES (342-2383)

The American Dietetic Association

To speak with a dietitian, find a dietitian in your area, or order free information:

120 S. Riverside Plaza, Suite 2000
Chicago, IL 60606-6995
800-877-1600

JOURNALS FOR PEOPLE WITH DIABETES

Diabetes Forecast (monthly magazine)
American Diabetes Association; subscription included with ADA membership
800-806-7801
http://www.diabetes.org

Diabetes Interview (monthly newspaper)
800-473-4636

Diabetes Self-Management (bimonthly magazine)
800-234-0923   (Customer Service)

Voice of the Diabetic (magazine)
573-875-8911

INFORMATION ABOUT EDUCATIONAL MATERIALS

American Diabetes Association
(to order publications)
800-232-6733

National Diabetes Information Clearinghouse (NDIC)
1 Information Way
Bethesda, MD 20892
301-654-3327

DIABETES IDENTIFICATION

Medic Alert Foundation U.S.
2323 Colorado Ave.
Turlock, CA 95382
800-432-5378

Goldware
P.O. Box 22335
San Diego, CA 92192
800-669-7311

Identifind
(iron-on labels for clothing)
Rt. 4, Box 420A
Canton, NC 28716
828-648-6768

Medic ID's
800-926-3342

INSULIN SUPPLIES

Hypoguard
7301 Ohmes Lane, Suite 200
Edina, MN 55439
(diabetes supplies, pumps, and medications)
800-888-5957

continued

Medicool
(manufactures and sells insulin cases)
800-433-2469

Medi-ject Corporation (manufacturer of a needle-free insulin injector)
800-328-3074

MII Medical Technologies
(Freedom Jet needle-free insulin system)
800-662-2471

Terumo Medical Corporation
(insulin syringes)
800-283-7866

Whittier Medical, Inc.
(Tru-Hand insulin bottle holder)
800-645-1115

INSURANCE COVERAGE

John Hall and Associates
P.O. Box 14868
Shawnee Mission, KS 66285-4868
913-268-7878

LIVING WITH DIABETES

Health Journeys Image Paths
(relaxation tapes for people with diabetes)
800-800-8661

Humedico
(educational materials and programs)
800-736-7051

SENIOR CITIZENS

American Association of Retired Persons
National Headquarters
601 E Street, NW
Washington, DC 20049
1-888-687-2277

Children of Aging Parents
1609 Woodburn, Suite 302
Levittown, PA 19056
215-945-6900

National Association of Area Agencies on Aging
1112 16th Street, NW, Suite 100
Washington, DC 20036
202-872-0888

National Institute on Aging
Resource Directory for Older People
National Institute on Aging
9000 Rockville Pike, Rm 5C27
Bethesda, MD 20898
301-496-1752

National Association for Home Care
519 C Street, NE
Washington, DC 20002
202-547-7424

SPORTS/ATHLETICS

International Diabetic Athletes Association
6829 North 12th Street
Suite 205
Phoenix, AZ 85014
602-433-2113
800-898-4322

TRAVEL

International Association for Medical Assistance to Travelers
417 Center Street
Lewiston, NY 14092
716-754-4883

INTERNET RESOURCES

A variety of diabetes resources are available on the Internet, primarily through the World Wide Web. Information on diabetes and its complications, chat rooms, and support groups can be found under "health and diabetes" through a variety of on-line services and search engines. Not all information found on the Internet is accurate or useful—be sure to check with your health care provider before making any changes in your care.

continued

American Diabetes Association (ADA)

http://www.diabetes.org

Listing of local and national Association events, general background on diabetes, selected articles from *Diabetes Forecast*, book ordering information, selected text from the medical journal *Diabetes Care*, and more.

The American Dietetic Association

http://www.eatright.org

Information about resources, news, and finding a dietitian.

Canadian Diabetes Association

http://www.diabetes.ca

Information about activities and an educational section.

Centerwatch

http://www.centerwatch.com/

Listing of clinical trials and information on FDA drug approvals. See the section on endocrinology.

Children with Diabetes

http://www.childrenwithdiabetes.com

Online community for kids, families, and adults with type 1 diabetes.

National Institute of Diabetes and Digestive and Kidney Diseases

http://www.niddk.nih.gov/ niddk_homepage.html

Information about DCCT results, diabetic eye disease, statistics, questions to ask your doctor, and a directory of diabetes organizations.

Online Resources for Diabetes

http://www.cruzio.com/~mendosa/faq.htm

Listing of and direct links to mailing lists and online resources; frequently asked questions about diabetes.

ADA REGIONAL OFFICES

New England Region
7 Washington Square
Albany, NY 12205
518/218-1755

Massachusetts Area Office
617/482-4580

Northern New England Area Office
603/627-9579

Rhode Island Area Office
401/738-6464

Pacific Northwest Region
2480 West 26th Avenue, Suite 120B
Denver, CO 80211
720/855-1102

Alaska Area Office
907/272-1424

Hawaii Area Office
808/521-1142

Idaho Area Office
208/342-2774

Montana Area Office
406/761-0908

Oregon Area Office
503/736-2770

Washington Area Office
206/352-7950

South Central Region
4425 West Airport Freeway, Suite 130
Irving, TX 75062
972/255-6900

Arkansas Area Office
501/221-7444

Louisiana Area Office
504/831-0278

Northeast Texas/Northern Louisiana Area Office
972/392-1181

continued

Oklahoma Area Office
918/492-3839

South Texas Area Office
210/829-1765

West Texas Area Office
806/794-0691

South Coastal Region
1101 North Lake Destiny Road, Suite 415
Maitland, Florida 32751
407/660-1926

Atlanta Metro Area Office
404/320-7100

Central Florida Area Office
407/660-1926

Northeast Florida/Southeast Georgia Area
Office
904/703-7200

Northwest Florida/Southern Alabama Area
Office
850/478-5957

Outstate Georgia Area Office
912/353-8110

Southeast Florida Area Office
305/477-8999

Southwest Florida Area Office
813/885-5007

Upstate Alabama Area Office
205/870-5172

Southern Region
2 Hanover Square
434 Fayetteville Square Mall, Suite 1600
Raleigh, NC 27601
919/743-5400

Central North Carolina Area Office
704/373-9111

Eastern North Carolina Area Office
919/743-5400

Greater Hampton Roads Area Office
757/455-6335

Kentucky Area Office
502/452-6072

South Carolina Area Office
803/799-4246

Tennessee Area Office
615/298-3066

Virginia Area Office
804/974-9905

Western Region
10445 Old Placerville Road
Sacramento, CA 95827-2508
916/369-0999

Los Angeles Area Office
213/966-2890

Nevada Area Office
702/369-9995

Sacramento Area Office
916/369-0999

San Diego Area Office
619/234-9897

San Francisco Area Office
415/777-4499

▶ ▶ ▶ ▶ ▶

PATIENT EDUCATION: METHODS AND PROGRAMS

Albisser AM, Harris MI, Sperlich M, Albisser JB. Getting referrals for diabetes education and self-management training. *The Diabetes Educator.* 1999;25:959–966.

American Association of Diabetes Educators. Diabetes Educational and Behavioral Research Summit. *The Diabetes Educator.* 1999; 25(Suppl):1–88.

AADE Position Statement. Individualization of diabetes self-management education. *The Diabetes Educator.* 2002;28:741–745.

American Diabetes Association. *Diabetes Education Goals,* 3rd edition. Alexandria, VA: American Diabetes Association; 2002.

American Diabetes Association. Position statement: third-party reimbursement for outpatient diabetes education and counseling. *Diabetes Care.* 1996;19(Suppl 1):48–49.

American Diabetes Association. Standards and Review Criteria: national standards for diabetes patient education and American Diabetes Association review criteria. *Diabetes Care.* 1990;13(Suppl 1):60–65; 1997; 20(Suppl 1):S67–69.

Betschart, JE, German, RR, Satterfield, D, Klein, RJ. Progress toward achieving Healthy People 2000 objectives for diabetes patient education. *The Diabetes Educator.* 1994; 20:391–392, 394, 396.

Brackenridge, BP. Diabetes education: a global perspective. *Diabetes Spectrum.* 1999;12:146–176.

Brown SA. Interventions to promote diabetes self-management: state of the science. *The Diabetes Educator.* 1999;25(Suppl):52–61.

Daly A, Leontos C. Legislation for health care coverage for diabetes self-management training, equipment and supplies: past, present, and future. *Diabetes Spectrum.* 1999;12:222–236.

Davis ED. A quality improvement project in diabetes patient education during hospitalization. *Diabetes Spectrum.* 2000;13:228–231.

Davis ED, Midgett L, Gourley S. Teach less, teach better at every opportunity. *The Diabetes Educator.* 1994;20:236–240.

Fain JA. Diabetes patient education research: an integrative review. *The Diabetes Educator.* 1999; 25(Suppl)7–15.

Funnell MM, Anderson RN, Burkhart NT, Gillard ML, Nwankwo R. *101 Tips for Diabetes Self-Management Education.* Alexandria, VA: American Diabetes Association, 2002.

Funnell MM, Haas LB. National standards for diabetes self-mangement education programs: a technical review. *Diabetes Care.* 1995;18: 100–116.

Funnell MM. Lessons learned as a diabetes educator. *Diabetes Spectrum.* 2000;13:69–70.

Funnell MM. Reimbursement for diabetes self-management education. *Practical Diabetology.* 2001;20(2):45–46.

Gagnayre R, Traynard PY, d'Ivernois JF, Slama G. An analysis of the teaching techniques used in diabetic specialist consultations. *Patient Education and Counseling.* 2000;39:163–167.

Gary TL, Genkinger JM, Guallar E, Peyrot M, Brancati FL. Meta-analysis of randomized educational and behavioral interventions in type 2 diabetes. *The Diabetes Educator.* 2003;28:488–501.

Gillard ML, Nwankwo R, Fitzgerald JT, Oh M, Musch DC, Johnson MW, Anderson R. Informal

PATIENT EDUCATION METHODS AND PROGRAMS *continued*

diabetes education: impact on self-management and blood glucose control. *The Diabetes Educator.* 2004;30:136–142.

Glasgow RE. Diabetes education research. *The Diabetes Educator.* 1999;25(Suppl):5–6.

Gagliardino JJ, Etchegoyen G, PEDNID-LA. A model educational program for people with type 2 diabetes. *Diabetes Care.* 2001; 24:1001–1007.

Izquierdo RE, Kundson PE, Meyer S, et al. A comparison of diabetes education administered through telemedicine versus in person. *Diabetes Care.* 2003;26:1002–1007.

Jones PM. Quality improvement initiative to integrate teaching diabetes standards into home care visits. *The Diabetes Educator.* 2002;28:1009–1020.

Kanzer-Lewis G. *Patient Education: You Can Do It!* Alexandria, VA: American Diabetes Association, 2003.

Lorig K, Gonzalez VM. Community-based diabetes self-management education: definition and case study. *Diabetes Spectrum.* 2000;13:234–238.

McKay HG, King D, Eakin EG, Seeley JR, Glasgow RE. The diabetes network internet-based physical activity intervention. *Diabetes Care.* 2001;24:1328–1334.

Mensing C, Boucher J, Cypress M, Weinger K, Barta P, Hosey G, Kopher W, Lasichak A, Lamb B, Mangan M, Norman J, Tanja J, Yauk L, Wisdom K, Adams C. National standards for diabetes self-management education. *Diabetes Care.* 2000;23:682–689.

Norris SL, Engelgau MM, Naranyan KMV. Effectiveness of self-management training in type 2 diabetes: a systematic review of randomized controlled trails. *Diabetes Care.* 2001;24:561–587.

Norris SL, Lau J, Smith SJ, Schmid CH, Engelgau MM. Self-management education for adults with type 2 diabetes. *Diabetes Care.* 2002; 25:1159–1171.

Norris SL. Self-management education in type 2 diabetes. *Practical Diabetology.* 2003;22(1):7–13.

Patterson SM, Graf HM. Integrating complementary and alternative medicine into the health education curriculum. *J Health Ed.* 2000;31:346–351.

Peragallo-Dittko V. Insulin resistance: a model for patient education. *Practical Diabetology.* 2000;19(4):37–41.

Piette JD, Glasgow RE. Strategies for improving behavioral and health outcomes among patients with diabetes: self-management education. In: Gerstein HC, Haynes RB, eds. *Evidence-Based Diabetes Care.* Ontario, CA: B.C. Decker, Inc., 2000.

Polonsky WH, Earles J, Smith S, Pease DK, Macmillan M, Christensen R, Taylor T, Dickert J, Jackson RA. Integrating medical management with diabetes self-management training. *Diabetes Care.* 2003;26:3094–3053.

Rickheim PL, Weaver TW, Flader JL, Kendall DM. Assessment of group versus individual diabetes education. *Diabetes Care.* 2002; 25:269–283.

Rosheim, KM, Fowles, JB. Where do people with diabetes obtain information about their disease? *Diabetes Spectrum.* 1999;12:136–140.

Roter DL, Hall JA, Merisca R, Nordstrom B, Cretin D, Svarstad B. Effectiveness of interventions to improve patient compliance: a meta-analysis. *Medical Care.* 1998;36:1138–1161.

Skinner TC, Cradock S, Arundel F, Graham W. Lifestyle and behavior: four theories and a philopshy: self-mangement education for individuals newly diagnosed with type 2 diabetes. *Diabetes Spectrum.* 2003;16:75–80.

Testa MA, Simonson DC. Health economic benefits and quality of life during improved glycemic control in patients with type 2 diabetes mellitus: a randomized, controlled, double-blind trial. *JAMA.* 1998;280:1490–1496.

Sarkisian CA, Brown AF, Norris CK, Wintz RL, Mangione CM. A systematic review of diabetes self-care interventions for older, African American or Latino adults. *The Diabetes Educator.* 2003;28:467–479.

PATIENT EDUCATION METHODS AND PROGRAMS *continued*

Satterfield D. Stories connect science to souls. *The Diabetes Educator.* 2002;27:176–19.

Sprague MA, Shultz JA, Branen LJ, Lambeth S, Hillers VN. Diabetes educators' perspectives on barriers for patients and educators in diabetes education. *The Diabetes Educator.* 1999; 25:907–916.

Thackery R, Neiger BL. Using social marketing to develop diabetes self-management education interventions. *The Diabetes Educator.* 2002; 28:536–544.

Walker EA. Characteristics of the adult learner. *The Diabetes Educator.* 1999;25(Suppl):16–24.

Weinger K. Group interventions: emerging applications for diabetes care. *Diabetes Spectrum.* 2003;16:86–112.

Whitlock WL, Brown A, Moore K, Pavliscak H, Dingbaum A, Lacefield D, Buker K, Xenakis S. Telemedicine improved diabetic management. *Military Medicine.* 2000;165:579–584.

Williams GC, Zeldman A. Patient-centered diabetes self-management education. *Current Medicine.* 2002;2:145–152.

Young-Hyman D. Provider impact in diabetes education. *The Diabetes Educator.* 1999; 25(Suppl):34–42.

PATIENT EDUCATION— EVALUATION AND EFFECTIVENESS

Anderson RM, Funnell MM: Theory is the cart, vision is the horse: reflections on research in diabetes patient education. *The Diabetes Educator* 1999;6(Suppl):43–51.

Bonomi AE, Wagner EH, Glasgow RE, VonKorff M. Assessment of chronic illness care (ACIC): a practical tool to measure quality improvement. *Health Services Research.* 2002;37(3):791–806.

Fitzgerald JT, Funnell MM, Hess GE, Barr PA, Anderson RM, Hiss RG, Davis WK: The

reliability and validity of a brief diabetes knowledge test. *Diabetes Care.* 1998;21:706–710.

Funnell MM, Anderson RM: Putting Humpty Dumpty back together again: reintegrating the clinical and behavioral components in diabetes care and education. *Diabetes Spectrum.* 1999;12:19–23.

Glasgow RE. A practical model of diabetes management and education. *Diabetes Care.* 1995;18:117–126.

Glasgow RE, Osteen VL. Evaluating diabetes education. *Diabetes Care.* 1992;15:1423–1432.

Glasgow RE. Outcomes of and for diabetes education research. *The Diabetes Educator.* 1999;25(Suppl):74–88.

Harris MA, Wysocki T, Adler M, Wilkinson K, Harvey LM, Buckloh LM, Mauras N, White NH. Validation of a structured interview for the assessment of diabetes self-management. *Diabetes Care.* 2000;23:1301–1304.

Mainous AG III, King DE, Hueston WJ, Gill JM, Pearson WS. The utility of a portable patient record for improving ongoing diabetes management. *The Diabetes Educator.* 2002;28:245–257.

Mulcahy K, Tomkey D, Peeples M, Weaver T. An educator guide to the Diabetes Outcomes Measurement System. *The Diabetes Educator.* 2001;27:830–848.

Mulcahy K, Peeples M, Tomky D, Weaver T. National Diabetes Education Outcomes System: application to practice. *The Diabetes Educator.* 2000;26:957–964.

Ovalle KB, Mullooly CA. DO IT: Diabetes outcomes for educational intervention and treatment. *The Diabetes Educator.* 1999;25:431.

Paddock LE, Veloski J, Chatterton ML, Gevritz FO, Nash DB. Development and validation of a questionnaire to evaluate patient satisfaction with diabetes disease management. *Diabetes Care.* 2000;23:951–956.

Peyrot M. Evaluation of patient education program: how to do it and how to use it. *Diabetes Spectrum.* 1996;9:86–93.

PATIENT EDUCATION—EVALUATION AND EFFECTIVENESS *continued*

Toobert DJ, Hampson SE, Glasgow RE. The summary of diabetes self-care activities measure. *Diabetes Care.* 2000;23:943–950.

COMPLIMENTARY AND ALTERNATIVE MEDICINE

Payne C, O'Connell BS. Complementary and integrative medicine: emerging therapies for diabetes, part 2. *Diabetes Spectrum.* 2001;14:196–226.

Roberts SS. Herbs and supplements. *Diabetes Forecast.* 2002;55(10):95–97.

Sabo CE, Michael SR, Temple LL. The use of alternative therapies by diabetes educators. *The Diabetes Educator.* 1999;25:945–956.

Shane-McWorter L, Geil P. Interactions between complementary therapies or nutrition supplements and conventional medications. *Diabetes Spectrum.* 2002;15:262–266.

Yeh GY, Eisenberg DM, Kaptchuk Tj, Phillips RS. Systematic review of herbs and dietary supplements for glycemic control in diabetes. *Diabetes Care.* 2003;26:1277–1295.

SPECIAL POPULATIONS: CHILDREN AND ADOLESCENTS

Almeida CM. Grief among parents of children with diabetes. *The Diabetes Educator.* 1995; 21:530–532.

American Diabetes Association. Consensus statement: management of dyslipidemia in children and adolescents with diabetes. *Diabetes Care.* 2003;26:3333–3341.

American Diabetes Association. Consensus Statement: type 2 diabetes in children. *Diabetes Care.* 2000;23:381–38.

American Diabetes Association. *The Take Charge Guide to Type 1 Diabetes.* Alexandria, VA: American Diabetes Association, 1996.

Bernstein G. Type 2 diabetes in children and adolescents. *Practical Diabetology.* 2000; 19(3):37–41.

Brackenridge BP, Rubin RR. *Sweet Kids: How to Balance Diabetes Control & Good Nutrition with Family Peace.* Alexandria, VA: American Diabetes Association, 1996.

Campbell RK. Marijuana and diabetes. *The Diabetes Educator.* 1985;11:54.

Clarke WL, Cox DJ, Gonder-Frederick LA, Kovatchev B. Hypoglycemia and driving. *Practical Diabetology.* 2002;21(2):20–23.

Coffman S. Community partnerships for parent-to-parent support. *The Diabetes Educator.* 2001;27:36–44.

Cook S, Aikens JE, Berrry CA, McNabb WL. Development of the diabetes problem-solving measure for adolescents. *The Diabetes Educator.* 2001;27:865–873.

Cook S, Solomon MC, Berrry CA. Nutrient intake of adolescents with diabetes. *The Diabetes Educator.* 2002;28:382–388.

Dickinson JK, O'Reilly MM. The lived experience of adolescent females with type 1 diabetes. *The Diabetes Educator.* 2004;30:99–107.

DuPasquier-Fediaevsky L, Tubiana-Rufi N, The PEDIAB Collaborative Group: Discordance between physician and adolescent assessments of adherence to treatment. *Diabetes Care.* 1999;22:1445–1449.

Frencher S, Soroudi N, Wylie-Rossett J, Alencherril J, Gandhi R, Sheren J, Alm M. Math curriculum: an innovative approach to address weight issues in children. *The Diabetes Educator.* 2003;29:248–252.

Gray M. Teaching teens to cope. *Practical Diabetology.* 2003;22(2):26–29.

Guthrie DW, Bartsocas C, Jarosz-Chabot P, Konstnantinova M. Psychosocial issues for children and adolescents with diabetes: Overview and recommendations. *Diabetes Spectrum.* 2003;16:7–12.

Haire-Joshu D, Nanney MS. Prevention of overweight and obesity in children: influences on the food environment. *The Diabetes Educator.* 2002;28:415–423.

SPECIAL POPULATIONS: CHILDREN AND ADOLESCENTS *continued*

Hanna KM, Guthrie D. Adolescents' behavioral autonomy related to diabetes management and adolescent activities/rules. *The Diabetes Educator.* 2003;29:283–291.

Hesketh KD, Wake MA, Cameron FJ. Health-related quality of life and metabolic control in children with type 1 diabetes. *Diabetes Care.* 2004;27:415–420.

Kaufman FR. What a child's health care team needs to know about federal disability law. *Diabetes Spectrum.* 2002;15:63–64.

Kadohiro JK. Diabetes and adolescents: from research to reality. *Diabetes Spectrum.* 2000;13:81–106.

Libman IM, Peitropaolo M, Araslanian SA, LaPorte RE, Becker DJ. Changing prevalence of weight in children and adolescents at onset of insulin-treated diabetes. *Diabetes Care.* 2003;26:2871–2875.

Loy S, Loy B. College bound. *Diabetes Forecast.* 2003;56(5):75–76.

Mellinger DC. Preparing students with diabetes for life at college. *Diabetes Care.* 2003; 26:2675–2678.

Mohn L: You take the wheel. *Diabetes Forecast.* 1996;49(12):26–29.

Nichols PJ, Norris SL. A systematic literature review of the effectiveness of diabetes education of school personnel. *The Diabetes Educator.* 2002;28:405–414.

Nordfeldt S, Ludvigsson JP: Severe hypoglycemia in children with IDDM. *Diabetes Care.* 1997; 20:497–503.

Plotnik LP, Clark LM, Brancati FL, Erlinger T. Safety and effectiveness of insulin pump therapy in children and adolescents with type 1 diabetes. *Diabetes Care.* 2003;26:1142–1147.

Roemer JB. Raising a baby with diabetes. *Diabetes Forecast.* 2003;56(12):64–68.

Schilling LS, Grey M, Knafl KA. A review of measures of self-management of type 1 diabetes by youth and their parents. *The Diabetes Educator.* 2002;28:796–808.

Siminerio L, Betschart J. *Guide to Raising A Child with Diabetes,* Second Edition. Alexandria, VA: American Diabetes Association; 2000.

Siminerio LM, Charron-Prochownik D, Vanion C, Schreiner B. Comparing outpatient and inpatient diabetes education for new diagnosed pediatric patients. *The Diabetes Educator.* 1999;25:895–906.

Siminerio LM. On kids, injections and maintaining trust. *Diabetes Forecast.* 1996;49(9):59–60.

Stenger PD. Grandparents stay in touch. *Diabetes Forecast.* 1995;48(12):49–52.

Thernlund GM, Dahlquist G, Hansson K, Ivarsson SA, Ludvigsson J, Sjoblad S, Hagglof B. Psychological stress and the onset of IDDM in children. *Diabetes Care.* 1995;18:1323–1329.

Touchett N. Kids and type 2. *Diabetes Forecast.* 2000;53(11):79–84.

Vetiska J, Glaab L, Perlamn K, Daneman D. School attendance of children with type 1 diabetes. *Diabetes Care.* 2000;23:1706–1707.

Wdowik MJ, Kendall PA, Harris MA, Kelm KS. Development and evaluation of an intervention program: "Control on Campus." *The Diabetes Educator.* 2000;26:95–104.

Weissberg J, Glasgow AM, Tynan WD, Wirtz P, Turek J, Ward J. Adolescent diabetes management and mismanagement. *Diabetes Care.* 1995; 18:77–82.

Wilson MA, Smith CB. Nutrient intake, glycemic control, and body mass index in adolescent using continuous subcutaneous insulin infusion and those using traditional insulin therapy. *The Diabetes Educator.* 2003;29:230–236.

Wiltshire EJ, Hirte C, Couper JJ. Dietary fats do not contribute to hyperlipidemia in children and adolescents with type 1 diabetes. *Diabetes Care.* 2003;26:1356–1361.

Wysocki T, Greco P, Harris MA, Bubb, J White NH. Behavior therapy for families of adolescents with diabetes. *Diabetes Care.* 2001;24:441–446.

SPECIAL POPULATIONS—CHILDREN AND ADOLESCENTS *continued*

Wysocki T, Harris MA, Mauras N, Fox L, Taylor A et al. Absence of adverse effects of severe hypoglycemia on cognitive function is school-aged children with diabetes over 18 months. *Diabetes Care.* 2003;26:1100–1105.

Wysocki T, Harris MA, Wilkinson K, Sadler M, Mauras N, White NH. Self-management competence as a predictor of outcomes of intensive therapy or usual care in youth with type 1 diabetes. *Diabetes Care.* 2003;26:2043–2047.

Wysocki T: *The Ten Keys to Helping Your Child Grow Up with Diabetes.* Alexandria, VA: American Diabetes Association, 1998.

SPECIAL POPULATIONS: CULTURAL CONCERNS

AADE Position Statement. Cultural sensitivity: definition, application, and recommendations for diabetes educators. *The Diabetes Educator.* 2002;28:922–927.

Ahmed AM, Jaber LA. Islamic pilgrimage. *Practical Diabetology.* 2003;22(2):41–43.

Ahmed AM. Ramadan fasting. *Practical Diabetology.* 2001;20(3):7–11.

Anderson LA, Janes GR, Ziemer DC, Phillips LS: Diabetes in urban African Americans: body image, satisfaction with size, and weight change attempts. *The Diabetes Educator.* 1997;23:294–300.

Anderson-Loftin W, Barnett S, Sullivan P, Bunn PS, Tavakoli A. Culturally competent dietary education for southern rural African Americans with diabetes. *The Diabetes Educator.* 2002;28:245–257.

Anderson RM, Barr PA, Edwards GJ, Funnell MM, Fitzgerald JT, Wisdom K. Using focus groups to identify psychosocial issues of urban black individuals with diabetes. *The Diabetes Educator.* 1996;22:28–33.

Anderson RM, Funnell MM, Arnold MS, Barr PA, Edwards GJ, Fitzgerald TJ. Assessing the cultural relevance of an education program for

Urban African Americans with diabetes. *The Diabetes Educator.* 2000;26:280–289.

Anderson RM, Herman WH, Davis JM, Freedman RP, Funnell MM, Neighbors HW. Barriers to improving diabetes care for blacks. *Diabetes Care.* 1991;14:605–609.

Blanchard MA, Rose LE, Taylor J, McEntee MA, Latchaw LL. Using a focus group to design a diabetes education program for an African American population. *The Diabetes Educator.* 1999;25:917–924.

Brown SA, Garcia AA, Kouzekanani K, Hanis CL. Culturally competent diabetes self-management education for Mexican Americans. *Diabetes Care.* 2002;25:259–267.

Brown SA. Gender and treatment differences in knowledge, health beliefs, and metabolic control in Mexican Americans with type 2 diabetes. *The Diabetes Educator.* 2000;26:425–438.

Burke DJ. Diabetes education for the Native American population. *The Diabetes Educator.* 2001;27:181–196.

Burnet D, Plaut A, Courtney R, Chin MH. A practical model for preventing type 2 diabetes in minority youth. *The Diabetes Educator.* 2002; 28:779–795.

Cook CB, Erdman, DM, Tyan GJ, Greenlunnd, KJ, Giles, WH et al. The pattern of dyslipidemia among urban African-Americans with type 2 diabetes. *Diabetes Care.* 2000;23:319–324.

Cook CB, Zeimer DC, El-Kebbi IM, Gallina DL, Dunbar VG, Ernst KL, Phillips LS: Diabetes in urban African-Americans: overcoming clinical inertia improves glycemic control in patients with type 2 diabetes. *Diabetes Care.* 1999;22:1494–1500.

Edwards GJ, Coleman-Burns P: A culturally sensitive approach to patient care. *Practical Diabetology.* 1996;15(3):4–9.

Egede LE, Bonadonna RJ. Diabetes self-management in African Americans: An exploration of the role of fatalism. *The Diabetes Educator.* 2003;29:105–115.

SPECIAL POPULATIONS: CULTURAL CONCERNS *continued*

Epple C, Wright Al, Joish VN, Bauer M. the role of active family nutritional support in Navajors' type 2 diabetes metabolic control. *Diabetes Care*. 2003;26:2829–2834.

Fisher, L, Chesla, CA, Skaff MM, Gilliss C, Mullan et al. The family and disease management in Hispanic and European-American patients with type 2 diabetes. *Diabetes Care*. 2000;23:267–272.

Fitzgerald JT, Anderson RA, Funnell MM, Arnold MS, Davis WK, Aman LC, Jacober SJ, Grunberger: Differences in the impact of dietary restrictions on African Americans and Caucasians with NIDDM. *The Diabetes Educator*. 1997;23:41–47.

Fitzgerald JT, Gruppen LD, Anderson RA, Funnell MM, Jacober SJ, Grunberger G, Aman LC. The influence of treatment modality and ethnicity on attitudes in type 2 diabetes. *Diabetes Care*. 2000;23:313–318.

Gary et al. Depressive symptoms and metabolic control in African Americans with type 2 diabetes. *Diabetes Care*. 2000;23:23–29.

Harris MI. Racial and ethnic differences in health care access and health outcomes for adults with type 2 diabetes. *Diabetes Care*. 2001;24:454–459.

Hogue VW, Babamoto KS, Jackson TB, Cohen LB, Laitinen DL. Pooled results of community pharmacy-based diabetes education programs in unerserved communities. *Diabetes Spectrum*. 2003;16:129–133.

Hu D, Henderson JA, Welty Tk, Lee ET, Jablonski KA, Magee MF, Robbins DC, Howard BV. Glycenic control in diabetic American Indians: Longitudinal data from the Strong Heart Study. *Diabetes Care*. 1999; 22:1802–1807.

Hughes HE. Love A. Peabody K, Kardong-Edgren S. Diabetes education programs for African-American women: What works? . The *Diabetes Educator*. 2001;27:46–54.

Jaber LA, Brown MB, Hammad A, Nowak SN, Zhu Q et al. Epidemiology of diabetes among Arab Americans. *Diabetes Care*. 2003;26:308–313.

Jaber LA, Brown MB, Hammad A, Zhu Q, Herman WH. Lack of acculturation is a risk factor for diabetes in Arab immigrants in the US. *Diabetes Care*. 2003;26:2010–2014.

Jaber LA, Slaughter RL, Grunberger G. Diabetes and related metabolic risk factors among Arab Americans. *The Annals of Pharmacotherapy*. 1995;29:573–577.

Jayne RL, Rankin SH.L Application of Leventhal's self-regulation model to Chinese immigrants with type 2 diabetes. *Image*. 2001;33:53–56.

Jefferson VQ, Melkus DG, Spollett GR. Health-promotion practices of young black women at risk for diabetes. *The Diabetes Educator*. 2000; 26:295–302.

Kulkarni K: Nutrition counseling for Indian and Pakistani patients. *Practical Diabetology*. 1996;15(2):19–20.

Magnus MH. What's your IQ on cross-cultural nutrition counseling? *The Diabetes Educator*. 1996;22:57–62.

Maillet NA, D'Eramo-Melkus G, Spollett G. Using focus groups to characterize the health beliefs and practices of black women with non-insulin-dependent diabetes. *The Diabetes Educator*. 1996;22:39–46.

McBean ZM, Huang Z, Virnig BA, Lurie N, Musgrave D. Racial variation in the control diabetes among elderly medicare mangeed care beneficiaries. *Diabetes Care*. 2003 26:3250–3256.

Montague MC. Identifying and treating African-Americans with diabetes and low health literacy. *Practical Diabetology*. 2002;21(4):7–13.

Philis-Tsimikas A, Walker C, Rivard L, Talavera G, Reimann JOF, Salmon M, Araujo R. Improvement in diabertes care of underinsured patients enrolled in Project Dulce: A community-based, culturally appropriate, nurse case

SPECIAL POPULATIONS: CULTURAL CONCERNS *continued*

management and peer education diabetes care model. *Diabetes Care.* 2004;27:110–115.

Pichert JW, Briscoe VJ: A questionnaire for assessing barriers to healthcare utilization, Part I. *The Diabetes Educator.* 1997;23:181, 183-184, 187-188, 190–191.

Pichert JW, Briscoe VJ: Strategies for over-coming barriers to healthcare utilization, Part II. *The Diabetes Educator.* 1997; 23:251–252, 255–256.

Quinn MT, Cook S, Nash K, Chin MH. Addressing religion and spirituality in African Americans with diabetes. *The Diabetes Educator.* 2001;27:643–655.

Quinn MT, McNabb WEL. Training lay health educators to conduct a church-based weight-loss program for African American women. *The Diabetes Educator.* 2001;27:231–237.

Rankin SH, Galbraith ME, Huang P: Quality of life and social environment as reported by Chinese immigrants with non-insulin-dependent diabetes mellitus. *The Diabetes Educator.* 1997;23:171–177.

Robideaux YD, Moore, K, Avery C, Muneta, B, Knight M, Buchwald D. Diabetes education materials: Recommendations of tribal leaders, Indian health professionals and American Indian community members. *The Diabetes Educator.* 2000;26:290–294.

Sabo LD, Davis SM: Native American diabetes project: designing culturally relevant education materials. *The Diabetes Educator.* 1997; 23:133–134, 139.

Samuel-Hodge CD, Headen SW, Skelly AH, Ingram AF, Keyserling TC, Jackson EJ, Ammerman AS, Elasy TA. Influences on day-to-day self-management of type 2 diabetes among African-American women. *Diabetes Care.* 2000; 23:928–933.

Schorling JB, Saunders JT. Is "sugar" the same as diabetes? A community-based study among rural African-Americans. *Diabetes Care.* 2000; 23:330–334.

Skelly AH, Smauel-Hodge C, Elasy T, Ammerman AS, Headen SW, Keyserling TC. Development and testing of culturally sensitive instruments for African American women with type 2 diabetes. *The Diabetes Educator.* 2000; 26:769–777.

Stamler LL. Developing and refining the research question: Step 1 in the research process. *The Diabetes Educator.* 2002;28:958–962.

Thaler, LM, Ziemer, DC, El-kebbi, IM, Gallina, DL, Cook, CB, Phillips LS. Diabetes in Urban African-Americans. XIX. Prediction of the need for pharmacological therapy. *Diabetes Care.* 2000;23:820–825.

Thaler, LM, Ziemer, DC, Gallina, DL, Cook, CB, Dunbar, VG, Phillips, LS, El-kebbi, IM. Diabetes in Urban African-Americans. XVII. Availability of rapid HbA1C measurements enhances clinical decision-making. *Diabetes Care.* 1999; 22:1415–1421.

Trevino RP, Marshall RM Jr., Hale DE, Rodriguez R, Baker G, Gomez J. Diabetes risk factors in low-income Mexian-American children. *Diabetes Care.* 1999;22:202–207.

Van Goeler DS, Rosal MC, Ockene JK, Scavron J, de Torrijos F. Self-management of type 2 diabetes: A survey of low-income urban Puerto Ricans. *The Diabetes Educator.* 2003;29:663–672.

Wang C-Y, Abbott L, Goodbody AK, Hui W-TY, Rausch C. Development of a community-based diabetes management program for pacific Islanders. *The Diabetes Educator.* 1999; 25:738–746.

Wing RR, Anglin K. Effectiveness of a behavioral weight control program for blacks and whites with NIDDM. *Diabetes Care.* 1996;19: 409–412.

SPECIAL POPULATIONS: LOW LITERACY

Gazmaraian JA, Baker DW, Williams MV, Parker RM, Scott TL, Green DC, et al. Health literacy among Medicare enrollees in a

SPECIAL POPULATIONS: LOW LITERACY *continued*

managed care organization. *JAMA*. 1999; 6:545–550.

Health Literacy. Report on the Council on Scientific Affairs. *JAMA*. 1999;281:552–556.

Kuklierus A, Mayer G. Using low literacy writing and formatting techniques to make health care materials more effective for patients. *Managed Care Advisor Newsletter:* July 21, 2001.

Mayer GG, Rushton N. Writing easy to read teaching aids. *Nursing*. 2002;32(3):48–49.

Nath CR, Sylvester ST, Yasek V, Gunel E. Development and validation of a literacy assessment tool for persons with diabetes. *The Diabetes Educator*. 2001;27:857–864.

Schillinger D, Piette J, Grumbach K, Wang F, Wilson C, Daher C, Leon-Grotz K, Castro C, Bindman AB. Physician communication with diabetic patients who have low health literacy. *Archives of Internal Medicine*. 2003;63:83–90.

Schillinger D, Grumbach K, Piette J, Wang F, Osmond D, Daher C, et al. Association of health literacy with diabetes outcomes. *JAMA*. 2002; 288:475–482.

Stanley K. Low-literacy materials for diabetes nutrition education. *Practical Diabetology*. 1999; 18(2):36–44.

SPECIAL POPULATIONS: OLDER ADULTS

Ahroni JH. Strategies for teaching elders from a human development perspective. *The Diabetes Educator*. 1996;22:47–53.

American Association of Diabetes Educators. Special considerations for the education and management of older adults with diabetes. *The Diabetes Educator*. 2003;29:93–96.

Asimakopoulou K, Hampson SE. Cognitive functioning and self-management in older people with diabetes. *Diabetes Spectrum*. 2002; 15:116–121.

Brown JB, Nichols GA, Glauber HS, Bakst AW. Type 2 diabetes: incremental medical care costs

during the first 8 years after diagnosis. *Diabetes Care*. 1999;22:1116–1124.

California Healthcare Foundation/American Geriatrics Society Panel on Improving Care for Elders with Diabetes. Guidelines for Improving the Care of Older Person with Diabetes Mellitus. *Journal of the American Geriatrics Society*. 51:S265–S280; 2003.

Chau DL, Edelman SV. Osteoporosis and diabetes. *Clinical Diabetes*. 2002;20:153–157.

D'Arrigo T. Diabetes and aging. *Diabetes Forecast*. 2001;54(2):54–58.

Deakins DA. Teaching elderly patients about diabetes. *American Journal of Nursing*. 1994; 94:38–42.

De Rekeneire N, Resnick HE, Schwartz AV, Shorr RI, Kuller LH, Simonsick EM, Vellas B, Harris TB. Diabetes is associated with subclinical functional imitation in nondisabled older individuals. *Diabetes Care*. 2003; 26:3257–3263.

Dye CJ, Haley-Zitlin V, Willoughby D. Insights from older adults with type 2 diabetes: Making dietary and exercise changes. *The Diabetes Educator*. 2003;29:116–127.

Ehmann K. Over sixty and newly diagnosed. *Diabetes Forecast*. 1995;48(5):34–39.

Fielo SB. The mystery of sleep: How nurses can help the elderly. *Nursing Profile*. 2001; February:10–14.

Finkelstein EA, Bray JW, Chen H, Larson MJ et al. Prevalence and costs of major depression among elderly claimants with diabetes. *Diabetes Care*. 2003;26:415–420.

Gilden JL: Nutrition and the older diabetic. *Clinics in Geriatric Medicine*. 1999;15:371–390.

Good CB. Polypharmacy in elderly patients with diabetes. *Diabetes Spectrum*. 2002; 15:240–248.

Gregg EW, Engelgau MM, Narayan V. Complications of diabetes in elderly people. *BMJ*. 2002;325:916–917.

SPECIAL POPULATIONS: OLDER ADULTS *continued*

Gregg EW, Mangion CM, Cauley JA, Thompson TJ, Schwartz AV et al. Diabetes and incidence of functional disability in older women. *Diabetes Care.* 2002;25:61–67.

Katajura M, Naka M, Kondo T, Nishii N et al. Prospective analysis of mortality, morbidity, and risk factors in elderly diabetic subjects. *Diabetes Care.* 2003;26:638–644.

Morley JE, Coe RM: Advances in the care of older people with diabetes. *Clinics in Geriatric Medicine.* 1999;15:211–423.

Parker MT, Leggett-Frazier N, Vincent PA, Swanson MS. The impact of an educational program on improving diabetes knowledge and changing behaviors of nurses in long-term care facilities. *The Diabetes Educator.* 1995;21: 541–546.

Piette JD, Heisler M, Wagner TH. Problems paying out of pocket medication costs among older adults with diabetes. *Diabetes Care.* 2004; 27:384–391.

Resnick HE, Vinik AI, Schwartz AV, Leveille SG, Brancati FL, Balfour J, Guralnik JM. Independent effects of peripheral nerve dysfunction on lower-extremity physical function in old age. *Diabetes Care.* 2000;23:1642–1647.

Roberts SS. Senior care. *Diabetes Forecast.* 2003;56(6):42–44.

Schwartz AV, et al. Older women with diabetes have a higher risk of falls. *Diabetes Care.* 2002; 25:1749–1754.

Schwartz et al. Older women with diabetes have an increased risk of fracture: A prospective study. *J Clinical Endocrinology and Metabolism.* 2001;86:32–38.

Sinclair AJ, Gadsby R, Penfold S, Croxson SCM, Bayer AJ. Prevalence of diabetes in care home residents. *Diabetes Care.* 2001;24:1066–1068.

Urban AD, Rearson MA, Murphy K. The diabetes center home care nurse: an integral part of the diabetes team. *The Diabetes Educator.* 1998;24:608–611.

Weisberg-Benchell J, Pichert JW. Counseling techniques for clinicians and educators. *Diabetes Spectrum.* 1999;12:2103–107.12–245

Willey KA, Singh MAF. Battling insulin resistance in elderly obese people with type 2 diabetes. *Diabetes Care.* 2003;26:1580–1588.

SPECIAL POPULATIONS: PRISONERS WITH DIABETES

American Diabetes Association. Position statement: management of diabetes in correctional institutions. *Diabetes Care.* 2004;27(Suppl. 1): S114–S121.

Steinberg C. Diabetes behind bars. *Diabetes Forecast.* 1995;48(9):20–25.

HEALTH CARE SYSTEM ISSUES FOR DIABETES EDUCATION

Barnes CS, Ziemer DC, Miller CD, Coyle JP, Wakins C Jr, Cook CB, Gallina DL, El-Kebbi I, Banch WT, Jr, Phillips LS. Little time for diabetes management in the primary care setting. *The Diabetes Educator.* 2004;30:126–135.

Chin MH, Cook S, Drum ML, Jin M, Guillen CA, Humikowski AC, Koppert J, Harrison JF, Lippold S, Schaefer CT. Improving diabetes care in Midwest community health centers with the health disparities collaborative. *Diabetes Care.* 2004;27:2–9.

Clancy DE, Cope DW, Magruder KM, Huang P, Salter KH, Fields AW. Evaluating group visits in an uninsured or inadequately insured patient population with uncontrolled type 2 diabetes. *The Diabetes Educator.* 2003;29:292–302.

Fain JA. Protecting patients' health information: Overview of the health insurance Portability and Accountability act. *The Diabetes Educator.* 2003;29:186.

Fleming BB, Greenfield S, Engelgau MM, Pagach LM et al. The Diabetes Quality

HEALTH CARE SYSTEM ISSUES FOR DIABETES EDUCATION *continued*

Improvement project. *Diabetes Care*. 2001; 24:1815–1820.

Funnell MM, Anderson RM. Changing office practice and health care systems to facilitate diabetes self-management. *Current Diabetes Reports*. 2003;3:127–133.

Glasgow RE, Orleans CT, Wagner EH. Does the chronic care model serve also as a template for improving prevention? *The Milbank Quarterly*. 2001;79:579–612.

Graber AL, Elasy TA, Quinn D, Wolff K, Brown A. Improving glycemic control in adults with diabetes mellitus: Shared responsibility in primary care practices. *Southern Medical Journal*. 2002;95:684–690.

Herman WH. Evidence-based diabetes care. *Clinical Diabetes*. 2002;20:22–24.

McDiarmid T, Chambliss ML, Koval PB, Houck S. Improving office-based preventive care for diabetes. *NCMJ*. 2001;62:813.

Meigs JB, Cagliero E, Dubey A, Murphy-Sheehy P, Gildesgame C et al. A controlled trial of web-based diabetes disease management. *Diabetes Care*. 2003;26:750–757.

Montori VM, Dineen Sf, Gorman CA, Zimmerman BR, Rissa RA et al. The imipact of planned care and a diabetes electronic management system on community-based diabetes care. *Diabetes Care*. 2002; 25:1952–1957.

Renders CM, Valk GD, Griffin SJ, Wagner EH, et al. Interventions to improve the management of diabetes mellitus in primary care, outpatient, and community settings (Cochrane Review). In: *The Cochrane Library*, Issue 3, 2002.

Renders CM, Valk GD, Griffin SJ, Wagner EH, et al. Interventions to improve the management of diabetes in primary care, outpatient, and community settings: A systematic review. *Diabetes Care*. 2001;24:1821–1833.

Tabei BP, Burke R, Constance A, Hare J, et al. Community-based screening for diabetes in Michigan. *Diabetes Care*. 2003;26:668–670.

Taylor CB, Miller NH, Reilly KR, Greenwald G et al. Evaluation of a nurse-care management system to improve outcomes in patients with complicated diabetes. *Diabetes Care*. 2003; 26:1058–1063.

Trento M, Passera P, Borgo E, Tomalino M, Bajardi M, Cavallo F, Porta M. A 5-year randomized controlled study of learning, problem solving ability and quality of life modification in people with type 2 diabetes managed by group care. *Diabetes Care*. 2004; 27:670–675.

Trento M, Passera P, Tomalino M, Bajardi M, Pomero F, Allione A, Vaccari P, Molinatti GM, Porta M. Group visits improve metabolic control in type 2 diabetes. *Diabetes Care*. 2001;24:995–1000.

Wagner EH, Glasgow RE, Davis C, Bonomi AE, Provost L, McCulloch D, Carver P, Sixta C. Quality improvement in chronic illness care: A collaborative approach. *Journal on Quality Improvement*. 2001;27:63–80

Wagner EH, Groves T. Care for chronic diseases. *BMJ*. 2002;325:913–914.

Wagner EH. The role of patient care teams in chronic disease management. *BMJ*. 2000; 350:569–572.

Wasson JH, Godfre MM, Nelson EC, Mphr JJ, Batalden PB. Microsystems in health care: Planning patient-centered care. *Joint Commission Journal of Quality and Safety*. 2003;29:227–237.

Yawn B, Zyzansky SJ, Goodwin MA, Gotler RS, Stange KC. Is diabetes treated as an acute or chronic illness in community family practice? *Diabetes Care*. 2001;24:1390–96.

PROFESSIONAL ISSUES FOR DIABETES EDUCATORS

Balz JC. Office-based diabetes educators. The *Diabetes Educator*. 2004;30:40–42.

Brown AW, Wolff KL, Elasy TA, Graber AL. The role of the advanced practice nurses in shared

PROFESSIONAL ISSUES FOR DIABETES EDUCATORS *continued*

care diabetes practice model. *The Diabetes Educator*. 2001;492–502.

Burson R. The advanced practice diabetes educator. *The Diabetes Educator*. 2002; 28:182–184.

Daly A. Advanced practice care in diabetes. *Diabetes Spectrum*. 2003;16:24–26; *The Diabetes Educator*. 2003;29:592–594.

Hinnen D. Why should I take one more exam? *Diabetes Spectrum*. 2002;15:140.

Jones PM, Clark LL. Developing education materials for teaching diabetes standards of care to home care nurses. *The Diabetes Educator*. 2002;28:712–728.

Lenz ER, Mundinger MO, Hopkins SC, Lin SX, Smolowitz J. Diabetes care processes and outcomes in patients treated by nurse practitioners or physicians. *The Diabetes Educator*. 2002;28:590–598.

Metzger SM. Parish nursing: Integrating body, mind and spirit. *Nursing*. 2000;30(12):64–65.

Spollett GR. Ten tips for becoming a Certified Diabetes Educator. *The Diabetes Educator*. 2001; 27:657–660.

Valetine V, Kulkarni K, Hinnen D. Evolving roles: From diabetes educators to advanced diabetes managers. *Diabetes Spectrum*. 2003;16:27–31; *The Diabetes Educator*. 2003;29:598–610.

Wagner EH. More than a case manager. *Annals of Internal Medicine*. 1998;129:654–655.

Zriebec J. A national job analysis of Certified Diabetes Educators by the National Certification Board for Diabetes Educators. *The Diabetes Educator*. 2001;27:694–702.

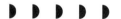

The following pamphlets are part of *The ADA Channel* Series, a low-literacy education resource for patients. They can be ordered in lots of 50 by calling the American Diabetes Association at 800-232-6733 or by visiting the online bookstore at http://store.diabetes.org

A Guide For Adults With Type 1 Diabetes

Diabetes care, including insulin, eating, activity and monitoring. Available in Spanish.

A Guide For Adults With Type 2 Diabetes

The differences between type 1 and type 2 diabetes, and caring for type 2 diabetes with meal planning, activity, and taking diabetes medicines (if needed). Available in Spanish.

A Guide To Eating and Diabetes

Basic diabetes meal planning using "Rate Your Plate" and simple carb counting. Available in Spanish.

A Guide To Factors Affecting Blood Sugar

Ways to figure out what makes blood sugar levels go up or down. Available in Spanish.

A Guide To Checking Your Blood Sugar

The importance of keeping blood sugar levels in the target range using blood sugar checks (a snapshot of your blood sugar level at that moment) and the hemoglobin A1C (a blood sugar check "with memory"). Available in Spanish.

A Guide For You and Your Diabetes Care Team

Who's on the diabetes team (the person with diabetes, family, friends, and the diabetes health care team) and the roles they each play. Available in Spanish.

A Guide To Changing Habits

Choosing and setting goals and making changes using "Let's Make a Plan." Available in Spanish.

A Guide To Emotions and Diabetes

Diabetes, feeling sad and blue, serious depression, and when and how to get help. Available in Spanish.

A Guide to the ADA Standards of Care

The ADA Standards of Care and how to use them to improve diabetes care and reduce the risk of diabetes complications. Available in Spanish.

All About Food Myths and Diabetes

Information about how to include sugars, carbohydrates, and favorite foods in meal plans; also, food myths and popular diets. Available in Spanish.

A Guide to Type 2 Diabetes and Exercise

Ways to become more active and how physical activity helps to look and feel your best.

Treating Type 2 Diabetes for Life

The many ways to treat type 2 diabetes throughout the life span.

A Guide to Long Term Complications

Helpful information about how to prevent, delay, or detect diabetes complications.

A Guide to Taking Care of Your Feet

Information on how to protect and care for your feet (checking your feet daily, buying shoes that fit well, using a monofilament, and having foot exams).

A Guide for Women With Diabetes

How diabetes can affect pregnancy, and sexual health throughout the life cycle.

A Guide For Men With Diabetes

How diabetes can affect men's sexual health.

Are You Ready to Quit Smoking?

Strategies to stop smoking.

A Guide to Intensive Management and Type 1 Diabetes

The advantages, disadvantages and how-tos of intensive management (taking insulin 3 or 4 times a day using a syringe, insulin pen, or a pump) to help you decide if it's right for you.

A Guide for Coping with Stress and Diabetes

Information on how feeling stressed can affect your blood sugar levels and ways to manage stress in your life.

Someone You Love Has Diabetes

Information on what it means to care for someone with diabetes.

Are You Ready to Lose Weight?

The benefits of losing weight and gives tips on doing it.

A Guide for Older Adults with Diabetes

Information targeted to the older adult who is dealing with diabetes care and other issues of growing older.

Make the Link! Diabetes, Heart Disease and Stroke

The higher risk of a heart attack or stroke with diabetes, and how you can help lower your risk by keeping your ABCs of diabetes on target. Available in Spanish.

Sample Educational Objectives

▶ ▶ ▶ ▶ ▶

The following sample illustrates how one program cross-referenced their educational objectives to the curriculum content of *Life with Diabetes*. This documentation is not a requirement for programs applying for Recognition. For Recognition requirements, please visit www.diabetes.org/recognition/ education or call 1-800-DIABETES.

Learning and Skill Objectives	Outline
A. Overview/Understanding of Diabetes	
1. States:	1
a. excess glucose in blood due to too little insulin in relationship to body needs.	
b. lifelong condition requiring treatment.	
c. which type of diabetes they have.	
B. Stress and Psychosocial Adjustment	
1. Identifies self as having diabetes.	2
2. Identifies thoughts, feelings, and areas of concern about diabetes.	
3. Identifies personal meaning of diabetes.	
4. Identifies effects of stress on blood glucose.	12
5. Identifies one strategy for coping with stress/feelings related to diabetes.	
6. Identifies signs and symptoms of depression.	
7. Identifies personal diabetes care goals.	15
C. Family and Social Support	
1. Identifies desired level of support from family/friends.	2
2. Informs others of ways they can be supportive.	

Learning and Skill Objectives	Outline
3. Identifies local sources for diabetes support.	16
D. Nutrition and Meal Planning	
1. States:	3
a. reasons for meal planning.	
b. rationale for eating meals on time.	
c. rationale for eating bedtime snack.	
d. rationale for reaching/maintaining desirable weight.	3, 17
e. rationale for eating less fat.	3, 18
f. awareness of types of fat and effects of each.	18
g. awareness of need to change diet with activity changes.	3, 7
2. Has a meal plan.	5
3. Is able to:	
a. describe personal meal plan.	5, 19
b. use meal plan to plan meals.	5, 19, 20, 21
c. use meal plan when eating away from home.	
d. identify behaviors that help control weight.	17
e. identify eating behaviors that help reduce risk of heart disease.	18
f. plan a sick-day diet.	11
g. explain how alcohol affects blood glucose.	

Learning and Skill Objectives	Outline
h. use product labels to choose foods that fit meal plan.	6
i. explain the benefits and cautions of a high-fiber diet.	18
j. plan eating/behavior changes that work toward personal goals.	15
k. calculate exchange values from a recipe or a product label nutrition panel.	22
4. Referral to a dietitian.	3
E. Exercise and Activity	
1. States that exercise/activity lowers blood glucose.	7
2. Identifies personal exercise plan.	
3. Identifies when not to exercise.	
4. Describes exercise snack, if needed.	11
5. Identifies insulin adjustment for exercise if needed.	
6. Identifies monitoring needed for exercise.	
F. Medication	
■ ORAL HYPOGLYCEMIC AGENTS	
1. States:	8
a. name and dose of agent.	
b. when to take.	
c. effect on blood glucose.	
d. side effects.	
e. precautions	
■ INSULIN	
1. States:	9
a. type(s) and dose to take.	
b. when to take.	
c. onset, peak, and duration.	
d. effect on blood glucose.	
e. when low blood glucose is most likely to occur.	11
f. insulin adjustment plan.	
g. how to store insulin.	9

Learning and Skill Objectives	Outline
2. Prepares and administers own insulin correctly.	
a. gently rolls insulin to mix.	
b. injects air into bottle.	
c. checks for/removes bubbles.	
d. draws up correct dose.	
e. disposes of syringes/lancets correctly.	
3. Selects appropriate injection site.	
a. selects suitable sub-Q tissue.	
b. states rotation plan.	
4. If using intensive therapy, states:	9
a. benefits of intensive therapy.	
b. type of insulin that affects specific blood glucose levels.	
c. need for frequent blood glucose testing.	
d. personal insulin plan and blood glucose goals.	
G. Monitoring and Use of Results	
■ BLOOD GLUCOSE	
1. Demonstrates ability to test blood glucose.	10
a. uses appropriate site to obtain blood samples.	
b. uses correct testing technique.	
c. accurately tests blood glucose.	
d. cares for meter and stores strips properly.	
2. States:	
a. need for monitoring.	
b. plan for monitoring blood glucose and record keeping at home.	
c. that normal blood glucose is 70–115 mg/dl.	
d. personal goal or target range.	
e. appropriate decisions to make about glucose regulation based on results.	11
f. where to obtain glucose meters and supplies.	10

Learning and Skill Objectives	Outline
3. Defines A1C.	
a. states normal value.	
b. states personal goal.	
■ **URINE KETONE TESTING**	
1. States purpose of urine ketone testing.	10
2. Tests urine ketones:	
a. if blood glucose >300 mg/dl.	
b. if ill or unable to eat.	
c. as otherwise prescribed.	
3. Interprets test results correctly.	
4. States proper action to take for ketonuria.	
5. Stores strips properly.	
H. Regulating Blood Glucose	
■ **GLUCOSE CONTROL RELATIONSHIPS**	
1. Identifies factors that influence blood glucose levels.	11
2. Identifies personal behaviors that influence blood glucose levels.	
a. relationship of food intake to blood glucose.	4, 11
b. relationship of diabetes medications to blood glucose.	8, 9, 11
c. relationship of exercise to blood glucose.	7, 11
3. States benefits of improved glucose control.	11, 14
4. States risks of improved glucose control.	11
5. Identifies treatment methods to improve glucose control.	
■ **HYPOGLYCEMIA**	
1. States:	11
a. meaning and other names.	
b. personal/common symptoms.	
1) occurring while awake.	
2) occurring while asleep.	
c. causes and how to prevent.	

Learning and Skill Objectives	Outline
d. when to contact health professional.	
e. proper action to be taken to treat hypoglycemia.	
2. Family member/roommate is able to give glucagon.	
3. Wears/carries diabetes identification.	
■ **HYPERGLYCEMIA**	
1. States:	11
a. meaning and other names.	
b. personal common symptoms.	
c. causes and how to prevent.	
d. states proper action to take and when to contact provider.	
e. relationship of ketoacidosis to high blood glucose.	
I. Personal Health Habits	
1. States:	13
a. body areas most susceptible to infection.	
b. signs/symptoms of infection and treatment measures.	
c. effects of smoking on circulation.	
d. need for foot care.	
e. plan for personal foot care.	
f. need for skin care.	
g. plan for personal skin care.	
h. need for regular dental care.	
i. benefits of regular medical care.	
J. Long-Term Complications	
1. States:	14
a. awareness of potential long-term complications and target organs.	
1) cardiovascular.	
2) peripheral vascular.	
3) sensory neuropathy.	
4) autonomic neuropathy.	
5) retinopathy.	
6) nephropathy.	

Learning and Skill Objectives	Outline
b. symptoms indicating onset of complications and importance of early diagnosis.	
c. ways to prevent, delay, or detect complications.	
d. common diabetes-related sexual concerns, dysfunctions, and treatment methods.	23
K. Problem-Solving and Behavior Change	
1. Identifies problem-solving strategies.	15
2. Identifies personal long-term diabetes care goals.	
3. Identifies personal short-term diabetes care goals.	
4. Identifies personal behavior-change goals.	
5. Identifies strategies to achieve goals.	
L. Health Care Systems	
1. States importance of plans for regular health monitoring.	13
a. diabetes management.	
b. ophthalmological exams.	
c. dental care.	
d. regular physical exams.	
e. other as indicated.	
2. Identifies personal risk factors for complications/health problems.	14
3. States how to obtain driver's license and insurance, and employment rights.	16
4. States awareness of community resources.	16
5. States name(s) and phone number(s) of health professional(s) to contact.	
a. stop smoking.	
b. weight control program.	
c. social worker.	
d. visiting nurse/home health.	
e. dietitian.	

Learning and Skill Objectives	Outline
f. diabetes support group.	
g. education program.	
h. other.	
M. Pregnancy	
1. Preconception.	
a. states importance of normal blood glucose levels before pregnancy.	9
b. states need for thorough medical exam before pregnancy.	
2. Preexisting diabetes.	
a. identifies importance of frequent care for changing insulin/dietary needs.	
3. Gestational diabetes.	
a. defines as hyperglycemia related to hormonal changes during pregnancy.	
b. states importance of follow-up care after delivery.	
4. Blood glucose control.	
a. states need to maintain glucose levels in the target range throughout pregnancy.	
b. lists symptoms of hyperglycemia and when to call a physician.	
c. states symptoms of hypoglycemia and how to treat.	
5. Prenatal care.	
a. lists danger signs during pregnancy; when to call a physician.	
b. identifies tests to monitor health of mother and infant.	
N. Pump Therapy	
1. States:	25
a. correct name of pump used.	
b. correct type of insulin used.	
c. advantages/disadvantages of pump therapy.	

Learning and Skill Objectives	Outline
d. definition of *basal* and *bolus*; how they relate to normal body physiology.	
e. that bolus insulin is given intermittently throughout the day based on:	
1) meals.	
2) blood glucose levels at time bolus is given.	
3) glucose values out of target range other than at meal times.	
f. how pump will affect lifestyle.	
g. proper equipment to be used.	
h. how often to change equipment.	
i. signs/symptoms/treatment of irritation/inflammation/infection.	
j. what to do with the pump for the following activities: sleeping, sexual activities, bathing, swimming, sports, traveling.	
k. awareness of alarms and how to handle.	
l. hotline phone number for appropriate company.	
m. how to obtain pump supplies.	
n. various ways the pump can be worn.	
o. usual battery life	

Learning and Skill Objectives	Outline
2. Demonstrates ability to:	
a. administer bolus dose three times.	
b. change basal rate three times.	
c. change battery.	
d. fill pump syringe/cartridge with insulin; place in pump.	
e. attach tubing; check for secure connection.	25
f. prime tubing with insulin.	
g. select and prepare suitable infusion site.	
h. correctly insert infusion needle and secure.	
i. check pump for correct/current basal rate program.	
j. program bolus dose based on blood glucose reading.	
k. activate pump to deliver bolus dose.	
l. terminate bolus delivery once dose is activated.	
3. Able to recognize signs of possible pump malfunction, and steps to address:	
a. change site; administer bolus with syringe.	
b. telephone pump manufacturer for technical help.	
c. monitor ketones for glucose over 240 mg/dl; respond appropriately.	

➔ About the American Diabetes Association

The American Diabetes Association is the nation's leading voluntary health organization supporting diabetes research, information, and advocacy. Its mission is to prevent and cure diabetes and to improve the lives of all people affected by diabetes. The American Diabetes Association is the leading publisher of comprehensive diabetes information. Its huge library- of practical and authoritative books for people with diabetes covers every aspect of self-care—cooking and nutrition, fitness, weight control, medications, complications, emotional issues, and general self-care.

To order American Diabetes Association books: Call 1-800-232-6733. Or log on to http://store.diabetes.org

To join the American Diabetes Association: Call 1-800-806-7801. www.diabetes.org/membership

For more information about diabetes or ADA programs and services: Call 1-800-342-2383. E-mail: AskADA@diabetes.org or log on to www.diabetes.org

To locate an ADA/NCQA Recognized Provider of quality diabetes care in your area: www.ncqa.org/dprp/

To find an ADA Recognized Education Program in your area: Call 1-888-232-0822. www.diabetes.org/recognition/education.asp

To join the fight to increase funding for diabetes research, end discrimination, and improve insurance coverage: Call 1-800-342-2383. www.diabetes.org/advocacy

To find out how you can get involved with the programs in your community: Call 1-800-342-2383. See below for program Web addresses.

- *American Diabetes Month:* Educational activities aimed at those diagnosed with diabetes—month of November. www.diabetes.org/ADM
- *American Diabetes Alert:* Annual public awareness campaign to find the undiagnosed—held the fourth Tuesday in March. www.diabetes.org/alert
- *The Diabetes Assistance & Resources Program (DAR):* diabetes awareness program targeted to the Latino community. www.diabetes.org/DAR
- *African American Program:* diabetes awareness program targeted to the African American community. www.diabetes.org/africanamerican
- *Awakening the Spirit: Pathways to Diabetes Prevention & Control:* diabetes awareness program targeted to the Native American community. www.diabetes.org/awakening

To find out about an important research project regarding type 2 diabetes: www.diabetes.org/ada/research.asp

To obtain information on making a planned gift or charitable bequest: Call 1-888-700-7029. www.diabetes.org/ada/plan.asp

To make a donation or memorial contribution: Call 1-800-342-2383. www.diabetes.org/ada/cont.asp